your pregnancy

your pregnancy

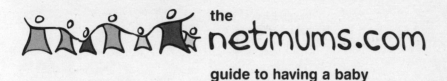

the netmums.com

guide to having a baby

with Hilary Pereira

headline

Copyright © 2009 Netmums Limited

The right of Netmums Limited to be identified as the Author of the Work has been asserted by them in accordance with the Copyright, Designs and Patents Act 1988.

First published in 2009 by
HEADLINE PUBLISHING GROUP

1

Cataloguing in Publication Data is available from the British Library

Trade paperback ISBN 978 0 7553 1800 1

Design by Viv Mullett

Typeset in Clearface by Palimpsest Book Production Limited, Grangemouth, Stirlingshire

Printed and bound in the UK by
Clays Ltd, St Ives plc

Headline's policy is to use papers that are natural, renewable and recyclable products and made from wood grown in sustainable forests. The logging and manufacturing processes are expected to conform to the environmental regulations of the country of origin.

HEADLINE PUBLISHING GROUP
An Hachette Livre UK Company
338 Euston Road
London NW1 3BH

www.headline.co.uk
www.hachettelivre.co.uk

Contents

Introduction

Finding yourself pregnant for the first time can leave you feeling scared, thrilled, surprised, shocked, exhilarated – or any of a whole raft of different emotions. One thing you won't be, though, is indifferent! Whatever you're feeling, we're here to support you, empathise with you and rejoice with you week by week throughout your amazing journey towards parenthood.

This uniquely interactive book is crammed full of all the information you'll need to cope with the emotional and physical upheaval of the next 280+ days, set alongside personal, intimate accounts from real mums of the joys and anxieties, niggles and very special privileges that come with the territory of expecting a baby. You'll read about the different aspects of pregnancy, from adapting to your changing body to undergoing diagnostic tests; alleviating back pain to celebrating your newly radiant skin (if you're lucky!); making all the practical preparations for having a new baby in your home to getting your head round the fact that you're soon to become a parent (yikes!). You'll learn loads about what's actually happening to your baby and your body each and every week; how to recognise any warning signs; how to stay healthy and give yourself a head start for labour; what the different tests in pregnancy mean; what to pack in your hospital bag; how to get the birth you want and lots, lots more.

In each chapter you'll find loads of quotes from Netmums all over the UK who are happy to share their many, varied experiences with you so you'll know you're not alone in pregnancy. You'll also feel equipped and empowered to ask the relevant questions of your medical team; push for your rights (full of confidence that you know just what they are); make lots of useful contacts to see you through the next 40+ weeks and examine all your options for labour and birth.

We've included a chart at the end of each chapter, where you can record your physical and emotional feelings throughout your pregnancy: you'll be amazed to see how much you've changed as the months go by and you look back over each chart – and you'll also have a lasting reminder to compare with any subsequent pregnancies, when the time comes. There's a quick quiz in each chapter, too, designed to help you monitor how much information you've taken on board (or not!) as you read along.

Your pregnancy could be a smooth ride or a rather more bumpy journey (excuse the pun), but it's sure to be a great adventure – so strap yourself in, hold tight and let's go. We're holding your hand through every twist and turn, and we won't let go until you're happily cuddling your very own newborn. Good luck.

NB: We have elected to refer to your baby as a 'he' throughout the book, to avoid the rather cumbersome use of 'he/she', 'his/her', and so on, but are keen to acknowledge that you are just as likely to give birth to a 'she'!

Meet the Team

Hilary Pereira is a journalist and author with a special interest in parenting. A former deputy editor of *Mother & Baby* magazine, she writes for a wide range of media including magazines and websites. She is also a mum with a vivid memory of pregnancy and the birth of her daughter. Hilary is married and lives in south London.

Margaret Haysom is an experienced midwife who has lost count of the number of babies she has delivered but guesses it's around 500. The number of pregnant women she has cared for during the course of her career is conservatively estimated at 4,500. She is extremely proud to have touched so many lives and hopes that many of the families with whom she has worked remember her as a friendly mentor.

Siobhan Freegard was raised in a small town in Ireland and came to London when she was 18. She worked her way up the corporate ladder to become a marketing director and had her first child at 29. After struggling with the work/life balance, she decided to have a stint as a full-time mum. She is now 41, with three children age 12, eight and five. She started Netmums as a result of feeling isolated and overwhelmed by the experience of being a new mum. Netmums is now the UK's fastest-growing online parenting website. There are 40 staff, all mums (and one dad). The website has over 500,000 members, with between 15,000 and 20,000 new members joining every month. Netmums receives over a million visits every month.

Part One

The First Trimester:
Months 1–3

Chapter 1
Weeks 1–8

Here's a funny thing: during the first two weeks of your pregnancy you weren't even pregnant! This is because the 40 weeks of pregnancy are calculated from the first day of your 'last menstrual period' (LMP): so for the first week or so you were bleeding, and for the remaining days your body was preparing to conceive. You would have conceived on or around the 14th day after the start of your LMP – assuming that your cycle is regular – so after one month of pregnancy, your baby will have been growing for just about two weeks. All of which means you've notched up your first fortnight of pregnancy without even knowing it – well done you!

Weeks 1 and 2 *280 days to go!*

That was then...

Even if you already know you're pregnant, it's kind of interesting to know what was going on in your body in the run-up to conception – and, as pregnancy is considered to last for 40 weeks, it would be a shame to miss out that first fortnight!

During the seven days that counted as Week 1, you had your last period. At the end of this week, the lining of your uterus (the endometrium) started to thicken up to receive a fertilised egg, should one happen to turn up. Meanwhile several eggs were maturing in your ovaries, and one or other ovary (it's completely arbitrary which) was busy preparing to release an egg.

You might have noticed a few twinges on the left or right side of your groin at around the time you ovulated. And do you remember noticing a thin, egg-white-like discharge in your underwear or on the toilet paper? That was cervical mucus, which becomes runnier than usual at ovulation time, to give sperm a better chance of making it through to the cervix. (Sometimes these little indicators are easier to spot retrospectively.)

Once the egg was released, it was helped on its journey down the nearest Fallopian tube by tiny tail-like projections called cilia – and not long afterwards it would have met up with one, single, manly sperm, found itself fertilised and taken a leisurely jaunt (of around seven to ten days) down to your uterus. If, however, this happy meeting hadn't actually taken place, you'd have had your period as usual and that would have been the end of this chapter!

Weeks 3 and 4 *266 days to go!*

...this is now

By now your pregnancy is a done deal, and the fertilised egg (which we can now call an embryo) has taken up residence in your uterus. This is your first week of 'gestation', which means the length of time your baby will spend inside you between conception and birth. Although you'll most likely have been blissfully – or maybe nail-bitingly – unaware of it, the most fantastic things have been going on.

From around 12 days after conception, for instance, the inner bit of the embryo has started growing into your baby; the outer part is developing into two membranes known as the 'amnion' and 'chorion'. The amnion will become the amniotic sac that produces and contains the warm amniotic fluid that will provide your baby with some of the nutrients he needs, as well as carrying away waste and forming a fantastic cushion against knocks and bumps throughout your pregnancy. The chorion will surround the amnion and become the placenta. (It won't be until around Week 8 that your placenta is sufficiently formed to sustain your baby.) This part also puts out minute finger-like projections called 'villi' to help the embryo to secure itself to the wall of the uterus. It all sounds very technical – and it is – but you don't need to worry about any of it; these miraculous-sounding developments happen automatically and are, in any case, out of your control.

Week 5 252 days to go!

Don't forget: Buy a home pregnancy-testing kit!

This is the week you'll confirm your pregnancy with a home testing kit – but don't be too disappointed if an early test gives a negative result; try a second one in another couple of days' time – first thing in the morning is best, when levels of the hormone called human chorionic gonadotropin (or hCG), which indicates the presence of human life, are at their highest.

Hey baby!

So you're actually pregnant then, are you? Brilliant! Incredible as it might sound (and you have to admit it's a bit hard to imagine with your baby currently about the size of a grain of rice!), during this week the development of your baby's brain and central nervous system get underway. He mostly resembles a little tadpole, with a longish tail; tiny eye sockets are already appearing like grooves either side of the developing brain. There's also the beginnings of an umbilical cord connecting your baby to your developing placenta (see *What's my placenta for?* on p. 16). Your baby's heart and a network of blood vessels is starting to sprout – and as all of this is happening to your tiny baby, he's floating around quite oblivious in his cosy amniotic sac.

All about *you*

Early signs of pregnancy to look out for

You might be a bit alarmed if you get a little light 'spotting' – small amounts of blood in your pants – a few days after implantation, but this can be quite normal (see *Is some light bleeding OK?*, on p. 14). If the bleeding stops after a day or two and you don't have a full period, you may have other signs of early pregnancy, too:

- sore, tender or tingly boobs
- overwhelming tiredness and sleepiness
- a sudden dislike of some of your fave foods, drinks or smells
- nausea and/or vomiting
- the need to pee more often than usual.

Some of these symptoms are similar to those you might get just before a period, although going off food and drink, nausea and excessive tiredness are not commonly associated with coming on, so if you have any or all of these, the chances are you're expecting! On the other hand, you may not notice any of the early signs – and if you escape pregnancy sickness altogether, lucky you.

What the netmums say

'Finding out I was pregnant'

Looking back the signs were all there, but it just didn't occur to me that I was pregnant. It slowly dawned on me when I started to get a bit of morning sickness that something wasn't right and then someone on the TV was talking about smoking in pregnancy and how the smell makes you feel sick. The penny dropped, because suddenly I couldn't stand my fiancé smoking any more so I took a test. At the dating scan soon after, I discovered I was already three months gone!
Mary from Merseyside, mum to Jamie, 18 months

I found out I was expecting Ollie by chance, six days before my period was even due! I'm a staff nurse on a gynaecology ward, and during a quiet time on night shift I volunteered to let one of the healthcare assistants practise taking blood on me as she'd just done the course but was nervous about taking a real patient's blood. She sent the blood off for basic hormone testing as that just happened to be the type of vial she'd chosen and I came on shift the next night to find that the sample had come back testing positive for pregnancy! The level was so low at that point that if the blood had been taken 24 hours earlier it would have

come back negative. Because of my own gynaecological history I'd been told I was unlikely to conceive again so it was a huge shock!
Jeanette from Southend, mum to Luke, 14, Andrew, nine and Ollie, six months

My periods were always regular, so when I was a week overdue and suffering from heavy, aching breasts, I knew straightaway I was pregnant. I did a test and it was positive.
Heidi from Ashford, mum to Kyran, 10 months

I had missed two periods and the smell of cooking made me feel sick. My favourite meal is spaghetti bolognese and each time I ate it, I felt sick – so I strongly suspected I was pregnant before I even took the test.
Lindsey from west Lothian, mum to Aaron, two-and-a-half

We'd been trying to conceive for about five years and had tried fertility drugs and IUI (intra-uterine insemination). A couple of months after that, while we were having a break from treatment, my period was late. On day 37 of my cycle, I started to let myself believe just a tiny bit that I might be pregnant. I had a funny feeling in my tummy which wasn't quite nausea, more like a really excited 'butterfly' feeling and my boobs had become really tender. I was reluctant to do a test because I didn't want another disappointment, but I remember being at work one day, completely unable to concentrate on anything but the thought that I might be pregnant. I bought a test on the way home, ran upstairs the minute I got in and did it. Positive! I just stared at it for about 10 minutes before I yelled down to my hubby.
Catherine from Billingham, mum to Matthew, three

Finding out and how you might feel
Hopefully, having your pregnancy confirmed will be one of the most joyful moments of your life – but sometimes the news, even if it's expected or

longed for, takes us mums by surprise. It's one thing to anticipate any completely new experience and another to go through it for real, and who can predict how you'll feel when you're actually in that life-changing moment?

Knowing it's all happening can be something of a turning point: you might feel a sudden burden of responsibility and start to fret about the inevitable, permanent life changes you'll have to adapt to; hopefully, though, you'll feel so elated that any changes will seem a minor price to pay for parenthood. Perhaps you'll feel a mixture of both emotions – let's call that a good balance.

You and your partner may not feel the same about the pregnancy, either, and this can put a bit of a strain on a relationship, especially if you don't get your true feelings out in the open from the start. You might worry that you'll hurt your other half's feelings if you don't feel the same way they do, particularly if you are more anxious than happy. One thing to bear in mind, though, is that whatever you feel at the point of discovering you're actually having a baby is unlikely to be how you'll feel throughout the whole pregnancy or after the birth, so use this as a starting point for discussing your thoughts and feelings.

What the netmums say

'How I felt once I knew'

Shock, disbelief, like I was in a dream! We'd been trying for a baby for nearly nine years and had been through various tests. We'd discovered that the only way we could have a family was to use donor sperm. After four failed IUI attempts and one cancelled IVF (due to a complication called Ovarian Hyper-Stimulation Syndrome [OHSS] from taking ovulation-stimulating drugs), in our hearts we knew our chances were slim. We decided to give IVF one more last try. I got OHSS this time around, too, and we assumed that we'd again failed. We hadn't! My call to the clinic was one of the best phone calls ever – I even asked the nurse if she was joking. Until my first scan I didn't actually believe that we were having a baby – and, in fact, we were having two! We are now the very proud parents of Matthew and Phoebe, and life couldn't get any better.

Sarah from Wigan, mum to twins Matthew and Phoebe, 20 months

When I found out I was pregnant with Damir I was very happy but also very scared to lose him. This was my second pregnancy: I miscarried in my first and only found out the baby had died when we went for the 12-week scan. As soon as I found out I was pregnant again I started worrying like crazy. At first I did two or three pregnancy tests every single week to check I was still pregnant and that this little baby was still alive – it was like an addiction. I didn't tell my husband as he'd have thought I'd gone bonkers! At 14 weeks the midwife let me listen to the baby's heartbeat and this reassured me enough to stop taking the tests. We were so relieved when Damir arrived safe and well.

Irma from Oldham, mum to Damir, 13 months

So when's it due?

One of the first questions us mums want answered is 'When's it due?' You can calculate this quite simply by counting 280 days from the first day of your last period, but you can make an approximation, accurate to within a few days, by using a much quicker method: find the date of the first day of your last period; add on exactly a year; go back three months and add on one week – hey presto, you have your estimated due date (or EDD).

So, if your last period started on 18 March:

18 March this year + 1 year = 18 March next year
Minus three months = 18 December this year
Plus one week = 25 December (in which case, how do you feel about 'Holly' or 'Nicholas' as names?).

The chances of you delivering your baby during the Queen's Christmas Day address to the nation are pretty low, however, as only around 5 per cent of babies are born on their EDDs.

Breaking the news

You can have your pregnancy confirmed for free at some health clinics, GPs' surgeries or pharmacies, but you might want to buy an over-the-counter test so that you can make the discovery in private; most GPs will accept a positive home test result as proof of your pregnancy anyway.

If you've taken the plunge and bought a home test to use secretly so you can get used to the news yourself before sharing it, you certainly aren't alone in doing so. Even if you've been trying to get pregnant, it can still be a bit mind-blowing to have it confirmed, and you might find it hard to believe for a little while.

How you share the news with your partner depends on how you're expecting him to react. If, for instance, you think he'll be in shock (or perhaps less than delighted at first), you'll probably want to avoid going down the balloons-and-fireworks route! People do come up with lots of different creative ways to break the news, as some of us Netmums describe below. You could take some inspiration from us – but, on the other hand, you might just prefer to show your partner the test result over a quiet cup of tea. Go with the flow.

If he does seem a bit overwhelmed by your news, give him a hug and tell him it feels weird to you as well, and that you'll be able to help each other get used to the idea over the coming weeks and months. After all, having a new baby in your home isn't something you'll have to cope with for a long while yet, and by the time the remaining weeks are up you'll most likely be bursting with eagerness to meet your new baby.

What the netmums say

'How I broke the news to my partner'

My husband was in bed on the morning I did the test, as he'd been on a night shift. He knew I thought I might be pregnant, but not that I was going to test. So I left a book on the joys of fatherhood and the positive test beside the bed for him to see when he woke up.
Emma from Bedford, mum to Geordan, two

I broke the news over the phone both times. With our first son, I did a test in the loos at work then phoned him in my lunch break. He was in total denial and kept saying 'Just because you're pregnant it doesn't mean we're having a baby'! The second time round he was in Paris when I phoned, which was far more romantic.
Jen from Hertfordshire, mum to Jack, four and Theo, 17 months

We started trying to conceive last September as we really liked the idea of a May or June baby. I have long, irregular cycles, so thought it would take a long time. We were due to go away at the end of September, and I took a test just before we left even though I knew it was too early. I was very disappointed when it was negative, but my husband comforted me and told me we'd try again next month. While we were away I felt bloated and had very sore boobs, but thought this was just my period on its way, as it was due the day we were flying home – on our first wedding anniversary. As soon as we got home, I sneaked upstairs and did a test even though my husband had advised waiting another week or so. I sat and waited for the result, and when the lines appeared I ran downstairs with my heart pounding. I said, 'I know you told me not to, but I just did a test... and it's positive!' and I waved the stick at him. Our baby's due on 30th May, which just happens to be my birthday. My husband's is in early June, so one of us could be sharing our birthday with the little one!
Claire from West Sussex, eight months pregnant

We'd been trying for a second baby for nine months, but as I sometimes go a year without a period I was terrified it would take years to conceive. One evening, all the signs were there so I rang my other half, Matthew, and told him to get back from work early. It turned out to be too early to test, but about two weeks later I tested positive! I was so excited, I ran into the living room, picked up my then three-year-old and danced around the room with him. I couldn't ring Matthew at work, so I took a picture of the test result on my phone and sent it to him. It wasn't long before he was home early again to celebrate!
Holly from Truro, mum to Benjamin, four and Milo, six months

Conceiving twins – or more!

Twins are conceived naturally in around one in 90 pregnancies. They result either from two eggs being released simultaneously and both becoming fertilised (known as 'dizygotic' or non-identical twins) or through the blastocyst dividing to form 'monozygotic' (identical) twins. When the twins are 'dizygotic', which literally means from two fertilised eggs, each baby has its own placenta and amniotic sac; when the twins are 'monozygotic', from a single fertilised egg, the babies share a placenta and may have a shared or separate amniotic sac. Non-identical twins are twice as common as identical twins, occurring in around two-thirds of twin pregnancies.

Extra care for multiple pregnancies

Having two or more babies in one pregnancy means you'll be monitored more closely than someone with a single pregnancy. You'll have extra antenatal appointments, probably extra scans and will be under the care of a consultant obstetrician throughout pregnancy. This is because there are added risks in carrying two or more babies: sometimes one baby can fail to thrive as well as the other; sometimes the extra strain of carrying more than one baby can make your own blood pressure rise or make other complications more likely, such as bleeding before or after the birth and pre-eclampsia (a dangerous disease of pregnancy characterised by high blood pressure, water retention and protein in the urine).You're also likely to feel the less positive effects of pregnancy (backache, varicose veins, nausea) more strongly and for longer than other mums, so take care of yourself. For more information on pre-eclampsia, see p. 274.

Mums carrying two or more babies are likely to gain weight faster and in greater quantity than those of us with just the one on board, and a closer eye will be kept on your weight gain and the babies' growth rates.

In over half of twin pregnancies, mums go into labour before 37 weeks (38 is considered full term for twins), and their babies have a low birth weight (less than 2.5kg/5.5lb). The statistics are more extreme for triplets, who have a 90 per cent chance of being born before 37 weeks, and of having a low birth weight. Quite a few twin and multiple births result in Caesarean deliveries, which are better all round if they are elective, which means pre-planned (see p. 290). That's not to say that a Caesarean is inevitable if you're carrying twins, especially not if both babies are head down at the start of labour.

We mums don't want to come over all negative about twins and multiple births, though – far from it. There are loads of advantages to having two babies at once:

- your children will be at the same age and stage simultaneously, and may be good company for each other
- it's great to get two lots of nappies and potty training out of the way in one go!
- you may consider your family to be complete after only one pregnancy
- if your family is complete with the twins' birth, you won't have to go through the anxiety of trying to conceive and early pregnancy again.

We know there are tons more great things about having more than one baby at once, and that you'll find out all about them after the birth. Lucky you!

Who'd have thought?

Because sperm can survive inside you for up to five days, you might not have become pregnant on the day you and your other half got frisky!

Your mission this week: Give your baby a head start

Ideally, if you've been planning to try to conceive, you'll have been taking a folic acid supplement (available from chemists and supermarkets) for at least the past six months. But not all pregnancies are planned quite so far ahead, so if you haven't, don't worry – just start right away. It's pretty crucial to the first 12 weeks of your baby's development, which is when all the major organs and limbs form, as well as the nervous system, the respiratory system and all the paraphernalia needed for proper circulation. Studies have proven that taking folic acid during this critical time – and before if possible – helps prevent birth defects like spina bifida.

Although you can get some folic acid from foods rich in folate (see *Fabulous folate – and where to find it*, p. 24), on its own it may not be enough to protect your baby, so ask your pharmacist to recommend a good one-a-day supplement. The usual dose is 400mcg (micrograms) per day, so check the label before you buy.

Look no further

We mums know just what's likely to be on your mind at each stage of pregnancy, so we've leapt in and answered your worries and queries each step of the way.

Is some light bleeding OK?

In many cases, yes. A little spotting (very light bleeding) around four to seven days after ovulation can happen as the fertilised egg implants in the wall of the uterus. You might find that it feels slightly uncomfortable, although you might just as easily be someone who is completely unaware of any symptoms at all.

If, though, the bleeding is more than light spotting, and is continuous, it's likeliest that you are starting your period, either because you haven't conceived after all, or because you did conceive, but the fertilised egg failed to implant, triggering your period.

Should I tell my GP I'm pregnant?

Yes, it's a good idea to make an appointment as soon as you have a positive test result so that you can get your general health and fitness checked out. If you have any existing medical conditions that could be affected by pregnancy, or if you're taking any prescription drugs, your GP will need to assess whether your current treatment is compatible with pregnancy and whether or not you'll need more frequent antenatal health checks than usual.

If you don't know whether or not you are immune to rubella (German measles which, in pregnancy, can have devastating effects on the foetus including blindness and deafness), ask your GP to check. Your status will be checked at your booking appointment but this may not happen until Week 10 or later, when a great deal of your baby's development has already happened, so it's a good idea to have it checked sooner rather than later. The check is made by a simple blood test. (Even if you had the jab in your teens, it doesn't always confer lifelong immunity, so it's worth making sure.) If you are not immune, you must take all steps to avoid rubella infection, especially in your first 12 weeks, after which time the danger of problems is reduced. After 20 weeks of pregnancy, there is very little risk of harm from rubella.

Other advice your GP will give you will include:

- stopping smoking. This is an absolute must, as smoking can have a very bad effect on your baby's development as well as on your own health
- cutting out alcohol. Current government advice is not to drink but, although you may have heard from other sources that one or two units once or twice a week is fine, you know what? – you'll probably find it easier just to stop drinking altogether while you're pregnant. It can't do your health any harm to have a bit of a break from booze either
- avoiding recreational drugs
- avoiding over-the-counter medicines, unless your GP advises otherwise.

Who'd have thought?

In order for you to have a good chance of conceiving, your partner must be producing adequate amounts of normal, healthy, good-quality sperm. This means an ejaculation of at least 2ml of semen, with at least 20 million sperm per 1ml of semen.

When will I know if I'm having a girl or boy?

No one can tell you yet what the sex of your baby is – but it was decided way back in that magical moment when your partner's sperm fertilised your egg. All eggs carry the X (female) chromosome, but each individual sperm may carry either an X or Y (male) chromosome. So if a sperm with an X chromosome meets your egg, your baby will be a girl, but if the successful sperm has a Y chromosome, you'll have a boy.

It might be months before you'll have an opportunity to find out whether you're carrying a little Amy or Ben (if you choose to, and if it's your hospital's policy to tell), but it's all academic in any case – boy or girl, your baby's gender is already a fact. If your baby is lying in a conducive position during your 20-week anomaly scan and your sonographer is willing to tell you the sex, you might have a chance to find out.

If you find yourself in the position of having diagnostic tests for Down's syndrome and some other conditions that involve sampling tissue or amniotic fluid, a by-product of the test itself is that the sex can be identified conclusively.

I was drinking every day right up until I found I was pregnant. Will I have harmed my baby?

Although in an ideal world you'd have given up tippling before trying to conceive, you're not alone with your worry: a great many of us who are surprised to find ourselves pregnant have this same thought. It's really unlikely your baby's been harmed by alcohol unless you've been drinking to the extreme.The really important thing to do is to stop drinking from now until after your baby's born or you've stopped breastfeeding.

What's my placenta for?

Your placenta is a really marvellous temporary organ that develops with your unborn baby. What it does is truly miraculous. The placenta links your baby's blood supply with your own, without the two supplies crossing; oxygen and food also pass from your blood supply into the placenta, from which the umbilical cord transports them to your baby. Waste products from the baby, such as carbon dioxide, are passed back along the umbilical cord to the placenta and then into your bloodstream. Antibodies, which protect your baby from most bacterial infections, pass from the placenta to your baby in the same way. Viruses, however, can cross the placenta, as can alcohol, nicotine and other drugs, which could damage your unborn baby. That's why it's so important to avoid these substances while you're pregnant.

Finally, the placenta produces hormones that help your baby to grow and develop. Towards the end of your pregnancy, more antibodies cross to your baby, giving further immunity for the first three months after birth.

Who'd have thought?

The current average age for a woman to give birth to a first baby in the UK is almost 30 (29.2 years*).

*Source: National Statistics

How are you feeling?

Throughout the book you'll find these *How are you feeling?* assessment charts. The purpose of these is to give you a point of reference to look back on as your pregnancy continues, so you can see how you're progressing physically and emotionally. It will also be a great record to compare any future pregnancies against.

Tick the box that most closely represents how you feel about the given statements.

Physically	Emotionally
I feel overwhelmingly tired Strongly agree ☐ Agree ☐ Neither agree nor disagree ☐ Disagree ☐ Strongly disagree ☐	I'm worried I'll be this tired throughout pregnancy Strongly agree ☐ Agree ☐ Neither agree nor disagree ☐ Disagree ☐ Strongly disagree ☐
I feel sick and sometimes actually throw up Strongly agree ☐ Agree ☐ Neither agree nor disagree ☐ Disagree ☐ Strongly disagree ☐	I'm anxious that I'll be sick in public Strongly agree ☐ Agree ☐ Neither agree nor disagree ☐ Disagree ☐ Strongly disagree ☐
I have had some light spotting Strongly agree ☐ Agree ☐ Neither agree nor disagree ☐ Disagree ☐ Strongly disagree ☐	I've been worrying about miscarrying my baby Strongly agree ☐ Agree ☐ Neither agree nor disagree ☐ Disagree ☐ Strongly disagree ☐
I feel 'different' but can't really describe how Strongly agree ☐ Agree ☐ Neither agree nor disagree ☐ Disagree ☐ Strongly disagree ☐	I'm not sure I'll make a good enough mum Strongly agree ☐ Agree ☐ Neither agree nor disagree ☐ Disagree ☐ Strongly disagree ☐
I had a healthy lifestyle before I got pregnant Strongly agree ☐ Agree ☐ Neither agree nor disagree ☐ Disagree ☐ Strongly disagree ☐	I feel I may have damaged my baby before I knew I was pregnant Strongly agree ☐ Agree ☐ Neither agree nor disagree ☐ Disagree ☐ Strongly disagree ☐
My boobs feel as if they're leading an independent life from me! Strongly agree ☐ Agree ☐ Neither agree nor disagree ☐ Disagree ☐ Strongly disagree ☐	I feel elated one minute and down in the dumps the next Strongly agree ☐ Agree ☐ Neither agree nor disagree ☐ Disagree ☐ Strongly disagree ☐

Quick quiz

How will you cope with pregnancy?

1 When faced with a long wait for anything:

a. I pace the floor, watch the clock and keep counting back from 100

b. I find something absorbing to do to pass the time

c. I sleep much more than usual so the wait doesn't seem as long!

2 How often do you like to paint your toenails?

a. Every week

b. Every month

c. Once a year

3 How do you keep in shape?

a. Lots and lots of contact sports

b. Daily aerobic exercise

c. Walking and swimming

4 How's your pelvic floor?

a. When I need to pee, I need to pee – now!

b. I try not to laugh too heartily in public but can hold on for the loo

c. Good. It doesn't usually bother me if I'm a mile or so from a loo

5 Fancy a drink?

a. Yes, please – a large G&T would hit the spot!

b. Half a lager and I'm anyone's!

c. Fruit smoothie or a cup of tea over booze any time

Mostly a: Being pregnant could take a bit of getting used to – but don't worry, you'll learn to adapt.

Mostly b: You won't have to make too many changes, and you'll take it in your stride.

Mostly c: It's pretty much 'situation normal' for you (bar the sickness and burgeoning bump!). Enjoy the journey.

Week 6 *245 days to go!*

Don't forget: Book antenatal classes early to avoid disappointment

If you already know that you will want or need certain services in pregnancy, at the birth or after your baby is born, mad as it may seem it's not too early to make enquiries about most of them. If, for instance, you want your antenatal care to be provided by an independent midwife, you'll need to start looking straightaway. If you're planning to attend National Childbirth Trust (NCT) classes and they tend to become over-subscribed in your area, put your name down now. Visit www.nct.org.uk to find your nearest branch. Typically a course of classes costs from around £120, depending on where you live. In London, it can be as much as £240. All other private classes, such as active birth classes, will also need to be booked in advance. NCT and the other classes will cover the emotional side of pregnancy, alternative therapies, self-hypnosis, breathing techniques and other more diverse and detailed aspects of labour and birth as well as breastfeeding and life in the early days of new motherhood. You'll probably attend around eight two-hour sessions and are encouraged to bring your birth partner with you. Classes usually start from around Week 27 of pregnancy.

Some mums choose to take the free hospital antenatal classes alongside more extensive private classes. The hospital classes, which you'll be offered automatically, will teach you about what labour is like, pain relief, interventions and Caesarean birth. You may also learn about skills you need as a parent, such as how to bath a baby and change a nappy. You'll also get the opportunity to visit the hospital and have a tour of the maternity unit. Typically you'll attend six to eight one- to two-hour sessions from Weeks 28–30 of pregnancy, although the timings might vary, depending on when the next available course falls in your pregnancy.

You might want to hire a 'doula' (a woman with previous experience of childbirth who offers practical and emotional support before, during and for a few days after the birth): their services can be very much in demand, so again it's worth looking around and booking now (check out www.doula.org.uk or www.britishdoulas.co.uk as a starting point).

Perhaps you know that you will be returning to work at the end of your maternity leave, and will need formal childcare: waiting lists can be very long for the best providers – some advisers even recommend securing a place before you're pregnant! – so get in there as soon as possible. All of these things can be cancelled or postponed if necessary, so there's no harm in sticking your name down now. You can find out about childcare services generally by visiting www.childcarelink.gov.uk and get details of your local providers from the National Association of Family Information Services website www.familyinformationservices.org.uk.

Check 'em out

Don't think it's too early to check out your chosen providers once you've got a shortlist. One good way of assessing a day nursery, for instance, is to just turn up and catch them unawares. Try to avoid mealtimes as they can be pretty chaotic (well, would you fancy feeding a roomful of 1- to 3-year-olds?). Maybe aim for mid-morning or afternoon: you should be able to get some sort of first impression that'll either reassure you or send you running for the hills!

Obviously you can't really do the same with a childminder, unless you dress up as a gas meter reader (and you don't mind at all getting marched off to the police station for illegal practice). Best advice here is to try to find someone by word of mouth: maybe some of your friends with kids have used one, or maybe they know of someone who has. It's a very hard decision to hand your baby over to the care of an unknown quantity. Although you won't necessarily know much about a nursery either, at least there are lots of staff members to keep an eye on each other, or to take a particularly tricky baby or child off a colleague's hands if they feel they're getting to breaking point.

Who'd have thought?

Around 20 per cent of women conceive within the first month of trying.

Hey baby!

It's a really important week for your baby's development as from now on and for the next few weeks all the foundations for his whole body are being laid down. This is the time when your baby is at greatest threat from 'foreign' substances such as chemicals in drugs, which could enter his bloodstream via the placenta.

Your baby's spine is starting to take shape now, and blood vessels are sprouting, forming a rudimentary umbilical cord. Now, instead of being the size of a grain of rice, your baby is already around the hearty size of a baked bean. (Come to think of it, your baby is kind of the shape of a baked bean as well!) It may sound teeny still, but imagine that amount of growth taking place in just one week and it's pretty awesome.

Little dents in your baby's outline are beginning to form, too, and these will become his chest cavity and abdomen. His tiny tummy is kick-started this week as well, and his intestines are hot on the trail!

There are the beginnings of a face this week (the very beginnings) with the jawline beginning to appear along with small dents for eyes and ears. Four little 'limb buds' are sprouting that will eventually become the arms and legs of your baby.

All about you

Telling other people

So are you going to hire a light aircraft and write your news across the sky for everyone to see? Or are you keeping it to yourselves until you start to show? Perhaps you'll compromise and tell just your closest family and friends until the most significant danger of miscarriage has passed after about 12 weeks, which is what many couples do.

There are two ways of looking at this conundrum: if you tell people early and then lose the baby, you'll have people around you to help you cope, whereas if you've been waiting for the danger of miscarriage to pass, you will have two sets of news to share – that you were pregnant and now you're not, which is a lot for other people to take in. You might prefer not to tell at all in these circumstances, but you must do whatever feels right for you. Bear in mind, though, that you can always turn to the Netmums for sharing confidences, finding advice and getting lots of warm and well-meaning support.

You might have other reasons for keeping your news to yourself for now: maybe you'd prefer not to be given 'special treatment' or told to 'take it easy' and not to do things 'in your condition'. Maybe you're wary of other people telling you their horror stories of threatened miscarriages or horrendous birth experiences – and tell you they will, that's for sure! Perhaps you're struggling to take the news on board yourself and don't feel ready to let anyone else know. Some of us just enjoy having the secret all to ourselves for a little while. In the end, though, the decision of when to reveal your pregnancy is a very personal one, and there's no right or wrong.

If you're employed, legally you don't have to announce the news until you give notice for maternity leave and pay in the fifteenth week before your baby is due. But as long as you're not worried about being sidelined for promotion or discounted as a valuable member of staff, it's in your interests to tell sooner so that you can benefit from other rights you're entitled to, such as paid time off for antenatal care, and health and safety protection. Maybe you could get some insight from a trusted colleague who's had experience of your company's attitude towards pregnancy, and gauge it from there.

What the netmums say

'When we told the world'

Even before I got pregnant, we had decided to wait until Week 12. However, I had a bleed in Week 9 and had a scan at the hospital. When we found out everything was fine and our little bean had a strong heartbeat, we thought it was safe to tell. So by Week 10 everyone knew.
Allison from Kent, mum to Edward, 12 months

With Will we didn't tell anyone until I started bleeding at seven weeks and had to stay in hospital. My husband realised that if it happened again he would have no support and so we decided to tell both mums and dads at that point. We did everything else by the book and didn't tell anyone else until 12 weeks. With Zac we told immediate family after a couple of weeks and then a few very close friends, but no one else until after 12 weeks. After Zac I had two secret early miscarriages and I just knew that I would have fared better if I'd had support, so this time we told everyone straightaway.

Natasha from Bristol, mum to Will, four, Zac, one, and expecting number three!

I told everyone straightaway. I think because it wasn't planned and I was very young, I needed as much advice and support from people as I could get. When we have another, we're hoping to keep it between me and my husband until 12 weeks, then surprise relatives and friends by giving them a scan photo.

Nicola from Norwich, mum to Jacob, three

I hadn't been feeling well for a couple of weeks – sickness, nightmares, migraines – so basically, we knew I was pregnant. We tried to wait until I could see a doctor as I had only been in the country permanently for three months and I hadn't got the correct paperwork to be on the NHS yet, but we couldn't stand it. We purchased a test on 23 December and took it the following morning – positive! It was perfect: we got to tell everyone on Christmas Eve! It really helped my parents and me to get through the holidays without each other.

Zoe, American living in Nottingham, mum to Leo and Lucas, 21-month-old twins

With Rhys and Siôn we told people before 12 weeks as we were just too excited! With Carys it was very different as a close friend was trying for her second baby and having problems conceiving. I really didn't want to upset her by telling her that I was pregnant, and I didn't want her to hear from anyone else, so we ended up telling practically no one until I was 20 weeks. I once even hid in a toilet on the way to a hospital appointment as I saw someone I knew in the corridor and didn't want them to find out and tell. As time passed I quite liked having 'our little secret' and I was quite sad when we finally shared the news!

Delyth from Wales, mum to Rhys, five, Siôn, three and Carys, two

Who'd have thought?

We Brits spend around £36 million per year on home pregnancy tests*.

*Research conducted by MINTEL

Fabulous folate – and where to find it

You can and should increase your intake of folate-rich foods throughout pregnancy: for the first 12 weeks they will help protect your baby from developing certain birth defects, and in any case they are all foods that will boost your own health and energy levels. Foods rich in folate include:

- green, leafy vegetables (the darker the better): spinach, spring greens, Savoy cabbage, broccoli, Brussels tops and curly kale are all good sources
- 'legumes' or pulses such as canned or dried beans and peas (try pinto, kidney, borlotti and haricot beans, as well as cans of mixed bean salad)
- asparagus (and don't worry that your wee will smell rather metallic after eating it – this is perfectly normal!)
- orange juice and whole oranges
- avocados
- strawberries (but don't leave them out of the fridge or in the light for any length of time as the folate content gets depleted).

Super snack ideas

- Keep a punnet of washed strawberries in the fridge and snack on them whole
- Whizz up some fresh strawberries with low-fat Greek yoghurt for a delicious dessert
- Mash avocado with a little lemon juice, paprika and crème fraîche for a delicious dip, and eat with raw broccoli florets
- Keep a small tub of mixed beans in low-fat vinaigrette dressing by you, and eat a spoonful whenever you get snackish

- Steam a few asparagus spears and top with a small knob of butter, a poached egg and ground black pepper for a delicious light lunch
- Use dark, leafy greens such as spinach in salads and sandwiches instead of lettuce or other salad leaves
- Keep some quartered and peeled orange segments in a tub for an instant pick-me-up
- Top your folate-fortified breakfast cereal with a few orange segments and halved strawberries for a folate boost.

For more information on your ideal pregnancy diet, see p. 74.

What not to eat

There are some foods us mums should avoid eating in pregnancy because of their potentially harmful effects on either ourselves or our babies. Here's what to avoid and why:

- **Vitamin A supplements** Unless you're advised to take them by a health professional, avoid supplements, including cod liver oil supplements, that contain vitamin A. Large amounts of vitamin A can cause malformations in a developing baby.
- **Liver and liver products** (such as pâté) These may contain large amounts of retinol, the animal form of vitamin A, and should also be avoided.
- **Raw or undercooked meat, unpasteurised milk or milk products** All could potentially contain the toxoplasmosis parasite, which can affect foetal brain and eye development.
- **Raw eggs, or foods containing raw or partially cooked eggs** These could potentially contain salmonella bacteria, which will make you very unwell with severe vomiting, diarrhoea and possibly dehydration. Although your baby won't be affected directly, your health is equally important, and a bad case of

salmonella poisoning may require hospitalisation. Cook eggs thoroughly until firm.

- **Pâté, blue-veined and mould-ripened soft cheeses, such as Brie and Camembert** Listeria bacteria, which is sometimes found in these cheeses, has been associated with miscarriage and even stillbirth.

- **Caffeine** Research suggests that consuming too much caffeine in pregnancy may be linked to an increased risk of miscarriage or low birth weight. To be on the safe side, switch to decaff beverages or cut out tea and coffee altogether for at least the first three months of pregnancy.

- **Alcohol** Recent advice from NICE (the National Institute for Clinical Excellence, which advises the government on best health practices) suggests that pregnant women should limit alcohol intake to less than 1.5 units per day and, if possible, should avoid alcohol completely in the first three months of pregnancy. Advice from the Department of Health now suggests that expectant mothers should avoid drinking alcohol at all; however, if you do choose to drink, don't down more than one to two units of alcohol once or twice a week. One unit is a small glass of wine, a half pint of ordinary strength beer, lager or cider, or a single 25ml (pub) measure of spirits.

Your mission this week: Spring in to action!

- Start making a video diary of your pregnancy, with weekly updates about how you're feeling, physically and emotionally. It will be a really special record to look back on in years to come.
- Get yourself measured for a bra (most department stores and branches of M&S will do this for free). It'll be very interesting to see how your size and shape changes as you go through pregnancy, so keep a record from now on. Go and get measured every couple of months.
- Make an initial list of boys' and girls' names so you can look back on it when you've named your baby after the birth. You might know exactly

what you want to call your baby already, but you might be surprised (or even horrified!) by your earliest ideas.

- Take some photos of your body as it is now – you might be one of the lucky mums who shrinks back to her pre-pregnancy shape quickly, but if you're not, you might want the proof that you were once, for example, the proud owner of an ironing-board tum.
- Note how many times a day you re-check your pregnancy test! You might not quite believe the reading right at this moment, but you sure will in a month or so's time!

Look no further

Can I choose where I go for antenatal care?
The most usual place to go for antenatal checks is at your local community clinic, which may or may not be in the same place as your GP's surgery. The aim is to make pregnancy seem less 'medicalised' and more natural, so the days of going to the hospital for checks are dwindling, and in many areas you'll only have to visit the hospital for your ultrasound scans and any other special tests. Exceptions are: if you have a complication of pregnancy; a pre-existing medical condition that can be affected by being pregnant; or a previous obstetric history that's unusual, when you'll probably be put under the care of a consultant obstetrician: this means you'll see a specialist doctor as well as a midwife at your checks. In fact, you can ask to see a consultant obstetrician at any time during your pregnancy in any case.

You might be offered 'shared care', which means you'll sometimes see your GP and sometimes your midwife – probably at alternate appointments. In some areas, you can go for midwife-only care, where you're looked after by a local midwife or team of midwives throughout pregnancy and for the birth. Many areas have a lovely community midwife service, but it's often a well-kept secret, so do a bit of asking around to find out if this is available to you. If not there's the option of hiring an independent midwife. It's quite a costly business at £1,800 to £4,000 for a package, depending on where you live, but it does mean that you'll know your midwife and her team intimately, that you'll always know the person who carries out your checks, and that you'll be attended by someone you know well when it comes to the birth. The aim, either way, is for you to be attended by the same midwife all the time, if it's possible. This might appeal to you particularly if you're planning a home birth (see p. 272). You can start checking out the options for hiring an independent midwife at www.independentmidwives.org.uk and www.homebirth.org.uk.

How many antenatal appointments will I have?

You'll start with your 'booking' appointment – a term that dates from the days when mums literally had to book a bed for labour! This should ideally take place before Week 12 of pregnancy, but the schedule does vary from place to place, so a lot depends on where you live. (For more information on what will happen at this appointment, see p. 70.)

After your booking appointment, you'll have an appointment about every four to six weeks – depending on whether it's your first pregnancy or not and your medical history – until the last few weeks of pregnancy when you should be seen more often.

What will happen at each antenatal appointment?

All mums have their blood pressure and urine checked at every antenatal appointment to test for the onset of problems such as gestational diabetes (see p. 212) and pre-eclampsia (see p. 274). Your midwife or doctor will also listen to your baby's heartbeat and palpate your bump (this means giving it a good feel around) to check your baby's size and position. She'll also take a measurement from the top of your pelvic bone to the top of your uterus (the fundus) as another check on your baby's growth rate.

Should I start eating for two now I'm pregnant?

Sounds good, doesn't it – but no! Opinion on whether or not to eat more seems to vary depending on what you read, with some sources advising you to take an extra 300 calories a day on board throughout your whole pregnancy, and others recommending just 50 for the first two trimesters (which, as it's the equivalent of half a small banana, is hardly worth the worry!). Because your baby will automatically take all the nutrients needed for healthy development from you, what you'll need to concentrate on is eating as healthily as possible so there are enough nutrients for both of you: you don't need to start stuffing back the pasties and stocking up the biscuit jar. And don't kid yourself that an extra dollop of mash is 'good for you' either! OK, you don't want to make an active decision to 'diet' when you're pregnant (unless you're advised to by your medical team), but there's no excuse for putting on half your original body weight either.

In your third trimester, when your baby is bulking up, you'll probably be advised to eat a bit more – but even then you'll only need to take in around an extra 200 calories per day – the equivalent of a small banana and half a pint of skimmed milk. And if you're still tempted to pack a few snacks now and try to lose the weight afterwards, bear in mind that being very overweight can put you at risk of developing health complications like gestational (pregnancy) diabetes, which has health implications for both you and your baby. It's also harder to get a good scan picture if you've got a dense layer of fat lying across your belly. *And* it's harder to lose 'baby weight' than you might imagine, so think on!

Why am I so tired?
At this stage it's down to the hormonal upheaval that's going on behind the scenes; later in pregnancy you'll feel exhausted again because your body's organs will be working harder than ever before. To allow this to happen, your metabolic rate will increase by a fifth; your heart is already pumping more blood more quickly around your body, and your breathing rate has also increased. It's a pretty exhausting business!

Five tips for combating tiredness

1 It may seem obvious to suggest getting more sleep, but one of the most helpful strategies for overcoming the exhaustion of early pregnancy is to try to catnap during the day. This is more feasible for some of us than others, of course: some workplaces are more ready to accept the need for a 'power nap' than others. If you have a rest room or common room – or if you work from home – you could try napping during your lunch break, but try not to sleep for longer than 30 minutes or you'll enter the really deep sleep phase that leaves you feeling doubly exhausted if you're woken from it before you're ready. And don't forget to set an alarm to wake yourself up...

2 Go for great quality sleep at night: start getting ready for bed half an hour earlier than usual; take a warm (not too hot) bath; have a small cup of warm milk; listen to a relaxation tape; put a few drops of lavender oil on your pillowcase and leave a window slightly open for good ventilation.

3 Avoid drinking too many liquids in the last hour before bedtime: you'll probably be up to the loo in the night at least once as it is, so don't make things worse for yourself by overloading your bladder.

4 See if you can negotiate with your employer to start work later and work through part of your lunch break (you'll need the rest for a kip!) or go home a little later. Explain that it will be better for you to travel off-peak so you're sure to get a seat on transport or don't get stressed in a traffic jam. Use the extra time for a lie-in.

5 Grab sleep whenever and wherever you can – even on the bus or train. (Just don't forget to set your mobile alarm to wake you!)

Who'd have thought?

Semen contains 100 times more zinc than is found in the blood. Your partner can improve the quality and quantity of his sperm by eating foods rich in zinc and folate. Zinc-rich foods include meat, dairy products, beans and lentils, yeast, nuts, seeds and wholegrain cereals. Pumpkin seeds provide one of the most concentrated vegetarian food sources of zinc, and there's no harm in buying your man a zinc supplement to take until you conceive.

Week 7 238 days to go!

Don't forget: Ask about screening tests

Your first pregnancy may not seem like the right time to be questioning the medical professionals and their practices, but you should know that you have options when it comes to antenatal testing (as well as your treatment throughout the whole 40 weeks and your birthing preferences).

This week is a good starting point for considering which antenatal screening tests (usually first performed at your booking appointment) you are happy to undergo, and which you'd really rather avoid. Why would you want to avoid any? Because, depending on the results, you might find yourself setting off down a road of further, more invasive testing; and unless you might consider a termination if you were to find that you are carrying, for example, a child with Down's syndrome – or unless you would be happier having advance warning that you are at high risk of having a child with a disability, so you have time to come to terms with the news before the birth – there wouldn't be any point in having such tests in the first place. When you're considering all this, bear in mind that the early tests only assess your risk factor and don't give you any conclusive answers.

So what are these tests and how are they done?

The numbers of antenatal screening tests you're offered will depend on where you live. Some authorities offer a full gamut of tests whilst others offer the bare minimum: whatever is on offer, though, should meet national standards.

Some screening tests are offered routinely, and involve a simple blood test. For example:

- alpha-fetoprotein (AFP) test. High levels of the substance called AFP – a protein produced by foetuses – can be associated with spina bifida in your unborn baby
- serum screening, which uses the AFP result and measures other chemicals in your blood to assess the risk of your baby having Down's syndrome
- tests for sickle-cell anaemia and thalassaemia (a disorder of the red blood cells).

Other screening tests are offered where there is a family history of a specific condition, such as cystic fibrosis or Tay-Sachs disease (a genetic condition affecting the nervous system). Some units offer further, more detailed blood tests. Ask your GP, midwife or hospital doctor for details.

In addition to the above screening tests, you'll also have your blood pressure and urine checked at each antenatal appointment. This is to test for the onset of potential problems such as gestational diabetes and pre-eclampsia (see p. 274).

Hey baby!

Your baby now measures around 9mm in length (from crown to rump – or top of the head to tailbone). This is how babies are measured throughout pregnancy, and the length will be recorded on your notes under CRL (crown-to-rump length). Would you believe that, even at this dinky size (roughly the equivalent of a pumpkin seed), your baby has already quadrupled in size since embedding in your uterus? He is now starting to move around within the amniotic sac. These movements can be detected by a monitor but you won't be able to feel them yourself until around Week 20, or a little later. This week your baby's lungs, liver and kidneys are developing.

All about you

What's that whiff?

Good grief, as if enough inconvenient changes aren't already going on, next you might find that your sense of smell goes into overdrive! Lots of mums at this early stage of pregnancy find certain aromas become really heightened and – wouldn't you know it? – some of the most commonly mentioned ones are also the stinkiest: cigarette smoke, burger stands, toilet blocks have all been cited. And, more cause for celebration (not!): those smells that used to be your favourites (bacon sarnies, coffee, your signature perfume and the like) will quite possibly begin to turn your stomach.

Lots of mums-to-be also report a metallic taste in their mouths (in fact, this is the sign for some second- and subsequent-time mums that they are pregnant again), so don't be surprised if your favourite pasta dish suddenly tastes more like a length of copper piping! Don't despair: the taste thing and the smell thing should get back to normal as your hormones level out in the second trimester of your pregnancy.

Are my scales deceiving me?

Because of disruptions to taste and smell, you could find that you actually lose weight in early pregnancy. Plenty of mums report being extra hungry but not fancying anything to eat (bummer!), but as long as you weren't seriously underweight at the outset, it won't hurt you or your baby if you shed a couple of pounds until this phase has passed. Just stick to bland foods for now: jacket spuds with cottage cheese; rice cakes with hummus; raw veg and a sour cream dip; plain omelettes and salad – anything you can stomach, but the more nutritious the better, especially as your intake has already taken a nosedive.

Overcoming pregnancy sickness

For 'pregnancy sickness' read 'morning sickness', because that's the misnomer this unpleasant, often humorously portrayed condition has been enjoying for decades. The reason it's inaccurate is that the overwhelming nausea, frequently accompanied by bouts of throwing up, that plagues some unfortunates can occur at any time of the day or night.

There are several tricks mums have used successfully to help combat the nausea and sickness associated with early pregnancy. Ginger, for example, has long been used as an anti-emetic (anti-sickness remedy), so drinking ginger tea or eating a ginger biscuit may help.

If you feel sick, you might find the acupressure wristbands used for travel sickness helpful – you'll find them at your local pharmacy or high-street chemist. Otherwise try eating small, regular, snack-sized meals rather than a full plate of food at a time, and always have a dry biscuit or something else bland before getting out of bed in the mornings. Check out the Netmums' tried-and-tested remedies, too (see pp. 33–6).

Who'd have thought?

Given that for the first two weeks of pregnancy you have yet to conceive, the average pregnancy actually lasts for 266 days – that's about eight-and-a-half months.

What the netmums say

'How I managed pregnancy sickness'

I was nearly six months' pregnant before I stopped feeling sick, although even after that whenever I cleaned my teeth it took me two or three attempts as it made me ill. I found that not eating much in the day – just having water, dry biscuits and ginger – was the only way to get through it. After about 6 p.m. I could usually cope with a meal.

Sarah from Wigan, mum to twins Matthew and Phoebe, 20 months

I felt queasy with both babies until about 14 weeks. It's a special type of queasy feeling – not like having a tummy bug. Cooking raw meat, the smell of smoke and travelling by car made it worse – the smoking ban hadn't been introduced and people still smoked in my office. I spent hours at work trying not to throw up. It makes me sick just thinking about it! I found ginger biscuits and flat lemonade really did help.

Jen from Hertfordshire, mum to Jack, four and Theo, 17 months

I lost half a stone in the first four months of my pregnancy because of pregnancy sickness. I couldn't stomach the smell of lots of things, including cucumber (I didn't realise it had a smell until this point!); rubbish bins; alcohol (which was a bit inconvenient as I work in a pub: I remember serving customers and then disappearing off into the loo to be sick!). I couldn't stand the sight, smell or feel of any meat, and was a bit worried that I could never have a bacon sarnie again. Luckily it wasn't permanent. I lived mainly on rich tea biscuits, eating from the moment I opened my eyes in the morning, which made things a bit better. Milk helped a lot: I would drink pints and pints, which also eased it. Sometimes, though, the only thing to do is just be sick and get it over with!

Georgina from Devon, mum to Charlotte, 17 weeks

I was sick every day from six weeks until the day before Tasha was born – and I only escaped that day because she was born at 9 a.m.

and I'd been in labour since midnight, but I still felt sick! Acupressure bands helped a bit, and so did just giving in to the vomit – it sounds disgusting but if I just got it over with when I got up in the morning, my day was better than if I tried not to be sick, as then I felt rough all day. I managed to go to work all through it, but I did have one memorable day when I was interviewing a woman at her shop and I realised I was going to throw up: I mumbled something about having left something in the car, ran out and was sick on the pavement. I'm sure she saw but she was kind enough not to say anything when I went back in!
Liz from Kent, mum to Tasha, 18 months

I felt nauseous for the first 10 weeks or so: I could only eat dry toast and sweets, and then eventually tinned spaghetti. I found I had more of an appetite in the morning than in the evening. I remember when I discovered I could eat Marmite, and my boyfriend mixed Marmite and spaghetti for me thinking I'd like it – I nearly killed him it was so disgusting. I think my hormones made me feel worse, although I was never actually sick.
Katie from Stoke-on-Trent, mum to Josh, four

I felt sick in both pregnancies, although I was only sick once or twice. The best thing I found for it – and still do if I feel queasy – was minty chewing gum. It seemed to work in three ways: it increased saliva which helped reduce heartburn; the mint helped any trapped wind along; and it also helped to clear my airways too, solving the problem of catarrh running down the back of my throat and making me feel sick.
Leslie from Taunton, mum to Katie, six and TJ, four

Who'd have thought?

Because your baby has his own self-contained blood circulatory system, his blood group may be different from yours.

When the sickness won't stop

Now don't be alarmed, but a very small number of pregnant women (around two per cent) experience severe vomiting attacks in pregnancy, sometimes to a debilitating degree. These women suffer from hyperemesis gravidarum – or HG, to give it its more manageable abbreviation. 'Hyperemesis' literally means 'excessive vomiting', and 'gravidarum' means 'of pregnancy'. The condition usually eases by around Week 16, but for an unhappy few it continues for the entire eight-and-a-half months. In very severe cases, where a woman cannot keep food or drink down and becomes underweight and dehydrated, hospitalisation is required.

Moody blues

No, we're not talking about the 1960s rock band but about why you might be the moodiest cow on earth just now. (Or is that a bit insensitive? OK then: why you're feeling a bit tearful and cross… and have perhaps developed a propensity for throwing things…)

Seriously, lots and lots of newly pregnant mums have succumbed to bouts of unexplained crying; panics that we don't know what we've got ourselves into; anxieties about the terrible world we're about to bring a new baby into, and general irritation with just about everything our partners try to do for us.

Hormonal influences

The good news is that you're not going crackers – you're just playing host to a whole wealth of hormones your body's not used to, and these are the little demons responsible in part for your mood swings. The main culprits are oestrogen and progesterone, which tend to do their worst between the sixth and tenth week of pregnancy, and in the final weeks before your baby is born. Their effect on the balance of your brain chemistry is what can alter your moods in a most irrational manner.

Getting back to the term 'mood swings': swings? Oh yes – just as you may well burst into tears as you read a neighbourhood poster about a 'lost, much-loved ginger tabby' (why are they always ginger tabbies?; and why are they never in your shed or garage?), you're also highly likely to have moments of pure elation which put a spring in your step and a big smile on your face. So quite a good balance then… Well, your poor other half might not know whether he's coming or going for a while, but as long as you explain to him that alternating between screaming banshee and cuddly kitten is perfectly normal, he'll probably not take it too personally.

Reality checks

As if blaming it on your hormones doesn't give you enough of an excuse for unpredictable behaviour, you do also have some very real reasons for feeling unsettled and, at times, grumpy. Let's not forget the extreme tiredness; physical discomforts including pregnancy sickness; new and permanent responsibility and concerns about the potential impact of parenthood on your relationship with your partner, let alone the nagging worry about giving birth: all these factors are not only very real, they're also pretty stressful. Stop beating yourself up: treat yourself to a little cry now and then, then take a look around at all the parents you know and ask yourself whether any of them would swap family life for a life without kids. In the vast majority of cases, the answer will be an overwhelming 'no'. Now try to look forward, past the immediate future and into your settled new life. That's better!

What the netmums say

'Crying over everything!'

I do remember being overly tearful about lots of things, but I also had an hysterical laughing fit watching *You've Been Framed* when I was pregnant with Joshua. I know you're supposed to laugh at the programme, but one clip that I don't even remember now set me off, and I was crying with laughter so much that I almost couldn't breathe. I just couldn't stop, much as I wanted to, and it got so bad that my husband started to panic: he could see that I was getting distressed and couldn't catch my breath properly. This hysteria went on for a good 15 to 20 minutes. When I eventually managed to pull myself together I was exhausted, shaking and quite scared at how I'd been so totally out of control of my emotions.

Lisa from Liverpool, mum to Joshua, five and Rose, three

I still cry at anything child related, especially the NSPCC ads – they make me want to take all the children home and look after them!

Georgina from Devon, mum to Charlotte, 17 weeks

Wait a minute – are these MY boobs?

By now you've probably noticed some changes to your boobs (although not all women's alter dramatically). In all likelihood they'll have got bigger already, as fat stores are laid down here throughout pregnancy in preparation for breastfeeding. You might observe what looks like a road map of Spaghetti Junction emerging just under the surface of the skin (nice!), and this is caused by the increase in blood supply that happens in pregnancy. Maybe the darker circles of skin around your nipples (the areolas) have become brownish pink due to increased pigment produced in pregnancy. Whatever: your boobs may seem to have taken on a life all their own, and are almost certainly going to demand a new bra some time soon – and at various times throughout pregnancy.

Tempting though it may be to encase your newly pumped-up pups in a sexy, push-up number and swan around town wearing a revealing décolletage, the best thing you can do for your own comfort – and to support your breasts well – is to invest in a more substantial, non-wired bra with broad straps and a deep panel of hooks. All right, so it might not be the look you (or your partner) have been aspiring to, but you'll thank us mums in the end when you're able to get on with life without your boobs making their presence felt every time you bend, stretch or hug your mates!

Join the dots...

Those were the days, weren't they, when we were footloose, fancy-free teenagers...? It's good to reminisce, but do any of us mums really want to re-visit our 'Spotty Herbert' period? Well sorry, but for many of us there's no option as those mischievous hormones do their worst, causing all sorts of skin eruptions, greasy patches and even unsightly skin pigmentation.

There's not a lot you can do about spot break-outs caused by hormones. Best advice is to follow a good skincare regime; steam your face whenever you can; use an oil-free moisturiser and invest in a great concealer! Also, step up your intake of water – around two-and-a-half litres a day is considered the optimum by nutritionists. Don't use acne creams or treatments unless your GP advises you to: some of them are dangerous to use in pregnancy as they can cause birth defects.

If you're one of the unfortunates who suffer from bad skin in pregnancy it can make those poster campaigns of 'blooming' expectant mums seem like a bit of a bad joke, but don't despair. Things could well settle down in your second trimester when hormone levels bottom out a bit, and – although there's no guarantee – you could still be the proud flaunter of gorgeous skin, hair and nails. In any case your skin should return to its pre-pregnancy condition a few weeks after your baby is born.

Breathe in!

Although you're almost certainly not showing yet, you might find this week that your clothes fit a little more snugly than they used to. It's an awkward time: too soon for maternity clothes but probably too late for your skinny jeans! You can help make clothes fit better with a few clever tricks: attach a loop made from elastic to your skirt or trouser buttonhole and use this as your new buttonhole: the elasticity and extra length will give you that extra half-inch or so you need for comfort; wear too-tight shirts open with a vest underneath; treat yourself to an Empire-line dress or kaftan in your usual size that you'll be able to wear after pregnancy too – the lack of waistband will be a welcome relief!

What the netmums say

'Early symptoms of pregnancy'

Before I even got a positive result with my first two pregnancies I used to get a stitch-like pain whenever I was rushing about. This time round it was the sort of pain you get when you're ovulating, but it lasted for quite a while every day.
Sharon from St Helens, mum to Lauren, 15, Robert, three, and 14 weeks pregnant

With my first and second pregnancies my earliest symptom was sore boobs. With this third pregnancy I felt sick very early on, was very tired, and kept needing to wee. I also had short, sharp pains in my belly that came and went in the first four to six weeks.
Maxine from Inverness, mum to Summer, three, Elsie, nearly two, and 12 weeks pregnant

From before even taking the test I was overwhelmed by total exhaustion and the ability to fall asleep anywhere, once memorably standing up at a bus stop! I also had aching, expanding, veiny boobs! I never felt sick once, though.
Kate from Cheltenham, mum to Jericho, 10, Bryn, three and Eleanor, one

Before I'd even done the test I knew I was pregnant because my sense of smell went really weird: I turned into a human bloodhound and could smell Chinese food from about a mile away! My partner's feet made me sick, too, even though they don't usually smell.
Gill from Warrington, mum to Nathan, four and Caitlin, 14 months

Your mission this week: Make a friend of your dentist

Now's the time to get a full MOT on your choppers, as dental care is free in pregnancy and for a year after the birth of your baby – yippee! OK, maybe you don't feel quite as elated as that, but at least you won't be paying for the privilege of seeing Dr Drill. The reason why dental care is free for you is that some of the hormones associated with pregnancy can cause all sorts of physiological changes, including spongy, inflamed or bleeding gums – and these nasties can, in turn, lead to gum disease. Believe us – that's the last thing you need to put yourself at risk of, given that there are a few other less avoidable discomforts looming on the horizon (but more of these later...).

Having said all that, the dental treatments open to you in pregnancy are somewhat limited. Medical procedure, such as root-canal work and even fillings, are best left until after the birth if at all possible because of the associated risk of infection. So don't worry too much about the reference to Dr Drill – it's thought that amalgam fillings might pose a threat to your unborn baby because of their mercury content, which could enter your bloodstream and cross the placenta, or pass to your baby via your breastmilk, so the worst you're likely to get is a temporary filling to tide you over (although if you have a permanent white filling instead, you're likely to be charged for it, as this is considered 'cosmetic').

X-rays are to be avoided at all costs in pregnancy – although if you are unfortunate enough to need emergency surgical work on your teeth you'll probably have to have at least one. There's a special barrier apron you'll be covered with if you do need any, which will protect you and your baby from the radiation, so there's no need to go into a state of panic if the word X-ray is mentioned – just remind your dentist that you're pregnant and that you'd prefer to avoid X-rays if at all possible.

The upside is that extra cleaning and polishing may be available to you, to help keep your teeth and gums in the best nick. And you'll be given advice on flossing and brushing to avoid bleeding gums – so don't mentally go 'Yeah, yeah, boring…': sit up, take notice and do as you're told. At the risk of sounding like your mum: 'It's for your own good'!

Look no further

How come toothpaste suddenly tastes so horrid?
Some mums experience wild cravings for toothpaste during pregnancy; others are completely turned off by it and feel sick whenever they use it. If you're one of the latter, cleaning your teeth effectively could be a bit problematic. How about trying out one of the fruit-flavoured gels on sale for kids? It might just be the change of flavour and/or texture you need. And make sure you have a good old sloosh of mouthwash, such as Corsodyl, twice a day, to reduce the risk of infection and keep your mouth smelling OK.

Why am I having these weird cravings?
If you're one of those expectant mums who's gone off all her favourite treat eats and drinks, you might also find that you've got some funny cravings for stuff you usually wouldn't touch with a bargepole! The Netmums have some weird and wonderful stories to share on this (see pp.43–4), and in most cases – as long as you're still eating a balanced diet and keeping to a sensible intake of calories – your GP or other healthcare provider won't interfere with food cravings. At worst, food cravings can be inconvenient, striking at all times of

the day and night, and nagging away at you until you can get your hands on whichever food you're fixated on.

There's a condition called 'pica', however, that isn't such a laughing matter – it's the term to describe cravings for inedible substances like soap or coal: some women even want to eat earth or clay. Although there has been some speculation that it's your body's way of telling you which essential minerals it needs, the truth is that we only need very tiny amounts of minerals – not the proportion contained in, say, a house brick! Associations have also been made between pica and iron deficiency, although not everyone agrees that there's a link.

You should see your GP if you are experiencing pica as it can put you and your baby in danger: for example, eating non-food substances can interfere with the absorption of the nutrients from food, and there's the danger that – if you have an extreme case – you might stop eating real food in favour of the craved item. Then there's the risk of lead poisoning… the list goes on. In short, the condition needs to be reported to your doctor or midwife. In some cases, mild aversion therapy – where you learn to make unpleasant associations with the substance you crave – can be helpful.

Some things women with pica have eaten

- soil
- coal
- ash
- chalk
- clay
- ice
- washing tablets
- toothpaste
- soap
- cigarette ends
- plaster
- wax
- hair
- paint chippings… YUM!

Who'd have thought?

The word 'pica' comes from the Latin for magpie – a bird that will eat almost anything!

What the netmums say

'My weirdest cravings'

When the sickness kicked in at about six weeks we were really tight for money, so it was the worst possible time to be craving raspberries: they don't come in large quantities and they're certainly not cheap!
Holly from Truro, mum to Benjamin, four and Milo, six months

I used to crave soap – and not just any soap, it had to be Dove soap for the taste!
Irene from Glasgow, mum to Nathan, three

During my pregnancy with Hannah I craved the smell of cleaning products! I loved the smell of washing powder, Dettol, washing-up liquid and bathroom sprays. It got to the point where I'd be sitting in the lounge craving the smells so much that I'd have to get up and find a cleaning product to sniff. I even put some washing powder to my lips once because the desire for it was so great!
Sarah from Bournemouth, mum to Hannah, two

I'm from Canada originally, and I had cravings for things I couldn't get here: it drove me nuts! I was thrilled to find Welch's Grape Jam at a speciality shop here and paid over £6 for it (it costs the equivalant of about £1.50 in Canada). Not only did I crave the jam, though – I craved it spread on meatballs! I enjoyed it once then the thought of it made me sick and I threw the rest of the bottle away.
Allison from Kent, mum to Edward, 12 months

I'm currently pregnant with baby number four, and with each pregnancy I've craved ice. I have at least three ice trays on the go

and if they run out I munch on frozen sweetcorn and peas. I've also taken to eating punnets of frozen fruit, and freezing fruit juice so it reaches that just slushy stage.
Kelly from Swindon, mum to Holly, seven, George, five and Mitchell, three

Through every pregnancy my craving was salad cream. I'd eat it on anything savoury and carried a bottle of it in my bag in case I ever needed it in an emergency!
Louvaine from Rickmansworth, mum to Josh, five, Caitlin, three, Isabel, two and Oliver, one

When I was pregnant with David I craved the smell of Domestos bleach (the pink bottle!). I just had to have it, and would sit down with a glass of it to smell. I really wanted to drink it, but I managed to stop myself. With Matthew it was Flash Pineforest. I'd sit sniffing it, then even clean the sideboards with it so I'd never be far from the smell.
Kerry from north Hertfordshire, mum to David, two and Matthew, one

With Andrew it was mayonnaise on everything including chocolate bars! With Stuart I ate lots of cheese, just on its own. With Jessica I had to have lemon-and-lime KitKats and with Sophie it was toast. The mayo was the weirdest!
Sharon from Aberdeenshire, mum to Andrew, 10, Stuart, nine, Jessica, three and Sophie, one

With Harley I craved dishwasher tablets in the last two weeks of my pregnancy! I didn't eat any, but I came close. My mum used to buy me giant Parma violets because of their chalky, powdery texture and they did the trick.
Marie from Oxfordshire, mum to Harley, two and Mason, six months

Who'd have thought?

The average number of children born to mums in England and Wales* has risen to 1.87 – the highest it's been in nearly 30 years.

*Source: National Statistics

Week 8 231 days to go!

Don't forget: Step up your fibre intake

Round about now you may start to experience some of the – shall we say 'less desirable' – effects of pregnancy, mostly caused by the hormone progesterone. Because its effect is similar to a muscle relaxant, it tends to slow down some of the more important functions of your insides: in other words, you could find yourself becoming somewhat constipated. The best way of trying to combat constipation is to step up the amount of fibre and water you consume daily. Choose wholegrain and wholewheat bread, pasta and cereals; stock up on fibrous vegetables such as asparagus, broccoli, cauliflower, Brussels sprouts, celery, and greens; and eat more fibrous fruit such as plums, peaches, nectarines, apples and pears. Make sure you're drinking the recommended two-and-a-half litres of water a day, as this really helps to ease constipation. Because your body absorbs more fluid during pregnancy, your stools can become dry and hard, so the idea is to keep them hydrated so they're softer to pass (OK, sorry about the graphic description, but there's no nice way of saying it!).

Not to put too fine a point on things, if you let the constipation take hold, the resulting straining on the loo is likely to give you another of the pregnancy nasties – piles. Now these little horrors can be really uncomfortable, so keep that fruit bowl handy and start working your way through it now! Don't beat yourself up if you start chugging back the fibre and still get piles, though: for some mums they're unavoidable, especially later in pregnancy when all your innards come under increasing strain from carting around the extra weight of your baby. Don't take laxatives without checking with your GP first, as they could be harmful to your pregnancy. (For more about piles, see *What can I do to help relieve my piles?*, p. 200.)

Seeing as you're now all prepared for constipation, you may as well know that later in pregnancy indigestion is also a common side effect of progesterone flooding your body (see p. 45). Heartburn is a more painful condition and is the result of the relaxation of the valve at the stomach opening, which allows acid to escape back up into the gullet (see p. 167).

Hey baby!

Your baby is about 2.2cm (just under 1in) long and rather resembles a cashew nut! He's able to open and close his mouth, and his tongue, top palate, ears, eyelids and nose are starting to form. The umbilical cord which connects him to you via the placenta is now formed and covered in a jelly-like substance, called Wharton's jelly, to help reduce the risk of it getting tangled.

Your baby's brain development is impressively fast, and you can help by swapping your daily jacket spud or ham sarnie for a tuna or mackerel salad, as the essential fatty acid DHA – which is fantastically good for brain growth – is found in oily fish such as these. Other good choices are salmon, trout, sardines, herrings, pilchards and kippers, so choose your fave and get stuck in.

All about you

How's your sex life?

Presumably it wasn't in bad shape until fairly recently, or you wouldn't have picked up this book in the first place. One of the anxieties lots of expectant couples have is that they're going to harm the baby if they carry on canoodling. Then there's the sudden mismatch of libido that sometimes accompanies pregnancy, with one or other of you feeling super-frisky while the other is more interested in a nice cup of chamomile tea and an early night. Plus you might be feeling anxious about whether or not your other half still fancies you enough to get it on (although at this stage, with burgeoning bosoms and not much else to show for it, he could perhaps be persuaded...).

Seriously, though, there's no need to abstain from lovemaking unless you've been advised to by your medical team – and this is only likely to happen if you've had repeated miscarriages or other previous problems in pregnancy. Your baby is safely tucked away inside his amniotic sac, cushioned from all external (and some internal!) movement and sound, well away from your vagina and cervix, so feel free to get sexy if you're in the mood. And although having an orgasm is thought to help trigger labour once you're at full term, it won't trigger a miscarriage in a healthy, uncomplicated pregnancy.

When one of you goes off sex

It's not unusual for one or other partner to go off the whole idea of sex in pregnancy – and it's not only the mums either. Some men feel they are intruding on the baby or that it's wrong to make love with a 'third party' involved. Other chaps regard their women in a whole new light once they're pregnant, focusing on the maternal side much more than the sex goddess side. If you're still feeling fruity but your other half isn't you might feel a bit rejected or neglected. Take some time out for an honest chat and the opportunity to come to some sort of a compromise: after all, there's plenty of lovemaking to be had without penetrative sex featuring on the menu; you'll have to settle for any close cuddles and quick snogs you can get! You might want to just remind him, though, that the boot might well be on the other foot for a while after your baby's born.

If it's you who's lost your libido, you won't be the first mum for this to happen to. Let's face it, you'd have to have a strong stomach to fancy a bit of the other whilst suffering from pregnancy sickness or chronic indigestion, although for some mums it's more of an emotional response than a physical one: either is understandable. It should help if you reassure your partner that you still fancy him but just can't get turned on right now; otherwise you could leave him feeling like a redundant baby-making machine. Try to keep the kisses, cuddles and closeness going, even if you don't feel like making love, and tell him that sex isn't necessarily out of the question for the whole nine months – in fact plenty of mums find themselves feeling all sexy again during those 'blooming' middle three months of pregnancy.

Who knows, the two of you might just find you're 100 per cent sexually compatible throughout pregnancy, feeling like rampant rabbits or confirmed celibates simultaneously at every stage. If this is you, then you're in a lucky minority – and hey, if you want to keep your friends, keep it to yourself!

What the netmums say

'Sex in pregnancy: turn-on or turn-off?'

In my first pregnancy I couldn't get enough sex: my poor hubby would barely get through the door from work before I would be pouncing on him. There was something very sexy knowing I was having his baby and that he was so delighted about it all. This was in the first, second and – yes – even the third trimester! The bigger I got, the sexier I felt! With my second baby I wasn't keen on sex at all, but for no specific reason. This time around I'm a bit of both: sometimes I feel sexy and in the mood, other times I'm just too tired. I'm sure having two toddlers doesn't help!
Maxine from Inverness, mum to Summer, three, Elsie, nearly two, and 12 weeks pregnant

Up until about Week 12, I couldn't bear the thought of sex. My poor hubby would snuggle up for a cuddle in the morning and I'd snap at him to go and brush his teeth first as the smell of morning breath made me feel queasy! After about Week 12 though, we couldn't get enough of each other, and even got up to some antics during labour! I think some of those hormones carried on flowing after the birth as well, as we had a very gentle bit of naughtiness just 10 days after our baby was born. I was soon too exhausted to think about it again for a while, though!
Julie from Bury St Edmunds, mum to Holly, 18 months

I did not feel sexy even the slightest, tiniest bit. My husband thought my curves were gorgeous, but I just wanted to bat his hands away, have a cup of tea and read a book. I did have some sexy dreams, but as soon as I woke up I was sick, and I just felt HUGE! It's funny, but even though I don't consider myself a prude, a part of me just felt sex was wrong during pregnancy, which is daft, I know. My poor, patient husband...
Sally from Northumberland, mum to Lily, 16 months

I'm embarrassed to admit it but my hubby and I haven't had sex for about five months: the thought of it repulses me. We do have

foreplay so that he doesn't feel left out and still feels loved, but sometimes even that is a challenge for me. I can't wait till we can have full sex again!
Clair from Portsmouth, due first baby any day...

For the first few weeks I felt really sexy, and tried everything to get my husband in the same mood. After a few weeks of failure he admitted that knowing his baby was in there put him off totally. By four months the morning sickness had worn me down and I had gone off it too and was grateful for his phobia. When I was seven months he got his drive back, but by then I was still feeling sick and wanted my bed for whatever sleep the kicks allowed me. Still, my drive came back almost straight after the birth and my husband had to barter me into waiting for four weeks!
Fiona from Surrey, mum to Deborah, three-and-a-half months

Shape up or slow down?

If you've always been active and are accustomed to hurling yourself around a squash court, thrashing up and down a swimming pool or working out in any other vigorous way, you're probably wondering what exercise is safe to continue in pregnancy. If, on the other hand, your sofa bears your permanent full-body imprint and you think 'gym' is the bloke from the chippy, you are probably not. Either way, you may want to change your behaviour just a little.

As long as you are otherwise healthy and know of no complications with your pregnancy (see *Look no further*, p. 51), then exercise is a good thing, and you should aim for a moderate level for around 30 minutes a day. For avid exercisers, the main rule is to stick to your normal exercise programme and not challenge yourself further for now. If you do want to swap something demanding for a more gentle class, don't forget to tell the instructor that you are pregnant so that she or he can advise you if there are any parts of the class you should avoid.

For non-exercisers, it's safer to start with something gentle like swimming, walking or aquanatal aerobics (gentle aerobic exercise in water), and stick with it. It's not advisable to start something you have never tried before, so don't be tempted to take up jogging or rollerskating with no previous experience. Although yoga and pilates can be fantastic exercise, and some classes are geared specifically towards pregnancy, they may not be right for you unless you've practised them before. Stretching muscles and ligaments you're unaccustomed to using may not be beneficial, especially now that your joints are generally more relaxed due to the effects of progesterone and other pregnancy hormones.

Whatever form of exercise you choose to do, make sure you take plenty of water and avoid getting too hot. Dehydration and overheating will impact on your baby, so drink plenty and stop exercising before you become uncomfortably warm.

Who'd have thought?

In 2006 a baby girl was born six weeks early during a transatlantic British Airways flight. Passengers and crew on flight BA215 from London to Boston worked together to deliver the tiny baby, who was named Nadine.

Your mission this week: Plan a holiday

It's worth thinking ahead about a possible last holiday as a twosome with your partner. Depending on where you were hoping to go this year, you may have to alter your plans as some vaccinations (if you're aiming for somewhere that requires them) cannot be given in pregnancy.

If you're heading off overseas, most airlines are happy for pregnant women with uncomplicated single pregnancies – and who have a 'fitness to fly' certificate from their GPs – to fly with them until the end of Week 35 of pregnancy, after which time you may find you have a problem (and rightly so: who wants to deliver an early baby 30,000 feet in the air?). With a multiple pregnancy the cut-off point is usually 32 weeks.

Despite being permitted to fly until relatively late in pregnancy, you might find, along with lots of us other mums, that you feel at your physical and emotional peak some time during your second trimester (Weeks 13–28). You will certainly be comfier on the flight without a huge bump to accommodate; you're less likely to feel exhausted before you even set off; you're unlikely to be as affected by heat and humidity as you might later on as you become bulkier; you're more likely to have time to spare in mid-pregnancy, as your final trimester will probably be taken up with preparations for the baby's arrival.

If you're planning a UK break, you can pretty much go whenever you like (antenatal appointments permitting). If you do go in your final trimester, however, it's an idea to make sure you're not miles and miles from a hospital with a maternity unit, just in case Baby Bump decides to put in an early appearance. (See *Late breaks*, p. 235.)

Look no further

Is there any exercise I should avoid?
It's generally thought that pregnant women should avoid high-risk activities, contact sports and exercise that relies on balance, such as horse-riding, so if your preferred method of exercise is squash, cycling, ice hockey or diving, you might want to have a re-think.

Exercise that wears you out to the point of exhaustion could leave your baby with a reduced oxygen supply as there's an increased demand from your own heart and lungs, so make sure you only push yourself to the point where your heart rate is raised but you can still converse.

Once you're into your second trimester of pregnancy and your bump is in evidence, you should avoid exercise that has you lying on your back because the weight of your uterus can press down on a main blood vessel called the vena cava, and this can affect your baby's oxygen supply.

Do I need to check with my GP before I exercise?
You should get clearance from your GP before you embark on any exercise if:

- you have experienced bleeding or a threatened miscarriage since you found you were pregnant
- you have suffered a previous early miscarriage or premature birth
- your placenta is low-lying
- you have any pre-existing medical conditions, including high blood pressure
- you have any joint problems or back pain
- you're carrying more than one baby.

Who'd have thought?
Around half of all pregnancies are unplanned.

How are you feeling?

Tick the box that most closely represents how you feel about the given statements. You'll find a chart at the end of each chapter, which will give you a good gauge of the changes in yourself as you progress through your pregnancy.

Physically	Emotionally
I can't stand smells and tastes I used to love Strongly agree ☐ Agree ☐ Neither agree nor disagree ☐ Disagree ☐ Strongly disagree ☐	I'm anxious about telling other people I'm pregnant Strongly agree ☐ Agree ☐ Neither agree nor disagree ☐ Disagree ☐ Strongly disagree ☐
I feel more ill than pregnant Strongly agree ☐ Agree ☐ Neither agree nor disagree ☐ Disagree ☐ Strongly disagree ☐	I'm so excited about telling other people Strongly agree ☐ Agree ☐ Neither agree nor disagree ☐ Disagree ☐ Strongly disagree ☐
I hardly feel any different from normal Strongly agree ☐ Agree ☐ Neither agree nor disagree ☐ Disagree ☐ Strongly disagree ☐	I can't wait to get a noticeable bump Strongly agree ☐ Agree ☐ Neither agree nor disagree ☐ Disagree ☐ Strongly disagree ☐
I feel 'different' but can't really describe how Strongly agree ☐ Agree ☐ Neither agree nor disagree ☐ Disagree ☐ Strongly disagree ☐	I'm worried about my body changing Strongly agree ☐ Agree ☐ Neither agree nor disagree ☐ Disagree ☐ Strongly disagree ☐
My back and other joints ache Strongly agree ☐ Agree ☐ Neither agree nor disagree ☐ Disagree ☐ Strongly disagree ☐	I'm anxious about antenatal tests Strongly agree ☐ Agree ☐ Neither agree nor disagree ☐ Disagree ☐ Strongly disagree ☐
I can't imagine ever wanting sex again Strongly agree ☐ Agree ☐ Neither agree nor disagree ☐ Disagree ☐ Strongly disagree ☐	I wish the first 12 weeks would pass more quickly Strongly agree ☐ Agree ☐ Neither agree nor disagree ☐ Disagree ☐ Strongly disagree ☐

Who'd have thought?

Your blood volume will increase by about 50 per cent during pregnancy, accounting for around 1.2kg (2.6lb) of your total weight gain.

Quick quiz

How clued up are you about pregnancy?

1 What is your placenta?
a. A Spanish cocktail
b. The lining of the uterus
c. A temporary organ that supports your unborn baby's life

2 What does 'gestation' mean?
a. An inability to digest something
b. The length of your baby from crown to rump
c. The length of time your baby spends inside you in pregnancy

3 What is an embryo?
a. A new type of sports car
b. Another name for sperm
c. The term given to a fertilised egg

4 What is a Fallopian tube?
a. A European underground train
b. The tube through which nutrients pass to your baby
c. A tube down which your egg travels on its journey to the uterus

5 Your pregnancy is scheduled to last 40 weeks, but for how long of that are you actually pregnant?
a. 40 weeks
b. 36 weeks
c. 38 weeks

Mostly a: You hardly know your amniotic sac from your handbag! You've done the right thing buying this book, which will help to clarify all the above and lots more.
Mostly b: You recognise these pregnancy terms, but are still a little unsure of what they mean. Read on to become highly enlightened.

Mostly c: You've done your homework. Good for you: the more informed you are, the better you can take control of your pregnancy, labour and birth. Keep reading to fill in any gaps and discover some intriguing facts.

Chapter 2
Weeks 9–12

Like lots of mums, you may regard the first 12 weeks of pregnancy as an almost 'breath-holding' time, because this is when you are at greatest risk of a miscarriage or of your baby developing a birth defect. About one in four pregnancies does end in miscarriage, but it's helpful to realise that this means you have a 75 per cent likelihood of carrying your baby successfully – and your risk decreases dramatically after Week 12, as 80 per cent of miscarriages occur during the first 12 weeks. Once you've gone through this next four weeks, you should be able to relax into pregnancy a bit more. Of course, your mind won't be entirely at rest until your baby is born, but there will be more opportunities for reassurance as you go along, depending on whether or not you choose to have antenatal screening and/or diagnostic tests and ultrasound scans.

Week 9 *224 days to go!*

Don't forget: Enquire about a dating scan

You'll probably be offered a dating scan some time between now and Week 12, during which your baby will be measured to ascertain or confirm just how far along your pregnancy you are. It's worth enquiring about this from your GP or midwife, as health authorities differ in what they offer in terms of scans and tests.

The dating scan will be the first of two which are routinely offered in pregnancy. The second one – the anomaly scan, which has a detailed look at your baby's physical development and the functioning of his vital organs – is usually performed at around 20–22 weeks (see p. 174 for more information).

Hey baby!

Your baby is doing his bit to move on from resembling a tiny piece of food (OK, so he's progressed from the size of a grain of rice, to a baked bean, to a pumpkin seed to a cashew nut so far) to taking on a more human-like form. Measuring around 23mm from crown to rump (same as the height of a postage stamp!), his little fingers, although still rather webbed-looking, are able to flex, his toes are becoming more defined and ankle and wrist joints are forming. In fact, so much fine tuning has been going on that he even has his own fingerprints in place, and his (or her) sex organs are also taking shape. Your baby currently weighs around 2g – that's less than a tenth of an ounce. (If only our weight gain in pregnancy was the equivalent of our babies'…)

All about you

Still feeling sick or even chucking up regularly? There is some hope on the horizon, you poor thing: lots of mums find that this is the peak of the sickness and things start to improve gradually from the end of this week onwards (fingers crossed).

As you may well be discovering by now, it's hard work being pregnant and you might find yourself getting more and more tired. Add in tingling, heavy breasts, possible headaches (see also p. 178) and perhaps the odd dizzy spell, and you might just be feeling a bit 'poor me'. Poor you!

It's not unusual to have the odd nosebleed either, because of the increase in blood supply and the impact of your hormones on your blood vessels, but hang in there, things are set to improve in a few more weeks. Don't forget, you've got a whole new human growing inside you, which is quite an achievement, so focus on the future, contain your bouncing boobs in a good sports bra, keep a good supply of tissues with you and sit tight.

Who'd have thought?

This time next year your baby will be 21 weeks old!

If you miscarry your baby

Whilst you have a very good chance (three in four) of carrying your baby successfully to full term, and whilst we don't want to dwell on the possibility of any other outcome, if you should find yourself amongst the mums whose pregnancy ends in miscarriage, it would be unfair to leave you with no further information, so here it is.

Miscarriage is most common in the first 12 weeks of pregnancy, but can happen up to Week 24, after which time if your baby dies you will be deemed to have suffered a stillbirth, and will be able to hold a funeral for your baby. Research has shown that babies who are miscarried often have some chromosomal or genetic abnormality. Although it's not understood what prompts a mum's body to recognise these signs and eject her baby, it seems that that is the most likely explanation for why these miscarriages (also referred to as 'spontaneous abortions') happen.

Other causes of miscarriage include the placenta failing to develop sufficiently; illness in the mum; an 'incompetent' cervix (where it fails to remain closed); an irregular-shaped uterus; fibroids (otherwise harmless tumours in the uterus); insufficiently high levels of pregnancy hormones, drug abuse or very excessive levels of smoking or alcohol drinking.

It's vital for your recovery that you don't blame yourself if you suffer a miscarriage. You might have read that a physical or emotional shock could have caused you to lose your baby, but the more likely explanation is one of those given above. Yes, in some rare cases a fall or other accident could 'dislodge' a baby, but it would have to be fairly severe – or the baby would have had to fail to implant fully – in order for miscarriage to occur. The sac of amniotic fluid that holds your baby provides sufficient cushioning for him to remain safe through most relatively minor knocks and bumps, so it's very unlikely you could have prevented the loss of your baby.

Missed abortion

For some mums, the discovery that their baby is no longer alive comes at their booking appointment or dating scan, when there is no evidence of a heartbeat or image of the baby. This is known as a delayed miscarriage, missed miscarriage or even missed abortion (abortion here meaning 'miscarriage'). This is a heartbreaking eventuality, especially as the first scan is an event that is usually anticipated with great excitement. If this happens to you, you may feel inadequate that you didn't recognise any signs that your baby was no longer alive, but at this stage of pregnancy there are no foetal movements for you to monitor or other outward signs to note, so it's unreasonable to feel guilty. Even if you'd noticed that your breasts no longer felt as full or tingly, or that whereas you had felt sick before you no longer had any symptoms, you would probably have assumed that you were simply progressing past these niggles. Whatever else you feel, you mustn't blame yourself: you couldn't have known about or prevented your baby's death.

What happens next?

You'll be given a scan to ascertain whether there are any remaining 'products of conception' (another rather cold-sounding medical term, which here means any remaining parts of your pregnancy), which need to be removed. If so, you'll be offered an operation known as an ERPC (Evacuation of Retained Products of Conception). It's performed under a light anaesthetic and is a simple, quick procedure. Some people still refer to this as a D&C (dilatation and curettage), but this is a slightly different operation which is no longer commonly performed. The alternative to having an operation is simply to wait for your body to expel any remains of your pregnancy, which will happen over time. Some women prefer this option to undergoing general anaesthetic; others feel uncomfortable about still carrying a dead foetus. Only you will know which option is better for you: the important thing is that you are given sufficient time in which to make the decision.

Getting support

If you have already shared the news of your pregnancy with friends and family, you'll need their support now more than ever, so allow them to rally around you if it's helpful. If you haven't told people yet and you'd rather not, there are other areas of support you can turn to, not least on Netmums where many mums have experienced miscarriage, and share their thoughts and feelings on the miscarriage support forum. You'll find extra support at The Miscarriage Association, too. Phone the helpline on 01924 200799 (Mon–Fri, 9 a.m.–4 p.m.); email them at info@miscarriageassociation.org.uk or visit the website at www.miscarriageassociation.org.uk.

What the netmums say

'Motherhood after miscarriage'

I had two miscarriages before we had Maya. The first was 10 years ago: I fell pregnant but didn't realise until I miscarried at 10 weeks. I was stuck in a room on the maternity ward and lost my baby whilst listening to all the babies crying around me. The second was three years ago: we were actively trying to conceive and we lost the baby again at 10 weeks. This second time was worse because it was very much a planned and wanted baby. Our local hospital was wonderful that time; we had a private room away from others and lots of support. When I fell pregnant for the third time, with Maya, we were given an early scan at seven weeks, where we saw the heartbeat, and another at 10 weeks, just to put our minds at ease. The miscarriages were awful but there is hope: you never forget, but it does get easier. A friend of mine is currently pregnant with twins after many years of trying and miscarriages so there is always hope.
Karen from northern Scotland, mum to Maya, two

After trying to conceive for six months I became pregnant. We were delighted, but at 11 weeks I started to have slight bleeding and went for a scan. I discovered I'd had a missed miscarriage and opted for an induction. I presumed my body would pass everything out but that was not the case as the baby and placenta had to be pulled from me. It was awful and I wish I'd opted for an ERPC [see p. 58]. We waited one cycle and then started to try for a baby again. I became obsessed with charting my temperature, cervical mucus and ovulation pain, and I was heartbroken each month when I wasn't pregnant. Sex became a chore and I was sure there was something wrong with me or that the miscarriage had damaged me. I started on the ovulation-stimulating drug Clomid and became pregnant. Everything felt different that month and our love life was like when we first met. We both had a positive feeling that we'd conceived that month and we had! Just as I was about to give up hope, it happened and we now have a beautiful baby boy.
Sarah from Lancashire, mum to Daniel, nine-and-a-half months

Chorionic villus sampling (CVS)

There's a test called chorionic villus sampling (CVS) that you may be offered this month if you've got a family history of inherited disorders, if a blood test is abnormal, or if you're over 35. CVS can detect serious abnormalities in your baby much as amniocentesis can except that a sample of placental tissue is analysed, whereas in amniocentesis a sample of amniotic fluid is taken for testing. The test, which involves a needle being passed through your abdomen, guided by ultrasound, takes around 20 minutes to perform.

Disorders which can be detected by CVS include:

- Down's syndrome
- Cystic fibrosis
- some types of haemophilia
- Duchenne Muscular Dystrophy (DMD)
- Sickle-cell anaemia
- Turner syndrome.

There are other disorders, too. Check with your medical team for details.

CVS is not entirely without risk. In around 2 per cent of cases, the procedure results in miscarriage, as compared with around 1 per cent of cases in mums who opt for amniocentesis. Your midwife or obstetrician should be able to offer you further advice on both tests, but the decision as to whether or not to go ahead with either is down to you. One question to consider before deciding is what you will do if you get a positive result, as your answer could well influence your decision.

Your age and Down's syndrome

Your age	Risk of having a baby with Down's syndrome*
25	1 in 1500
30	1 in 800
35	1 in 300
38	1 in 180
40	1 in 100
45	1 in 30

*With thanks to Guy's and St Thomas' Hospital NHS Trust

What the netmums say

'What CVS feels like'

I recently had a CVS test after I was found to have too much amniotic fluid. We went to St George's in London as our local hospital wasn't able to do it. The doctor we had was lovely, although he did say before the procedure that it felt like having an injection. I promptly asked him when was the last time he'd had a CVS that he knew what it felt like. My midwife was in stitches! The initial pierce with the needle was not too bad but then he said 'Deep breath' and with one short, sharp movement the needle was all the way through my tummy into placental tissue. It was a bit of a shock rather than being very painful, and when the doctor was removing the tissue it was very uncomfortable. The afterpains were worse than the procedure and felt a bit like contractions, but ibuprofen helped. I'd have CVS again if I needed to as I didn't find it too uncomfortable and it was in the interests of my baby's health.
Fiona from Cranleigh, 20 weeks pregnant

My partner and I decided to have CVS because my score for Down's was not good, and my partner and I have no family to care for a disabled child should anything happen to us. We'd decided that we couldn't bring a child with a disability into the world when it was avoidable. It sounds harsh, but it was how we felt. I was very nervous about the whole procedure but my consultant was fantastic and put me at ease. I found it quite painful – not the initial jab, but as the needle went through the final layer it brought a tear to my eyes. Then he said 'Cough, please' and the needle was removed, which was a great relief. Afterwards I found that although the pain in the local area subsided quite quickly I was in pain when I tried to walk. The consultant was extremely apologetic, but said it couldn't be avoided because of where he'd had to go in with the needle. I would definitely go through the whole procedure again if need be. Now that it's all over and our results were clear, we're patiently waiting to meet our baby.
Sam from Woking, seven months pregnant

Is home birth for you?

If you've been inspired by celebs like Charlotte Church, Davina McCall, Nellie Furtado and Lucy Lawless, maybe you'll be one of the increasing number of mums who choose to give birth at home. If you're keen on the idea of a home birth – or even if it's something you haven't considered before – it's a good idea to start doing a bit of research now. You might, for example, like the idea of your baby arriving straight into your own world rather than emerging into the comparatively stark environment of a hospital; maybe you think you'd feel more confident in your own space, with your own stuff around you; perhaps you're freaked out by hospitals in general. These are all good reasons to consider a home birth (whereas thinking 'I can't be bothered to pack a bag – I'll stay at home' probably isn't...).

Although home births in England shot up by 10 per cent to almost 17,000 between 2005 and 2006, they still only accounted for 2.5 per cent of all births; however, the rise might have been triggered by the number of horror stories circulating in the press about the lack of hygiene in hospitals. It's not really that surprising that lots of mums are worried about the risk of infection, but this on its own isn't reason enough to go for a home birth. If your pregnancy has been complicated in any way or if you have a pre-existing medical condition or family history of difficult births, it's probably best to opt, if you can, for a birth centre attached to a hospital so that you are close to medical and surgical facilities if you should need them. If there have been no complications, then a home birth might be a good choice for you. You'll need to keep an open mind, though, as around 30 per cent of women labouring at home end up being transferred to hospital because of concerns about pain relief, a long labour or the baby being in distress. Research also shows that if you do run into problems, the outcome is less good if you give birth at home.

In the end, it's your choice where you give birth, and the NHS is legally obliged to provide midwifery care if you opt for a home birth, so if you're determined but are meeting with opposition from your doctors that you think is unfair, you can insist on your own choice. We're not advocating that you go against all sound medical advice, though, so if there are any known or anticipated problems, you'll need to make an informed decision. The best place to make enquiries about a home birth is through your community midwives. For more advice and support about your rights in pregnancy, contact the Association for Improvements in the Maternity Services (AIMS) on 0870 765 1433 or visit www.aims.org.uk. For more info and opinions (but not medical advice) visit www.homebirth.org.uk.

The upsides of home birth

Advantages to giving birth at home include:

- being surrounded by your own familiar things and home comforts
- being assured of a comforting, warm bath whenever you want it during labour
- having your own bed to climb into after the birth – or any time during labour
- being able to use your phone when you want to without having to wander out to a corridor
- having control of the lighting and sound levels
- having a ready supply of your own food and drink to lay hands on (fridge-cold chocolate – yay!)
- the intimacy of having just your midwives attending you
- have a less 'medicalised' experience than you would do in hospital
- being assured that your partner is comfortable and can be with you throughout.

The downsides of home birth

Of course, there are downsides to consider, too: some mums aren't confident about having a home birth with a first pregnancy as they don't know how the labour and birth are likely to go, whereas mums who've had previous straightforward and uncomplicated labours might feel happier to go ahead with a home birth. Other disadvantages include:

- not having access to strong pain relief or an epidural – although Entonox (gas and air) can be brought to your home
- not being close to emergency medical facilities
- the danger of your midwife being delayed and you not being able to call on another
- the possibility of a medical emergency occurring
- the possibility that you will have to transfer to hospital whilst in strong labour
- the risk of having more intervention as a result of having to transfer to hospital than if you'd been in hospital all along.

Who'd have thought?

During pregnancy your heart and liver expand to cope with the extra demands of pregnancy.

'Domino' delivery

Some hospitals provide what's known as 'domino' care. This means you're cared for during your pregnancy by community midwives – just as you would be for a home birth – but that your midwife will attend you during the first stage and accompany you to hospital for the birth, then accompany you home from hospital around six hours later. It's a good compromise between home and hospital birth, and worth discussing if you're keen on being in your own surroundings as much as possible, but would welcome the reassurance of being in a hospital environment for the delivery of your baby. (And if you like the thought you can get a lovely cup of tea and a toasted sarnie whenever you fancy it during the first stage…!)

What the netmums say

'My home birth experience'

I wanted to have a home birth but my partner didn't, so we settled on a hospital birth. At Week 37 my midwife asked if I'd like a home birth and I told her my partner was against it. She joked with me to watch out that I didn't have an unplanned one on the kitchen floor. Well I ended up with my home birth when my mum and partner had to deliver my daughter in the living room! She came so suddenly that the paramedics didn't arrive until five minutes after she was born. We later got transferred to the hospital as I wanted to be checked over and make sure she was OK. Our first baby had had problems maintaining his temperature at birth, so we thought it would be for the best. I saw my midwife at the hospital and we had a joke about the birth. Looking back I think the only thing I'd change is that I'd have planned it as a home birth with my midwife and some gas and air, but I can't change that and I have a happy, healthy daughter, which is all that matters. If I have another baby I'm going for a planned home birth next time.

Julie from Leeds, mum to Morgan, 17 months and Paige, three months

My first delivery was meant to be a home birth, but I developed severe pre-eclampsia, so that put paid to that. The second home birth was refused on the grounds that I could get it again. However, by my third there was no excuse: the midwives in my area are very pro home birth, and I got a lot of support. I went into labour at 11 p.m. on a snowy February night. The midwife arrived at 4 a.m. and only examined me once. I gave birth in my own bedroom, in total peace with soft lighting and minimal interference. I was able to hold my daughter, Madeleine, straightaway, and within 15 minutes her two big brothers were able to see and hold her. It all felt very natural: I had no stitches as I wasn't rushed. When they opened my curtains there was snow on the rooftops and I felt incredibly emotional and happy. A hot bath later I was back in my newly made-up bed eating my own grub and laughing with my family. It was brilliant!

Julie from Southend, mum to Jude, nine, Leon, six and Madeleine, three

Having had a hospital birth first time round, I attended a different health centre for my second pregnancy and it was obvious they were pro home birth. The experience was great: I was relaxed to the point that I hadn't realised how strong or regular the contractions were! I went into labour at about 2 a.m., called the midwife about 4.30 a.m. and delivered my little girl, with just TENS and gas and air for pain relief, in my bedroom at 9.50 a.m. I was able to hold her for the first time in my own bed, and the midwives even let me find out the sex myself. I can't really describe how wonderful the experience was, although the words 'mind-blowing', 'amazing' and 'unforgettable' come to mind.

Liz from south Gloucestershire, mum to Alex, four and Amy, 14 months

Your mission this week: Decide on a birth partner

You might think you know exactly who's going to be there when you give birth, but although it sounds a bit obvious, it's best just to check they're going to be happy to be there!

Some mums are amazed and disappointed to discover that their partners feel really unhappy about the prospect of being at the birth – and it can certainly come as a bit of a blow if you'd planned it all out in your head. The simple truth is that lots of dads-to-be can't bear the thought of watching their partners in great pain – especially as some of them feel like they're responsible for it all because they got them pregnant in the first place!

There's no point pressurising a reluctant dad to be there if he's really reluctant, but it might help to have a good chat and find out what's on his mind. If he's squeamish about blood, you can tell him he won't have to see anything gory as long as he stays up at the head end of the bed and focuses on you (although you might well not want him focusing on you when the time comes). In any case, there won't be any blood until the delivery itself. Or how about choosing a second birth partner – someone who's practical, calm and not a bit squeamish – so your bloke has the option of legging it if he starts coming over all faint or if he just can't stand watching your pain and being unable to help much? There's also the very real prospect that you'll tell him in no uncertain (probably Anglo-Saxon) terms where to go once you're in the thick of labour. (Best warn him about this and tell him in advance not to take it to heart. It's surprisingly common!) Some men find this a bit hard to take and need to go for a break to compose themselves, so it's helpful to have someone on standby – maybe your mum or a friend with experience of labour – to take his place.

Whatever you decide, now's the time to discuss it all and run it by whomever you might want to be there. Apart from anything else, they might need to advance book a few days off work.

Who'd have thought?

Mums who plan a home birth are less likely to use pain relief than those who plan a hospital birth. According to a survey, only 53 per cent of mums who planned a home birth used gas and air as compared with 72 per cent who had a planned hospital birth.

What the netmums say

'My choice of birth partner'

I had my husband and my mum with me through labour and it worked really well. Of course I wanted my husband there for support, but having a woman there who has been through it made all the difference. I found that at the times when I felt like giving up, encouragement from my mum seemed to help more. Also it gave each of them a break and meant I wasn't left alone if one of them needed the loo. I also had to have stitches and when the midwife asked my hubby to dress our daughter, I thought he was going to cry as he didn't have a clue! Mum, of course, was on hand to show him the ropes. It has brought my husband and mum closer together too.
Steph from Southampton, mum to Olivia, two, and eight months pregnant

With my firstborn my partner decided he didn't want to be at the birth: he has an older son and was present at his birth, which had been complicated and affected him a lot. I decided to ask my older sister who, although she doesn't have children of her own yet, was fantastic! She was really calm, supportive and great at keeping the gas and air flowing. She was so proud to be a part of my first birthing experience and she has a great bond with Cameron. For my second birth my sister wasn't able to be there, but my mum and dad took me to the hospital and mum ended up staying. By that time I was 8cm dilated and didn't really care who was watching! Mum was a great help and my little sister even ended up in with us for the last stage – although I think it's put her off having kids for life! I do wish my partner had been able to be there for the births, but in reality he would have been no use to me at all. My births both ended up being relaxed, positive experiences and that's all that matters: 'Daddy' got to see his babies straight after, so didn't really miss out on bonding time.
Amy from Lincolnshire, mum to Cameron, three and Nathan, 11 months

I had my partner with me, who was fantastic and stayed very calm despite the drama. I did get quite frightened and then worried that I was scaring him. I think that made me look more to my midwife for support. When we have another (hopefully), I am toying with the idea of home birth, and may also consider having a second female there for support. I like the idea of having another woman there who has been through childbirth and can understand.
Kim from Norfolk, mum to Oli, one

For my first daughter's birth I had my then fiancé, Marc, there with me and he was fantastic. My mum and mother-in-law were hovering in and out of the room, but as she was born they left; had I been more with it I'd have asked them to stay. My mum-in-law asked if she could be present again at our second baby's birth. I didn't mind at all, and it was great because she was rubbing my lower back whilst Marc was in front of me holding my hands and giving me encouragement. I actually delivered standing up with my mum-in-law standing behind me. It turned out that our baby must have been in the wrong position all along as she came out looking at her grandmother! Next time I'm hoping for a home birth and would love both my mum and mother-in-law there again.
Amy from Fareham, mum to Bethany, four and Ella, one

What is a nuchal translucency scan?
It's a special scan offered in some hospitals, depending on your local NHS Trust, which is performed between Weeks 11 and 13 of pregnancy to screen for Down's syndrome. During the scan, a measurement is taken of the nuchal skin fold at the base of your baby's neck: babies with Down's syndrome have a thicker fold of skin here than other babies. If your hospital does offer a nuchal translucency test, it's likely to be carried out as part of your dating scan.

Look no further

What happens at a dating scan?
You'll be called into a darkened sonography (scanning) room and invited to lie down on a special table (this is great in itself – a lie-down in the middle of

the day – but if all is well, it just gets better from this point on!). Your sonographer (the scan technician) will ask you to lower your clothes past your hip bones so that your abdomen is exposed (don't worry, you'll be allowed a certain degree of modesty and won't be expected to expose all your bits at this stage). Then he or she will tuck some tissue into your lower clothes to protect them before dropping some special gel on to your tummy: be warned, it's often very cold! The gel helps the scanning instrument to glide smoothly over your tummy.

Next, the scanning instrument – which looks a bit like the scanning gun you see in supermarkets only straighter – will be passed over your belly until the sonographer gets an on-screen image of your baby. This is just thrilling for most mums, and can be the defining moment when the reality of pregnancy finally hits home.

If all's well, the sonographer will turn the screen so that you can see your baby; he or she should be happy to point out anything illuminating – although at this stage, depending on which week you have your scan performed, there might not be much for you to recognise. If yours is scheduled for Week 11 or Week 12, however, you should be able to see your baby almost fully formed, but in miniature!

How do ultrasound scans work?

The 3D – or in some units even 4D – images you see on screen are produced when sound waves are directed via the scanner head into your uterus, then reflected back to the scanning machine, which transmits them to the screen. This then allows the sonographer to take lots of measurements that help to assess how well your baby is growing and developing.

What's a transvaginal scan?

If you have an early scan (in the first 8–10 weeks) it will be performed by placing a probe inside your vagina close to your cervix. This is because it can give a much more detailed view of your uterus than an abdominal scan, and everything inside your uterus is so small and underdeveloped at this early stage that detecting anything via an abdominal scan would be impossible. You might be offered an early scan if you've had previous miscarriages or difficulty getting pregnant, or if you've been having fertility treatment.

How do I decide between CVS and amniocentesis?
One advantage of CVS is that it can be carried out 10 to 13 weeks after your LMP, whereas amniocentesis can't be performed until 15 to 18 weeks. As with amniocentesis, the results take around two weeks to come through, although a few preliminary results may be available after around 72 hours. It does mean that if your results confirm an abnormality in your baby, you will have more time in which to decide whether or not to progress with the pregnancy, and the pregnancy won't be as far advanced.

Week 10 217 days to go!

Don't forget: Get ready for your booking appointment

This is the week you're likely to meet your midwife for the first time, so make sure you go armed with any questions you might have. Don't forget she's an expert on pregnancy, so don't be afraid to ask about anything and everything, from the physical to the emotional as well as any worries that are playing on your mind. This is the appointment at which you'll have your first antenatal tests, too, so make sure in advance that you know your own mind about which you want and which you don't. Blood is likely to be taken for:

- a full blood count to be performed
- checking your blood group and rhesus factor
- checking your rubella status
- checking for hepatitis B
- checking for syphilis
- checking for HIV
- checking for thalassaemia
- performing a sickle cell screen.

At this appointment, you'll also be asked to sign a form called FW8, which entitles you to free prescriptions in pregnancy and for a year afterwards. You'll have your urine tested and your blood pressure checked too.

Although you might not see the same person throughout your pregnancy it's worth trying to get to know each midwife in case she's the one who ends up delivering your baby. Try to build a rapport if you can, and make a point of listening to what she has to say without interrupting unnecessarily. You might find it helpful to take a notebook and pen with you so you can write down anything you think you might forget. If your booking appointment is delayed until Week 12, you'll probably get to hear your baby's heartbeat transmitted through an amplifier called a Sonicaid; any earlier and it's unlikely to be heard yet: it's a really thrilling moment for lots of mums, and you might want to take your partner with you, if you have a later appointment, to share in the excitement.

Hey baby!

Your baby is somewhere between 27–35mm long now – so probably around the length of your top thumb joint. From this point on, he ceases to be an embryo and is now a fully fledged foetus (not that a label makes much difference to you, him or anyone else much…). The significant thing about this move from embryo to foetus, though, is that all his major organs have developed beyond the point when a birth defect would have occurred, as most happen before Week 10. Now all that remains is for the finer development of those organs to continue and for a whole lot of growing to go on.

Your baby's getting to be quite a buster, weighing 3–4g – roughly the equivalent of four paperclips! He's more active than ever, although you still won't be able to feel a thing. If you have a scan around now, though, you'll probably see him generally flinging his arms and legs around and limbering up like an Olympic gymnast. The webbing has gone from fingers and toes and he's even got the dexterity and sense of touch to be able to grab hold of things – not that there's much in your uterus to grab hold of, of course.

Your baby's eyelids are almost formed; soon they'll fuse shut, and they'll stay that way until around Weeks 25–27. His outer ears and upper lip are fully formed, as are his (or her!) genitals. And he's finally lost that cute little tail he started out with in his 'tadpole' phase.

Who'd have thought?

A US study in child development found that the children of mums who reported moderate stress levels in pregnancy were more advanced at age two than those of unstressed mums.

All about you

You might have noticed your waistbands tightening a bit more by now –
although for some mums it takes a few weeks more before they start to 'show'
at all. It's a tricky point in pregnancy, especially if you haven't shared the news
yet, as you're more likely to look like you've piled on a few pounds through
over-indulgence than look pregnant. Some mums really embrace the changes,
however small, as they happen, and see them as more proof (if it were needed!)
that their pregnancy is progressing; others find the prospect of losing their
figures harder to adjust to (see *You and your body image*, p. 76). If you're
unhappy about your changing shape, talk to a trusted friend or your midwife:
maybe your feelings are about something a bit deeper than just the superficial
changes that are happening, and it's far better to chat things through as they
arise than to let yourself slide into antenatal depression (see below).

Antenatal depression

Most of us have heard of postnatal depression, which affects between
70,000 and 100,000 mums in the UK every year, but antenatal
depression is less talked-about. According to a study carried out at
Bristol University in 2001, it's a condition that affects about 10 per cent
of mums-to-be. Although most of us experience some mood swings in
pregnancy, mums who are depressed feel more down than anything
for a lot of the time, and might find it hard to cope with being
pregnant. Other symptoms can include:

- lack of concentration
- extreme irritability
- excessive tiredness (and wanting to sleep all the time)
- sleeplessness at night
- the inability to enjoy things
- overeating or loss of appetite
- compulsive behaviour
- excessive crying.

If you are experiencing any or all of the above and are unhappy,
contact your GP or midwife so you can get the help and support you
need. Depression can have dramatic consequences if left untreated.

What the netmums say

'Depression in pregnancy'

I was supposed to be working full time in a busy retail shop. I just couldn't face it and would be up in the office with the managers crying my eyes out and I didn't know why. I had a week off, but when I got back I felt the same, so my employers arranged to have all my leftover holiday put in front of my maternity leave so that I finished work about three weeks earlier than the earliest you can usually leave. At the time I didn't realise I was depressed. I was diagnosed when Bethany was four months old, and only realised when I felt better how early it had started for me. My biggest fear was that I'd be depressed in my next pregnancy, but luckily I was fine with Ella.

Amy from Fareham, mum to Bethany, four and Ella, one

I was already depressed when I fell pregnant for the second time, although my depression had nothing to do with having had a baby, but more to do with my housing situation. When I found I was pregnant again I was really confused: part of me really wanted this baby, but another big part really resented the baby. I had so many negative thoughts and feelings throughout the pregnancy; I even had hot baths in the hope it would bring on a miscarriage. I never spoke about it to anyone, but if I'm truthful I just didn't want the baby to thrive. I feel really guilty about it now, especially when I look into my daughter's eyes, but at the time I was in a dark place in my mind. When I moved and returned to work I started to pick up, but it wasn't until a few weeks after my daughter's birth that I realised I did actually want and love my daughter.

Julie from Leeds, mum to Morgan, 17 months and Paige, three months

You and your appetite

Hungry? It's not surprising! With a bit of luck (and a following wind!) you'll have stopped feeling nauseous by around now and will have got back on track with your appetite. As long as you haven't suddenly developed a taste for coal dust or chalk (see *Why am I having these weird cravings?*, p. 41), go ahead and get stuck in: that is unless you've developed not-so-weird cravings for doughnuts, choc-nut sundaes or melted cheese with everything. The key is to eat little and often, choosing foods that take a while to digest. (See *Low GI Foods*, below, for what to include daily.)

Planning your pregnancy diet

There's a relatively new way of eating that's suitable for everyone and should suit you very well now you're pregnant. It's based on a dietary scale called the Glycaemic Index (GI). Foods with a low GI value take longer to digest, so keep you feeling full for longer; those with a high GI value give you a fast energy boost, but leave you feeling hungry again soon after. Low-GI foods keep your blood-sugar levels more or less constant throughout the day; high-GI foods mean your blood-sugar levels peak and trough throughout the day, which is not good for you and will encourage you to eat more and more of the 'wrong' foods every time you feel hungry.

Low-GI foods

Foods which have a low GI value tend to be those which are non-processed and don't contain added sugar. They include complex carbohydrates such as wholegrains and fibrous fruit and veg. Foods to include in your daily diet so that you are satisfied for longer, include:

- wholemeal bread, cereals and pasta
- oats and grains
- rye bread, sourdough bread and rice cakes
- no-added-sugar muesli
- unsalted, unsweetened nuts and dried fruits
- low-sugar, low-fat cereal bars
- mixed seeds, including sunflower, pumpkin and sesame
- fibrous fruit and veg: pears, apples, figs, plums, apricots, peaches, broccoli, asparagus, squash, peas, greens, runner beans

- legumes: lentils, chickpeas, black-eye beans, borlotti beans, broad beans
- wholegrain rice, red rice, couscous, bulgur wheat and quinoa
- strawberries, blueberries, raspberries, blackberries
- lean white meat and fish
- oily fish (but no more than two portions per week in pregnancy)
- low-fat bio yoghurt and fromage frais
- pasteurised goats' cheese, feta and halloumi
- eggs (cooked thoroughly in pregnancy)
- salad leaves, including spinach (well washed).

High-GI foods

The foods to avoid when eating a balanced low-GI diet are those which are typically high in added sugar and fat, and those which are heavily processed. They include:

- cakes, biscuits, chocolate
- pies, pasties, sausage rolls
- fat-fried chips
- battered fish (or battered anything else for that matter!)
- sweets
- high-sugar fruits such as watermelon, honeydew melon and grapes
- sugar-coated cereals
- white bread, white rolls, scones and crumpets
- white pasta and white rice
- high-fat, high-sugar desserts, including yoghurts
- crisps and other salty, oily snacks
- red meat
- processed foods such as hotdogs, processed cheese, most ready meals; burgers and sausages.

Getting the right balance

Try to include some protein at every meal, even if it's a little crumbled feta cheese on a bed of salad leaves. Choose complex carbohydrates like brown or red rice, wholegrain bread, wholemeal pasta and new potatoes in their skins, and carbohydrate vegetables such as broccoli, asparagus, carrots, peas, greens, beans and squash. As a rule of thumb, your protein (be it fish, lean white meat or cheese) should be roughly the size of the palm of your hand, and your vegetables should make up the greatest part of your meal, with carbs making up the smallest part.

Snacking without pigging out

Remember to eat little and often, so have a snack between meals – probably around two hours after eating. Choose a handful of berries topped with a tablespoon of natural bio yoghurt; an ounce or two of pasteurised, non-mould-ripened cheese with an oatcake or rye cracker; a banana; a no-added-sugar cereal bar; a small bowl (half a portion) of unsweetened cereal with semi-skimmed milk; a tablespoon of hummus spread on a rice cake or some carrot sticks dipped in low-fat soft cheese. If you're looking for a treat, have a small piece of fruit cake (without marzipan or icing unless it's Christmas), two or three squares (not four or five!) of good-quality dark chocolate (it's got iron in it, so that can be your excuse) or a scoop of fruit sorbet. You're not on a weight-loss diet – unless your medical team has told you otherwise – but you don't want to pile on excessive amounts of weight either. And if you do, don't expect it all to fall away with the birth of your baby.

You and your body image

You're still at the beginning of big physical changes, and how you feel about your body will play a part in how much you enjoy your pregnancy. Some mums absolutely love being pregnant and revel in not having to suck their tummies in for a few months! Others hate the feeling that their body is no longer under their control. Because society as a whole tends to take the view that long and lean is the only acceptable way to be, you might feel that putting on weight in pregnancy is a negative thing. If this rings true for you, it's important that you try to take a more positive view, because if you try to prevent a healthy weight gain by cutting down on your calories, you could be putting your health at risk. And things could get a whole lot worse later in pregnancy when unthinking individuals blurt out things like 'God, you're huge! Are you sure you haven't got twins in there?'

However you feel about your body, you're probably not alone. You'll find it helpful to share your feelings with the Netmums, who'll empathise and offer their thoughts on the subject. You'll soon see that pregnancy affects people in lots of different ways.

One thing's for sure: week by week – sometimes day by day – your body will undergo noticeable changes – and you might feel differently at different stages. Maybe you'll love having a little bump to show, but won't be so keen on an exercise-ball-sized belly a few months down the line! Perhaps you love your newly defined cleavage but don't like sporting a protruding tummy. Maybe you'll feel feminine and sexy today, but lumpen and dowdy tomorrow. Some mums alternate between rejoicing in being pregnant and wishing they weren't expecting at all. Whatever anyone says to you, it's important that you acknowledge your own feelings, take them seriously and talk to someone who can sympathise. Your emotional wellbeing is every bit as important as your physical health.

Remember, inside your new figure you're still you. And it may help to think that your body has become a beautiful haven for your growing baby and is on temporary loan as a mobile home!

Learn to love your body

Here are a few tips to help you get a more positive view of your changing body:

- focus on your best bits and try to accentuate these. If you love your new boobs, treat yourself to some Empire-line scoop-neck tops and show them off. This style also skims your bump, drawing attention away from your middle
- talk to your bump: find a quiet time, like last thing at night or in the bath and try to communicate with your baby. You could either chat gently, sing a nursery song or try to send thought waves
- treat your tum nicely: get a little baby oil or body cream and massage your belly in circular motions from your belly button outwards. Make it part of your daily routine to help you to feel more accepting of the changes
- if you are fit and reasonably supple, look for a yoga class that's specifically

for pregnant women: yoga focuses on the link between mind and body, and may help you to feel more serene

- eat healthily: it will make you feel that you are doing the best for your baby, yourself and your figure. Of course you will change shape in pregnancy, but you don't have to pile on loads of surplus fat through eating the wrong things
- buy cheap and cheerful clothes to suit your shape as you change: there's nothing like a new piece of gear to make you feel attractive.

What the netmums say

'Me and my changing body'

I hated the first three months. I'm normally quite skinny, and I just felt fat and bloated. I put on a layer of fat all over and felt really stodgy. I think it was actually just all the ginger biscuits I was eating to stop the nausea! I felt much better when I got a bump, and I loved my increased bust size. Best thing about being pregnant was the cleavage! Again, I'd had enough by the last couple of months and just felt like a whale. I didn't actually like looking at myself in a mirror.
Jen from Hertfordshire, mum to Jack, four and Theo, 17 months

I loved my bump and was quite sad when it went – well, just until I realised I had a baby instead! I am naturally very skinny, so putting on weight and growing this huge belly and boobs was a revelation, and I loved every minute: I also felt very attractive and sexy – that is until I could no longer reach my toes or do up my shoes!
Kirsty from Hereford, mum to Isla, six months

With both pregnancies I didn't really get much of a bump and mostly stayed in my normal clothes. With Paige I was more self-conscious, as under my bump I had a jelly-like bit of flesh hanging down – it was horrid. The great thing with both pregnancies, though, was that I lost about a stone in weight during the first few months so never really put much on, and was straight back into my normal clothes after each baby was born.
Julie from Leeds, mum to Morgan, 17 months and Paige, three months

Even though I'm very prone to stretch marks and I started getting them from about 20 weeks, I loved having a bump and it made me feel so special. Each pregnancy is unique, and with my first child I had a huge, round bump that took up all of my tummy! Craig was a big boy weighing in at 9lb 6oz. Second time around my bump was more compact and Georgia turned out to be a more modest 8lb 1oz. I missed my bump after both pregnancies, and I'd got so used to it being there that sometimes I'd forget I'd given birth and go to touch it and feel a big load of wobbly jelly where my bump once was! I think there's a part of you which almost grieves for your bump once your baby is born.

Terri from Liverpool, mum to Craig, five and Georgia, 17 months

Your mission this week: Revamp your store cupboards

Clear out your cupboards of any out-of-date foods and drinks and re-stock with healthier options: ditch the white pasta and rice for now and get in some brown or red wholegrain stuff; buy in some healthy snacks like a dried fruit-and-seed mix or some rice cakes or oatcakes. Have a look down the list of low-GI foods on p. 74 and go shopping for enough food to see you through the next few days – but don't buy up the whole shop or get everything on the list as you'll end up wasting food.

Try different food combos like poached egg on toasted rye bread or hummus in a salad sandwich. Experiment by mixing and matching so you don't get bored. Next time you go shopping, try to get different things from the list and ring the changes. You don't have to alter your eating habits so radically that you'll just revert back to 'normal' when your baby's born: by making more gradual changes you're more likely to stick to a healthier way of eating afterwards, too – and that can only be good news when you come to wean your baby. (OK, maybe we're jumping ahead of ourselves a little here, but it can't hurt to think ahead…)

Look no further

How much weight should I put on in pregnancy?
An acceptable weight gain, as long as you were at a normal weight at the outset with a body mass index (BMI) of 19–25, is something between

11–16kg (25–35lb) – slightly more if you were underweight to start with; less if you were overweight or obese – so putting on more will probably mean you've laid down fat you'll only be able to shift through diet and exercise: what a bore! Best to try not to gain too much in the first place. Talk to your midwife, GP or obstetrician to discover the ideal weight gain for you. You'll need to use a little bit of self-will to stay within acceptable limits as changes to antenatal care mean you probably won't be weighed at each antenatal appointment as you would have been a few years ago.

How do I calculate my BMI?

If you know your pre-pregnancy weight, you can work out your starting BMI by dividing your weight in kilograms by the square of your height in metres (or by dividing your weight in pounds by the square of your height in inches) then multiplying by 703.

How can I eat a low-GI meal in a restaurant?

Well, it will help if you can avoid the curry house and choose an Italian or English restaurant instead. There are a few simple rules: firstly, drink a glass of water before you go out so you won't feel starving hungry. When you get there, don't take any bread when it's passed round, however tempting, but do have a handful of olives instead. A good starter choice would be parma ham and melon, a small salad or a non-creamy soup such as minestrone or consommé. For a main course, go for anything lean and grilled, so a steak, chicken breast or grilled fish would all be fine. Supplement it with a large mixed salad or some roasted vegetables, but go easy on the spuds. If there's a choice, opt for boiled new potatoes in their skins rather than mash or roasties. The cheese board with a few oat biscuits or a bowl of fresh-fruit salad would be better choices than a stodgy pudding. Indulge in a chocolate with your coffee instead.

If you just can't resist a curry, try to avoid fried rice, naan, chapatis and poppadoms as well as curries cooked in creamy sauces. Dhansaks are a good choice as they contain lentils which will lower the GI of the dish; dahl is another lentil dish which would make a great accompaniment; bindi bhaji (okra) and sag (spinach) dishes are better than Bombay potato or onion bhaji. Most Indian restaurants will also provide salad if you ask.

Week 11 210 days to go!

Don't forget: Write things down!

Somewhere between 50 per cent and 80 per cent of mums notice that their memory suffers in pregnancy. The phenomenon even has a label – 'baby brain' – and can give rise to some funny mishaps as well as some really embarrassing or downright inconvenient lapses of memory. One mum parked her car in town to go shopping, then forgot whereabouts she'd left it and had to call her husband to drive her around looking for it! See *You and your 'baby brain'*, p. 82, for more info and advice on memory lapses.

Hey baby!

Your baby's making a great effort at growing now. His skin is still almost transparent but pretty much everything is in place, right down to his finger- and toenails. If you're carrying a boy, he'll start to produce testosterone this week. Boy or girl, the external genitals are growing fast now, although it may still be hard to tell the sex from a scan. Your baby's lungs, though formed, are still very immature. His heart has divided into right and left atria (chambers) and ventricles, and have developed valves. Little ribs can now been seen through his skin.

Your baby is busily mastering some new skills: he can suck and swallow, and his intestines can process the liquid that he is swallowing. He can also kick, punch and arch his body, flex his fingers, form a fist and wrinkle his forehead. Luckily for you, you can't yet feel his punches: but just you wait until your third trimester, by which time he might object to you balancing a book or magazine on your bump and promptly kick it off!

Your baby is approximately the length of your thumb by the end of this week, and half his weight is accounted for by his head.

All about you

With any luck you'll be feeling a lot more settled in your pregnancy. The end of the critical 12-week danger zone is just around the corner and news of your pregnancy will soon be out of the bag for all to know. If you've met your medical team you should be feeling reassured and better informed. Your uterus is about the size of a grapefruit now!

You and your 'baby brain'

There is plenty of anecdotal evidence from mums-to-be and those who've had their babies already that memory and concentration can go a bit haywire during pregnancy. There's not much scientific evidence to support this suggestion, though – in fact a few of the studies that have been carried out come up with opposite conclusions, with some agreeing that pregnancy does cause temporary brain impairment and others saying it can't. Well, whatever the boffins say, we know from experience that when you're expecting it can be almost impossible at times to repeat your own phone number, remember where you've parked the car or recall your mental shopping list! And that's why we suggest you carry a little notebook and pen with you wherever you go to record important information, and invest in a supply of sticky notes to post around the house. It's a great idea to get one of those 'family organiser' calendars too: they've got lots of space for you to record every move you need to make for the next few months! (See *Your mission this week*, p. 88.)

Some recent studies do suggest that the reason why we mums insist our brains don't work properly in pregnancy is because we're suffering from a 'neurological overload' – in other words, we've got so much new information to think about that everyday stuff goes out the window. Pregnancy is, after all, a far more important thing to get your head round than remembering your mum-in-law's birthday or paying the phone bill. It's interesting to learn that all sorts of stressful situations can result in a failing memory: according to one study, paying less attention to the more mundane events of life is also how we react to a bereavement, other major stress or just the demands of a hectic lifestyle. For some mums the forgetfulness starts early in pregnancy – when, coincidentally, the pregnancy hormones oestrogen and progesterone, which have been linked to memory function, flood in – whilst for others it affects them more in later pregnancy. Whatever your experience, you might as well get into good habits now.

Who'd have thought?

Squeezing lemon juice over your food can reduce the GI (Glycaemic Index) value of the entire meal. (But it doesn't mean you can justify a huge plateful of cheesy lasagne if you serve it with a lemon wedge!)

What the netmums say

'Me and my "baby brain"!'

I was shopping with Andrew on our first trip out after he was born. We were in the supermarket and my husband James had the trolley and I had the pram. I left the pram next to the shelf and went to reach something. James started to walk on with the trolley and I went to catch up with him and just left the pram. James looked at me and asked if I had forgotten something, and it took about ten seconds for me to realise. I honestly think having children damages short-term memory and common sense permanently – or maybe that's because I've got four of them!

Sharon from Aberdeenshire, mum to Andrew, 10, Stuart, nine, Jessica, three and Sophie, one

With all my pregnancies – and for a while after birth (probably due to no sleep) – my brain was a sieve. I couldn't and still can't remember where I put anything: I still keep leaving things like my travelcard and mobile in my pocket then putting them in the washing machine. I also forget my own mobile number and often find myself wondering why I dial half my partner's old mobile number and half his new number when trying to call him. No wonder why a few strangers have answered in the past!

Alicia from London, mum to Kyrus, two, Demiyah, one, and 14 weeks pregnant

I remember once when Alfie was very small, I came home after shopping and must have left my bank card on the windowsill; I walked into the kitchen and came back out again... and I couldn't remember where I'd put my card! I spent the next two days (no joking here!) looking for it, and when I finally found it I honestly had no recollection of putting it there!

Izzy from Wiltshire, mum to Alfie, two

Understanding your notes

You'll soon be the proud carrier of your own maternity notes (if you don't
have them already). They're given to you to bring to appointments so that,
should you need any maternity care from anyone other than your own
midwife or doctor, you can provide a full account of your pregnancy and
relevant medical history to date.

Your antenatal notes are for you to read as well as your medical team, but
you might find them a bit confusing, so here's a rundown of what's what.
Although different health authorities' notes might be presented slightly
differently, most will include:

- your name, address and hospital number
- your ethnicity and religion (if relevant)
- your medical history as well as any relevant family medical history
- a record of any medicines you're taking or have been prescribed in pregnancy
- a record of any previous pregnancies and whether they resulted in
  termination, miscarriage, stillbirth or a live birth
- your estimated due date (EDD)
- a write-up of each of your antenatal visits, including a record of your
  blood pressure, the results of any tests and some remarks about your
  baby's development and heart rate
- details of any complications or difficulties with your pregnancy
- measurements of your bump and details of how your baby is lying
- scan pictures and write-ups.

You'll also find a section on how you'd like the birth to go. Even if you can't
imagine giving birth yet, it's important you give it some thought and make
a few decisions ahead of time, especially as you might be in no fit state to
discuss the pros and cons of an epidural once you're in established labour.
Don't worry that your recorded thoughts will be taken as if written in
tablets of stone – you can always change your mind as you go along or on
the day. It's just helpful for your team to know your preferences about
things like pain relief and intervention so they can try to implement them
if you still feel the same way when the time comes. Some mums use this
section instead of a birth plan, but it's a good idea to write your own birth
plan and give a copy to all your medical team as you'll be able to include

much more detail (see p. 294). You'll also be able to give a copy to your birth partner(s) so they can speak up for you if you don't feel able to do so yourself.

Jargon busting

Reading your notes can feel a bit like trying to decipher some weird computer language, so here's a guide to what the blue blazes some of the abbreviations and bits of jargon mean:

Date
The date of each antenatal visit

Foetal heart
FHH or H – foetal heart heard
FHNH – foetal heart not heard – this isn't necessarily anything to worry about
FMF – foetal movements have been felt

Weight
Your weight is recorded at your first antenatal visit.

Weeks of gestation
The length of your pregnancy in weeks and days, from the first day of your last monthly period (LMP). Sometimes recorded as, for example, 10 weeks + 5, which would mean 10 weeks and five days of pregnancy.

Urinalysis (urine testing)
A urine sample will be tested at every antenatal visit for the following things:

Glucose (sugar)
This may be a sign of diabetes in pregnancy. If glucose appears repeatedly or there's a large amount present, a blood test will be carried out.

Albumin (Alb)
Albumin (protein) may be a sign of pre-eclampsia (a serious pregnancy condition affecting the placenta and threatening the wellbeing of mum and baby. See p. 274).

Ketones
These are chemicals produced by your body when your fat-burning mechanisms aren't working properly. This could indicate gestational diabetes

(see p. 212) or be a sign that you're not eating enough, or it could happen as a result of prolonged pregnancy sickness.

If glucose, albumin or ketones are detected in your urine, the quantity is recorded with plus signs: + means a trace, + + means more than a trace and + + + means a significant amount. You may also see the letters Tr, which means a small trace has been found. A tick, nil or NAD all mean the same – nothing abnormal detected.

Blood pressure

Your blood pressure will be written down as two numbers, one on top of the other: for example, 110/80. The top number is your systolic pressure (the pressure in the arteries when your heart contracts); the bottom number is your diastolic pressure (the pressure in the arteries when your heart relaxes between pumps). In pregnancy, a normal blood pressure range is between 95/60 and 135/85. Your blood pressure will be measured at your booking-in visit and this figure will be used as your normal level, against which future readings will be compared. If you blood pressure rises to 140/90 or above, you may be given medication which is compatible with pregnancy.

Height of fundus (FH)

The fundus is the top of your uterus (womb). The midwife will measure how far the top of your uterus has grown away from your pelvic bone and record this in centimetres. This gives a good indication of your baby's growth.

The lie

The 'lie' refers to the position of the crown of your baby's head within your pelvis:

* O (occiput) – this refers to the back of your baby's head, which could be facing:
* R – right
* L – left
* A (anterior) – to the front
* P (posterior) – to the back
* L (lateral) or T (transverse) – to the side

Presentation

The 'presentation' refers to which way up your baby is:

* C or Ceph (cephalic) or Vx (vertex) – head down
* Br (breech) – feet or bottom first

Relation of PP to brim

PP (presenting part) refers to the bit of your baby that will arrive first (usually the head). Your midwife will note down how much of your baby's head can be felt above the brim of your pelvis in fifths: 5/5 means that the head is not engaged (sitting in the pelvis) at all and is often described as being 'free'; 0/5 means that the head is fully engaged (your baby's head has dropped down into your pelvis ready to be born). E or Eng means engaged; NE means not engaged.

Oedema

The medical term for swelling, which most commonly occurs in your feet, ankles or hands during pregnancy. This is because your body retains more fluid, but it can also be a symptom of pre-eclampsia (see p. 274), so your midwife will always check this out.

Hb

This stands for haemoglobin, the substance found in red blood cells that carries oxygen around your body and to your baby. An essential ingredient of haemoglobin is iron. A blood test will determine your haemoglobin level, and if it's low you'll be prescribed iron supplements to raise it.

Remarks or notes

In this section, your midwife will record any other information, any medical history of concern, further blood tests you might need, or any medication you've been prescribed.

Natural therapies

If you're still bothered by pregnancy niggles and discomforts after this week, you could think about treating yourself to a natural therapy that's known to be safe for mums-to-be. Maybe you could use a really good pregnancy massage; perhaps you fancy trying aromatherapy. Some mums have reported great success with natural therapies in alleviating lots of things from nausea to heartburn and general aches and pains.

There's a whole raft of therapies to try, but make sure you let the relevant therapist know that you're pregnant and how far along you are – and do check out his or her credentials so you're confident you are dealing with someone competent who's had experience of treating pregnant ladies. Some practitioners prefer to wait until the second trimester of pregnancy, when the greatest danger of miscarriage has passed.

Some mums swear by acupuncture to help with sickness, constipation and piles. During acupuncture, hair-fine needles are inserted superficially into the skin. It sounds painful, but shouldn't be.

Reflexology can be very soothing, as you get a lovely foot massage as part of therapy. The principle is that different areas of your feet correspond with different organs in your body, and that gentle manipulation can help the relevant organs to work more efficiently.

Osteopathy involves gentle manipulation of your joints to help relieve pelvic pain, backache and joint strain.

Always check with your doctor or midwife before using a natural therapy, as any problem or symptom you're having could potentially need medical treatment.

Your mission this week: Get organised

Set aside a special place for storing all your important pregnancy paperwork: clear a drawer or space in a cupboard – or buy yourself a new storage box that can be used for baby toys or memorabilia afterwards. Make a point of storing everything – your medical notes, appointment cards and any hospital test forms you may have – in this new place. Record all your upcoming appointments, scan dates and other significant dates on your new family organiser (see *You and your 'baby brain'*, p. 82) and leave a sticky note permanently by the kettle, or anywhere you visit frequently, to remind you to check your organiser and/or pregnancy box daily.

It's probably a good idea to let your partner know where your special box or other place is, too, just in case he needs to find something in a hurry!

Look no further

Where does all the extra weight come from in pregnancy?
The thought of putting on an average two stone (12.7kg) in pregnancy can be a bit alarming, but when you take into account things like the final weight of your baby, the increase in your own blood volume and the weight of your

amniotic sac, it's easier to imagine where some of the weight goes.

Your baby will account for more than a quarter of your overall weight gain, with the average birth weight being around 3.4kg (7lb 8oz). Your placenta and amniotic sac will weigh about half that again – so around 1.7kg (about 3lb 7oz). The rest of your weight gain will be accounted for by fat laid down by your body in preparation for breastfeeding (plus any excess you put on through overeating!), the extra blood circulating around your body and the extra weight of your expanding uterus. So you can see that most of the weight should fall away after the delivery – unless you've accumulated lots of fat, in which case it'll be harder work to return to your pre-pregnancy size.

My boobs have hardly grown at all. Does this mean I won't be able to breastfeed?
Not at all. Some mums notice their boobs growing at an alarming rate; others like you hardly notice any change; and it might be that you'll get bigger a bit later in pregnancy in any case. The amount your breasts increase in size depends on how much fat is laid down there for breastfeeding, but this doesn't mean you'll produce less milk if you have less fat. There are very few mums who can't breastfeed because of some physiological problem: usually it's down to poor positioning of the baby at the breast, a lack of confidence, an aversion to the thought of breastfeeding or other psychological difficulties. Don't worry: if you want to feed your baby (and it's known to be the best start you can give him or her), with a little help and encouragement from your midwife, health visitor or a breastfeeding counsellor you'll manage just fine.

I keep having the weirdest dreams. Why?
Loads of mums report having the most bizarre dreams, often starting in their first trimester. It's hardly surprising that such a big life change has an impact subconsciously – and however you might interpret your strange dreams, it might help to remember that dreaming is your mind's way of mentally sorting and 'filing' your recent experiences and emotions. Dream experts believe that a combination of pregnancy hormones, mixed feelings, understandable anxieties and, hopefully, excitement stimulate the brain to come up with some weird and wonderful scenarios while we sleep. There's no need to worry, or to attach any significance to your dreams.

Week 12 *20½ days to go!*

Don't forget: Think about your birth plan

Even though there's ages to go yet before the birth (and you'd probably prefer not to give it too much thought just now) it's really useful to start thinking about the sort of labour and delivery you think might suit you best. If you're planning a home birth, your options will be somewhat limited, but if you're planning to go to a birth centre or hospital maternity unit, there are all sorts of things you'd be better off making a decision about in advance (whilst keeping an open mind on the day itself, of course!).

If you start to weigh up your options now, you'll have lots of time to discuss them with your partner and your medical team; no one is going to write anything down in tablets of stone, but it's a good idea to start getting some idea of the choices open to you. It might help to talk to other mums about what they would have changed if they could have on the day. Most mums start to think more seriously about committing things to paper about halfway through pregnancy (see p. 294), by which time you might also have changed your mind about some of your ideas. This is perfectly normal – you'll probably make more changes as the birth approaches, too. Don't forget to turn to the Netmums' forum for more discussion.

Hey baby!

Your baby is almost 2½ inches (7cm) long now and weighs about 14g (about half an ounce). This week, your placenta takes over the important task of hormone production. Your baby's external genitals are now formed and should be visible on an ultrasound scan (depending on whether or not your baby cooperates and lies in a conducive position for viewing!).

Now that your baby's eyes have come closer together from their original positions on either side of the head, and now that his chin is becoming more defined, his face looks decidedly more like a human baby's!

All the organs are functioning now: your baby's liver is making bile and his kidneys are producing urine. Important neurological pathways in your baby's brain (called 'synapses') are forming, and his reflexes are responsive.

Who'd have thought?

During pregnancy, your body makes collagen – that magical stuff cosmetics companies try to get us to buy to fill in our wrinkly bits! So expect to look more youthful than ever (at least for the time being).

All about you

By the end of this week, the greatest danger of miscarriage will have passed. Lots of mums find they relax into pregnancy a bit more once they've reached this important milestone. Now that your uterus has lifted up from behind your pelvic bone, you might be aware of a little bump, although unless you're wearing a lycra cycling suit, it probably won't be obvious to anyone who doesn't know you're pregnant. Spotting your bump for the first time yourself can be another turning point: it's evidence that your baby's growing and developing, and heralds the start of your new pregnancy shape. How you feel about the physical changes pregnancy brings will make a difference to how well you cope over the coming months – and may even have an impact on how you feel about your baby. See p. 76 for more about your new body image.

Your 12-week scan

If you haven't already had an early scan (usually only offered in special circumstances such as following repeated miscarriage or fertility treatment), or a booking scan, you'll probably have one around now. For most parents it's a defining moment of pregnancy and makes it all seem more real. Most hospitals can provide a printout of your scan picture, and some even offer a piece of video footage. In either case you'll probably be asked to pay a small charge. For more on scans, see *What happens at a dating scan?*, p. 68.

Who'd have thought?

Acupuncture is not only helpful in alleviating stress, nausea and other pregnancy niggles, it's also been shown to improve blood flow to the uterus and can boost your energy levels.

What the netmums say

'Having a dating scan'

I'd had an early scan at eight weeks as I'd become pregnant through IVF, and the scan confirmed it was twins. Then I had another at 10 weeks as I'd started bleeding, but thankfully everything was fine. My next scan was at 13 weeks, and I was so nervous, thinking that one or both babies were not going to make it and I would never be a mum. I breathed the biggest sigh of relief when they told me everything was fine, and then I could actually enjoy the scan. They showed me each baby in turn, and where their arms and legs were. I left the scan room walking on air: it was the most amazing feeling ever knowing that they were still there and growing nicely.
Sarah from Wigan, mum to twins Matthew and Phoebe, 20 months

With all three of my pregnancies my feelings towards my 12-week scan are still unforgettable. In each case I was excited for the week leading up to it until the night before, when I was nervous that they'd find something wrong or that they wouldn't even find a baby and my body was tricking me into thinking I was pregnant! I remember seeing the baby on the screen, and saying, 'Just the one, then?' (I have twins on my side of the family) and the sonographer saying, 'Yes, just one lonely baby.' I couldn't believe how well formed all my babies looked at this stage: I thought they were so big and developed considering I was hardly showing. I also remember the overwhelming feeling of relief after being told all was well.
Alicia from London, mum to Kyrus, two, Demiyah, one, and 14 weeks pregnant

Cassidy is my first baby, and I was incredibly nervous at my first scan. I suppose the 12-weeker is the confirmation that you really are pregnant and not just imagining it! I'd had a missed miscarriage the October before, so was frightened I'd be told something awful again; at the same time I was looking forward to seeing my little munchkin. The baby was fine, and I've never seen my husband look so amazed, choked and happy. But then, when I asked for a

picture, I was told they were no longer distributed at 12-week scans. I offered to pay, but was again told no. We were devastated. My husband is in the Army so we live away from all our family and friends, and we wanted to share this with them. I logged a complaint and was issued an apology and an invitation to go back for another scan a few weeks later to have some photos taken.
Sara, British Forces, Germany, mum to Cassidy, 20 months (born in England)

Pain relief options for labour

Making choices about your labour and delivery is dependent on getting yourself as well informed as possible, and one of the first things to consider is whether you're hoping to go for a 'natural' birth, without the aid of medical pain relief other than Entonox (gas and air) or whether you'll happily take what's on offer. Lots of mums are sensible enough to keep an open mind so that they don't feel like failures if they opt for pain relief on the day.

Analgesics and anaesthesia in labour can impact on you and your baby in different ways. Most cross the placenta, and can make your baby drowsy, as well as you, prolonging labour. That's not to say they don't have a place in modern labour, though – only that you need to know what's what before you can make an informed decision.

TENS (Transcutaneous Electrical Nerve Stimulation)

TENS is a portable machine that transmits electrical impulses via electrodes that you stick to particular points on your lower back in labour. It takes about 30 minutes before you really feel any effect, but then you can adjust the strength of the impulses yourself with a handheld control. Lots of mums find it particularly useful early in labour. TENS is a non-medical system that works by diverting pain messages away from the brain. The sensation it delivers has been described as feeling like pins and needles. Some mums have said that it's helpful just to have something they need to control, as it distracts them from the pain; others have just found it irritating or uncomfortable; lots have abandoned it as their labour pains have become more forceful; some have managed labour with nothing but TENS for relief.

You can hire a machine from some hospital units, National Childbirth

Trust branches and from Boots (visit www.bootsmaternityrental products.co.uk for details). They are relatively inexpensive and are usually rented for a four-week period from around 37 weeks, in case you go into early labour or your baby is overdue. Boots allows you to extend the rental period by a fortnight at no extra charge if you're more than a week overdue.

Gas & air (Entonox)

Entonox is a specially balanced mixture of oxygen and nitrous oxide (also known as laughing gas), delivered from a canister via a long plastic tube and breathing pipe. Lots of mums find that it suits them well in early labour as it makes them 'high' at the peak of a contraction, but doesn't have a lasting effect between times. Because Entonox takes about 30 to 45 seconds to have an effect, you start breathing it through the mouthpipe as each contraction builds but before it reaches its peak.

Some mums use Entonox in early labour and then have some more in order to deliver their babies. If there is a tear or cut (episiotomy, see p. 385) to the perineum (the area of skin between the vagina and anus), it's also useful for while you're being stitched. Entonox does cross the placenta but isn't known to affect babies adversely, probably because the effects are so fleeting. In fact, the extra oxygen is thought to be helpful to babies during labour.

Some of us mums have hilarious tales to tell about the effects of Entonox, probably because of the laughing gas that's in it. You might find yourself laughing hysterically or saying inappropriate things to your medical team or birth partner. No one will mind (except perhaps your birth partner unless you warn him or her in advance!): your medical team will have seen and heard just about everything, and will know that however badly behaved you are, it's not your fault!

Some mums share Entonox with their birthing partners, who willingly breathe in the heady mixture – but this isn't what it's for at all! Try to keep your partner's mitts off the mouthpipe, as he or she is supposed to be in full control during your labour!

Injectable pain relief

Most often used in the first stage of labour, pain relief given by injection can take up to half an hour to become effective, but can then give some welcome temporary respite from pain. But there are advantages and disadvantages to weigh up before you go down this route.

Meptazinol (also known as Meptid) can be given at any time during the first stage of labour, and is as effective as pethidine (see below). One advantage over pethidine is that Meptazinol doesn't affect your unborn baby's breathing as much. Disadvantages are that it can make you feel sick and dizzy, and that it's not widely available.

Pethidine is a muscle relaxant as well as a painkiller – in fact it's a synthetic version of morphine. Unlike some other analgesics, pethidine doesn't need to be signed off by a doctor, so your midwife can just go ahead and administer it. For this reason, it's also an option for pain relief during a home birth, although not all midwives are comfortable with this, so it's always best to check ahead of time. Because it's likely to make you sick, pethidine is usually given in combination with an anti-emetic (anti-sickness drug).

You're likely to feel quite woozy and 'out of it' if you choose pethidine – some mums give birth without even knowing it (which may appeal to you or not!). It's also well known to slow the breathing of both mum and baby; your baby will be left with the effects of pethidine for up to four days after the birth, and this could have a knock-on effect on how well you manage to establish breastfeeding.

Pethidine can be given as single injections into the top of your thigh, or intravenously through a catheter set up in your arm. If it's set up intravenously, you can sometimes control the dosage yourself: this is called Patient Controlled Analgesia or PCA, but it's not available everywhere.

Pethidine isn't a good choice later in labour because it can make you very drowsy and will mean progress is slowed down. Also, if it's given too close to birth it can have a bad effect on your baby, who may have to have an injection in any case at birth to reverse its effects.

Diamorphine is used in some hospitals, depending on individual policy. This acts in a similar way to pethidine, but can provide better pain control with less nausea or vomiting.

Who'd have thought?

Eating fish when you're pregnant can boost your baby's brain development. A US study found that babies of mums who ate at least one portion per week had better verbal skills at 15 months than those whose mothers ate no fish. The Food Standards Agency (FSA), however, recommends that pregnant women restrict their intake of oily fish (such as salmon, mackerel and sardines) to two portions a week because they contain high levels of mercury.

Epidurals

An epidural effectively numbs your lower body by bathing the nerves from the uterus and birth canal with local anaesthetic via an injection into a space in the spinal column. It takes about 20 minutes to set up, when an anaesthetist will insert a fine tube into this 'epidural space' so that the anaesthetic can be topped up as it wears off.

The advantage of an epidural is that, if it's working effectively, you can enjoy a more or less pain-free labour and any stitching after a cut or tear can be done while the epidural is still working.

The main disadvantage of a standard epidural is that you won't be able to walk, so will have to labour on a bed. It also means you won't be able to move around during labour, and will probably be strapped to a foetal heart monitor throughout.

There's also a greater risk of other intervention, such as ventouse, forceps or Caesarean delivery after an epidural (see *Assisted delivery*, p. 98). This is because it's hard to push effectively when you can't feel your contractions. Some mums also find that the epidural only numbs one side of their lower body.

Mobile epidural

Although you're not really mobile in the true sense of the word, you will have more freedom of movement than with an ordinary epidural. It's set up in the same way, with a thin tube passed through a hollow needle into the epidural space in your lower spine. The other end of the tube is attached to a pump, which administers a combination of anaesthetic and pain-killing drugs. Sometimes the pump is under your control: this is another example of

Patient Controlled Analgesia (PCA). The pain block is still good: the difference is that the dose of anaesthetic is less than with an ordinary epidural, so you may retain some movement in your legs, enabling you to move around more during labour. You're also less likely to have a ventouse or forceps delivery than with an ordinary epidural, and because the numbing effect is less widespread, you're more likely to be able to time the top-ups to wear off in time for the delivery. You'll still need constant monitoring of your contractions, foetal heart rate and blood pressure, though. You'll also have an intravenous infusion and intermittent catheterisation as you won't be able to feel when your bladder's full.

Spinal

A spinal block is administered in a similar way to an epidural, but the anaesthetic is injected into the sac containing spinal fluid, rather than into the epidural space around it. This means that the anaesthetic is simpler to administer and becomes effective more quickly, within 10 minutes; low blood pressure is more pronounced with a spinal, though, so this needs closer monitoring and treatment. A spinal block is given in one injection and can't be topped up as a catheter is not left in place. The effect lasts for up to three hours. Mums aren't usually offered a choice between spinal and epidural anaesthesia for a Caesarean section, since the decision is very much down to the anaesthetist's professional judgement.

Combined Spinal Epidural (CSE)

Some hospitals prefer to give you a spinal in the early stages of labour for quick pain relief and to keep you a bit more mobile than with an epidural. At the same time, an epidural is set up, but no drugs are passed down the tube. When the effect of the spinal injection wears off, epidural anaesthesia is given.

Who'd have thought?

The main hormone responsible for making your boobs pneumatic is human placental lactogen (HPL), and it's the same hormone that triggers the production of colostrum, the creamy substance your breasts produce to feed your baby in the first few days after birth.

Pros and cons of epidurals and spinals

A great advantage of an epidural over other injectable pain relief is that it won't have an adverse effect on your baby and you'll be fully alert yourself throughout labour and the birth:

- You'll also be completely pain-free for as long as it is working effectively, and you can help to control the top-ups.
- There's very little risk of harmful effects from epidurals, and recent research has shown that you are no more likely to get the backache commonly associated with epidurals than if you delivered your baby without one.
- If you end up having an emergency Caesarean, you'll be able to have it under your epidural rather than having to have a general anaesthetic. This means less risk to you, a quicker recovery and your partner can still attend the birth with you.

Many mums find that an epidural makes labour much more enjoyable, despite a few minus points:

- You can only have a mobile epidural if you haven't had other injectable pain relief for the previous three hours. You can, however, have a normal epidural.
- You'll be catheterised (have a tube passed up your urethra to drain urine from your bladder) because you'll be unable to feel when you need to pee once you're numb.
- Epidurals may cause low blood pressure, so a drip to counteract this effect is routinely set up beforehand.
- You're more likely to need an assisted delivery with an epidural or spinal, which also increases your risk of an episiotomy.
- In rare cases a slow leak of spinal fluid after the epidural has been taken out can cause a headache, meaning you have to lie flat for a day or so until the leak seals itself.

Assisted delivery

Assisted delivery – also known as 'intervention' – means having extra physical help to deliver your baby, whether by forceps, ventouse or

Caesarean. Caesarean deliveries are discussed elsewhere (see p. 289), but forceps and ventouse are both means of assisting a vaginal delivery. If you have to have an assisted delivery, you'll probably have to have your feet up in stirrups, which means you'll be immobile for the delivery of your baby. This can be uncomfortable, but allows the obstetrician or midwife maximum access to your vagina. You'll probably also need an episiotomy in order to create enough space for the instruments to enter the birth canal. Forceps are like a pair of large metal salad servers, which cup together around your baby's head once inside your vagina. Your midwife or obstetrician then pulls on the handles to ease your baby down the birth canal. A ventouse relies on vacuum suction to extract your baby via a plastic cup which fits over his head. The type of method used will probably depend on your baby's position. Ventouse is more flexible and considered gentler, but forceps are more efficient and less likely to slip off and need re-attaching. Babies born via assisted delivery often have slightly misshapen heads, but these return to normal within weeks or months of birth.

What the netmums say

'Pain relief: what I planned and what I actually had'

I was at home until I was 4cm dilated, so up until that point I had nothing apart from a warm bath to try to soothe the pain. In hospital I had gas and air, which I didn't find helpful, so I ended up with pethidine: it made my daughter drowsy at birth, which was scary, but did stop the pain!
Kari from Exeter, mum to Jennifer, 11 weeks

With my first baby I was at home with a TENS machine until I was 7cm dilated. Then at hospital I had gas and air, and then diamorphine, but as he was born 20 minutes after having it, I don't think it did much for the pain – it just made me sick. If I'd have known he was coming so soon, I wouldn't have bothered with the diamorphine. I had my second baby, William, at home and it was a short labour, so gas and air was fine.
Lynne from Newcastle, mum to Matthew, three and William, two

I had a few puffs of gas & air, but it made me feel really ill so I gave up. After that I basically just used relaxation techniques and breathing. I did ask for more towards the end, but by then I was too far along. Next time I'll consider pain relief earlier, but I'm reasonably happy to try again without, as I only really had pain when the midwives interrupted my relaxation. Amelie was only born when I was able to ignore their 'push coaching', relax and let my body take over.
Danie from Ipswich, mum to Amelie, five weeks

I had gas & air when I was finally told I could stay at the hospital, having been sent home twice already, but I didn't like it and kept being sick so I had pethidine. That made me feel very strange and spacey; I'd never have that again! Then I had an epidural which was great as I felt nothing and it let me have a little sleep, but what wasn't so great was that I couldn't feel the sensation to push. Next time I think I'd be more inclined to try for a natural birth, or at least try not to have as much pain relief.
Isabel from Westbury, mum to Alfie, two

After being induced, I managed for the first three hours with a TENS machine as the contractions were fairly mild and manageable. Then my waters broke and the contractions got worse. When I was 3cm dilated I had an epidural put in and I was in heaven! It was definitely the best thing since sliced bread! I read an entire book while dilating to 10cm and my son was born into a happy, relaxed room.
Ruth from Cheshire, mum to William, eight months

Who'd have thought?

Stimulating your baby during pregnancy by talking to him, thinking about him and stroking or massaging your belly has been proven to be beneficial to him. Not only can it help better prepare your baby for the outside world, studies have also shown that parents who stimulate their babies in the uterus have a closer and stronger bond with their children.

Tear or cut?

Some mums have difficulty delivering their baby's head and shoulders. Episiotomies used to be routinely performed when this happened because it was thought that the vagina wouldn't stretch sufficiently to allow them to pass through efficiently. In fact, with controlled pushing using breathing techniques the vagina should be elastic enough to allow your baby through. The only other circumstance when an episiotomy might be necessary is if you're going to have a forceps delivery – but these are relatively rare nowadays.

Some midwives and obstetricians are happy to allow mums to tear – where the perineum (the area between the vagina and anus) ruptures; others prefer to make an incision with sharp scissors for speed of delivery. It's generally thought that tears heal better because the skin 'knits' back together, whereas with a straight incision healing takes longer. Either way you're unlikely to be aware of the process at the time, but you might have a preference you'd like to record in advance. (For advice on massaging your perineum to avoid a tear or episiotomy, see p. 319.)

Options for the third stage of labour

The third stage of labour is the delivery of the placenta, and most mums are routinely given an injection into the upper thigh of Syntometrine to speed this up. This is known as a 'managed' third stage. You don't have to agree to having your third stage managed, though: some mums feel sick, dizzy and unable to hold their babies after the injection, and left to your own devices you will eventually deliver your placenta through a series of contractions. Sometimes hospital staff prefer to manage your third stage so that they can get on with the business of checking the placenta to make sure it has come away complete. Don't let staff shortages influence your decision, though: you can say no if you want to. For more about the three stages of labour, see p. 252.

Your mission this week: Plan baby's space

Try to plan out where your baby will sleep after the birth: it might seem a bit early to decide yet, but if it's going to involve redecorating a room or shifting things around, it's better to plan things before you get too big and uncomfortable, and while you've still got some time to make changes.

Of course, you won't know at this stage whether you're expecting a girl or a boy, and this might influence your choice of colour scheme if you're planning to redecorate a room as a nursery. The most important thing at this stage, though, is to check that a cot that's suitable for your baby for the first six months will fit into your bedroom, as current government advice is to keep your baby in your bedroom with you for this length of time.

For lots of mums, browsing round nursery shops is one of the great joys of pregnancy, and if the only products you ever used to fall in love with before you got pregnant were the Manolo Blahniks in the pages of your favourite celeb mag, you might be surprised at how exciting you find baby bedding and cot mobiles! You might as well mention to your other half, too, that clothes-shopping fever tends to transfer from mum to baby after the birth, so although you might not be looking to buy yourself many new clothes for a while (at least until you get your figure back) it's very likely you'll fall for some item of baby attire or other in every shop you visit!

Who'd have thought?

Sometimes you can get what's known as a 'false positive' result from an antenatal test. This means a result can suggest something's wrong when actually it isn't – but you'll need to have a diagnostic test to check for certain.

Look no further

If I do tear or have to have an episiotomy, won't it really hurt to be stitched up again?

No, for a couple of reasons: firstly, you'll be given an injection of local anaesthetic into your perineum before the stitching begins; secondly, the chances are that you'll be so overwhelmed with meeting your baby for the first time you'll hardly notice what's going on at the business end of things! You'll probably have to have your legs up in stirrups, which is somewhat less than dignified and might be a bit uncomfortable, but on the plus side you'll be admiring your newborn, counting fingers and toes (yes, lots and lots of mums actually do that!) and wondering at the intelligence in those trusting, curious little eyes (your baby's, not your partner's).

What if I ask for an epidural and I can't have one?
The most common reason for refusing an epidural is that you're too close to giving birth, and it would actually be detrimental to your progress. Sometimes, though, there just isn't an anaesthetist available to give you an epidural on the day – and this is why it's doubly important that you let your medical team know in advance if you're likely to want an epidural. That way, they can try to ensure that someone is on duty and available for when your time comes. It's got to be better to say you'll probably want one, then refuse it on the day than to say you don't want one, then be refused if you change your mind on the day.

Won't I lose control if I take gas & air?
Well, you might act a bit out of character for a minute or so after each dose you inhale, but you'll soon come back to yourself again – and don't worry: the medical team have seen just about all sorts of behaviour and heard the ripest possible language, so won't be shocked no matter how badly behaved you are! Some mums say they laughed all the way through the first stage of labour; others just feel sick after taking gas and air. The important thing to remember is that labour is a relatively short period of time (when taken in the context of the whole of your life!), so even if you do feel you've made a fool of yourself, you won't have to see the medical staff who attended you again if you don't want to.

Who'd have thought?

If you're one of the unlucky few who are still feeling sick by this week, try sniffing a cut lemon – some mums swear by fresh citrus smells as an anti-nausea remedy.

How are you feeling?

Tick the box that most closely represents how you feel about the given statements, then look back to the chart in the last chapter to see how you've changed in this past month.

Physically	Emotionally
I'm still feeling sick or vomiting Strongly agree ☐ Agree ☐ Neither agree nor disagree ☐ Disagree ☐ Strongly disagree ☐	I'm still worried I'll throw up in public Strongly agree ☐ Agree ☐ Neither agree nor disagree ☐ Disagree ☐ Strongly disagree ☐
I feel more fat than pregnant Strongly agree ☐ Agree ☐ Neither agree nor disagree ☐ Disagree ☐ Strongly disagree ☐	I love the fact that my 'bump' is beginning to show Strongly agree ☐ Agree ☐ Neither agree nor disagree ☐ Disagree ☐ Strongly disagree ☐
I feel better if I eat four or five small meals a day Strongly agree ☐ Agree ☐ Neither agree nor disagree ☐ Disagree ☐ Strongly disagree ☐	My brain seems to have gone to mush! Strongly agree ☐ Agree ☐ Neither agree nor disagree ☐ Disagree ☐ Strongly disagree ☐
I'm starting to feel sexy again Strongly agree ☐ Agree ☐ Neither agree nor disagree ☐ Disagree ☐ Strongly disagree ☐	I'm more focused on my baby than on my partner Strongly agree ☐ Agree ☐ Neither agree nor disagree ☐ Disagree ☐ Strongly disagree ☐
My boobs feel like cannon balls! Strongly agree ☐ Agree ☐ Neither agree nor disagree ☐ Disagree ☐ Strongly disagree ☐	I sometimes wonder what I've got myself into Strongly agree ☐ Agree ☐ Neither agree nor disagree ☐ Disagree ☐ Strongly disagree ☐
I feel less sleepy than I did at the beginning Strongly agree ☐ Agree ☐ Neither agree nor disagree ☐ Disagree ☐ Strongly disagree ☐	I'm so relieved the first 12 weeks are over Strongly agree ☐ Agree ☐ Neither agree nor disagree ☐ Disagree ☐ Strongly disagree ☐

Quick quiz

What have you learned about pain relief?

1 Which is/are most likely to make your baby sleepy at birth?
a. Pethidine and Meptid
b. Meptid
c. Epidural

2 How are pethidine and Meptid given?
a. By injection
b. Tablets or injection
c. Through a breathing mask

3 What is gas and air made up from?
a. Oxygen and laughing gas
b. Just laughing gas
c. Petrol and oxygen

4 How long do the effects of gas and air last?
a. It wears off almost as soon as you stop inhaling it
b. It lasts for 10 minutes after you've stopped using it
c. It can last for two to three days after the birth

5 Which of the following is a side effect of having an epidural?
a. You won't be able to feel when you need a pee, so will have a catheter
b. You won't be able to pee at all
c. You won't be allowed to eat

Answers: The answers to this quiz are all 'a'.

Mostly a: You've clearly been paying attention, so go to the top of the class! Getting properly genned up about pain relief does mean that you'll be in a good position to make a decision about what you think you'd prefer.

Mostly b: Have you been reading this chapter with one eye shut? You've got it all half right! It's worth reading the section on pain relief again when you're feeling at your most alert, as this is one of the areas of labour that you could have some control over if you know what you're talking about!

Mostly c: Oh dear: if this was a school report it would say 'Must try harder'! Did you read the pain relief section just as you were nodding off to sleep? Try to go through it again, then take the quiz a second time to be sure you've got the facts straight. Because it's an important area to have a say in, you need to be as well informed as possible.

Part Two

The Second Trimester:
Months 4–6

Chapter 3
Weeks 13–16

Now that Week 12 is a dim and distant memory (well, perhaps not quite, but it's a milestone nonetheless), you should be able to relax a bit more about being pregnant. That's not to say you won't encounter any problems along the way – or that there is no chance at all that you'll lose your baby; just that the worst danger of miscarriage has passed. Hopefully your pregnancy is well established and progressing beautifully.

This is the beginning of the trimester most mums-to-be enjoy the most: you'll have a neat bump to show off, but won't yet feel like a ship in full sail; you'll probably have more energy than you've had of late and may not opt for 'bed' if asked where you'd like to spend the evening; with luck any nausea or sickness you've been putting up with will have subsided and you'll feel energised enough to go shopping for any new furniture and other 'baby bits' you know you'll need. It might seem a bit soon – and maybe you'd rather leave it until more towards the end of this trimester at around Week 25 or 26 – but believe us mums that by your third trimester you're more likely to want a long sit down and a cup of tea than a traipse round a supersize shopping mall!

Who'd have thought?

Research has found that unborn babies are at their most wakeful at around midnight, which might also explain why they tend to be awake in the middle of the night for a few weeks after birth.

Week 13 196 days to go!

Don't forget: Tell people who don't know yet!

As this is a common time for couples to share their news with others, we're revisiting that subject this week. Even if you've told your nearest and dearest already, chances are there are others to let in on your secret. How and when you tell different people can have as much of an impact on them as it can be a release for you – and they won't all be filled with immeasurable joy either, so don't have too many expectations! With luck the majority will be thrilled for you. For more advice on breaking the news and the impact it might have, see *Breaking your news sensitively*, below.

Hey baby!

Your baby's continuing the good work, and is now pretty much fully developed in that his features and organs are all present and correct. His crown-to-rump length is around 11.5cm (4.5in) and he now weighs about 80g (around 3oz). It's going to be many weeks before his organs are capable of supporting him independently, though, as they need to strengthen and mature. This week he continues to practise breathing, drinking, swallowing and peeing – and he can even force a little smile! His liver continues to produce bile and his pancreas is producing insulin. His intestines are maturing and starting to work like yours. All 20 of his milk teeth are formed and his vocal chords are developing in readiness for that first cry.

All about you

It can be hard to time your announcement when you finally go public about your pregnancy: it's big news, and not exactly something you can slip easily into a conversation at the water cooler; on the other hand, you don't necessarily want to use it as a conversation opener either. You'll find the right time – just don't go blurting it out at an inappropriate moment to get it out of the way. Bear in mind, too, that once you've told colleagues, for instance, your boss will soon get to know secondhand, so it's probably best to start with him or her.

Breaking your news sensitively

Sometimes other people's reactions aren't quite what we mums are hoping for, and it can pay to tread carefully and consider different people's circumstances before deciding how to break the news. For instance, if you have a friend or colleague who has suffered a recent miscarriage or who is struggling to get pregnant herself, your announcement might not be met with quite the elation you were anticipating – and for good reason. In situations like this, however keen you are to blurt out your news, make an effort to look for the right moment: it's probably a much better idea to share it one-to-one in a private place where a few tears won't matter (whether of joy, shock or self-pity) than to announce it to a group of people where one or more are likely to be sensitive.

You might come across some jealousy and resentment, too – especially from those who'd like to be pregnant but aren't in a relationship, or are in a relationship but have partners who don't want kids just now. You may even have the odd bitchy comment made about you or to you: accept any unpleasantness for what it is – the green-eyed monster, not only of jealousy, but also insecurity. These people deserve your pity more than anything else (and doesn't that make you feel superior!).

How your relationships might change
You might feel a slight shift in your long-term personal relationships after you've told everyone about your pregnancy. If, for example, your best friend has chosen not to have children, she might have been secretly banking on you coming to the same decision – and it could either make her feel alienated, or make her question her own life choices once she knows you're going to be a mum. She's probably fearful that you won't be there for her any more; that you'll change completely; that your social life together will go out the window; that you'll only be able to talk babies from now on; that you'll make a new best friend at your postnatal group; or that you'll move away to get your child into the right school! All these fears are rational, so you might want to think about how you'll reassure her on each point – or whether you'll need to help her adapt to your changing relationship. It's worth pointing out that as she's always been your greatest support, you're going to need her more than ever now; that you understand that things are bound to change, but you hope that won't mean you can't be as close friends as ever; that you don't yet know how much of an impact your baby will have on friends and family but that you're going to make a real effort to keep your other relationships strong; that she's always welcome to drop in on you at home; and that you hope she'll be happy to be a big part of your baby's life too.

You and your mum

This very special relationship can't fail to be altered by your own impending motherhood. Whether or not you're very close to your mum, most mums-to-be find that they regard their own mothers in a new light during pregnancy and once they are new mums themselves. You might suddenly understand, for instance, why mums tend to feel so protective towards their children, even when they're grown up. Or, with all the decisions to make about whether or not to return to work, how to afford childcare and what provision will be best for your baby, you might come to a sudden realisation of what your mum went through or gave up to have you.

If you've lost your mum, be prepared for the grief to re-emerge during your pregnancy and with the arrival of your baby. Do give vent to it, even if it means having some bereavement counselling (and the waiting lists can be long, so take action via your GP as soon as you think you might benefit). Suppressing your feelings could make you feel much worse, and could potentially trigger antenatal or postnatal depression.

For your mum's part, it could be something of a shock to be faced with the evidence that her little girl is all grown up (and this will be the next thing that occurs to her and your dad after they've digested the fact that you've actually been having sex! Yes, we know – it can be a deeply uncomfortable moment!). But once she's accepted these feelings, she'll probably want to share your pregnancy and take the opportunity to mother you throughout. Try to resist the temptation to shout: 'What do you know about it? It's thirty years since you were last pregnant!' or worse, however moody you might be feeling. Let your mum offer you her advice – you don't have to take it!

Who'd have thought?

Unborn babies are usually inactive for no longer than around 13 minutes at a time between Weeks 8 and 19, and always return to the lowest part of the amniotic sac to rest!

What the netmums say

'Me and my relationships'

I've become even closer with my partner and feel like we have something so special. We're happier now than we've ever been. The relationship with my mother-in-law is not so good, though. I know it's mostly my fault as she's only trying to help, but I feel as if she's trying to take over and be my mother when I've already got one – and my mum is my best friend. I hardly see any of my friends any more as none of them have children. I do get the occasional text or email asking how I am, but that's about it.

Laura from east Hull, 28 weeks pregnant

My mum was very interfering after my first child was born. Throughout the pregnancy she kept saying that I had to breastfeed no matter what, and that I should buy a cat net to go over the Moses basket, even though it never got used as it clearly wasn't needed at all. She was also my birth partner, and as soon as my son was born she got him dressed for me and was cuddling him before I even had a chance to hold him: she certainly took advantage of me not being able to get up straight after my epidural! I found living with her a nightmare in the early months after birth: she'd come running as soon as she heard my son start to fuss, and would push me out of the way to look after him. Of course she did it all out of love for her first grandchild, but she still didn't take the hint when I said I'd *ask* if I needed any help!

Alicia from London, mum to Kyrus, two, Demiyah, one, and 14 weeks pregnant

My lovely mum had always been my very best friend but my feelings for her got even stronger once I'd had Natasha. I'm sure she'd have liked to come to the hospital with me, but she didn't push herself forward and I didn't ask her as I wasn't sure I wanted to risk shouting and swearing at her! She's since died, but in the short time she was able to be Grandma to Natasha, I so appreciated all she'd done for me when I was growing up. I'm only sorry Natasha's missing out on so much grandmotherly love, wisdom and humour, but we talk about her often to keep her memory alive.

Hilary from Carshalton, mum to Natasha, three

Who'd have thought?

Unborn babies have been shown to dodge away from needles invading the amniotic sac – during amniocentesis, for example – and have even been seen swiping at them.

You and your back

By now you might be starting to feel the low backache that afflicts lots of mums-to-be (although some mums escape this until later in pregnancy, and other lucky souls don't experience it at all!). It's caused by a combination of pregnancy hormones including progesterone and, more specifically, relaxin, a hormone that softens and loosens the ligaments that hold your joints together. Even this early in pregnancy, the softening and stretching of muscles and ligaments, especially in your lower back and pelvis, can cause your joints to become slightly misaligned, and the result is a nagging backache.

Unfortunately, you're probably not going to 'grow out of' backache in pregnancy: on the contrary, as the weeks go by and you increase in weight, the imbalance caused by your bump will mean you'll subconsciously try to compensate by increasing the curvature of your lower back – and this in itself can cause even more discomfort from trapped nerves, aching muscles and ligaments.

For some mums, the worst of the strain occurs in the lower back, but it's also common (sorry to be the bearer of more bad news) to suffer discomfort in the mid (thoracic) spine as it can get a bit hunched as your boobs grow heavier, resulting in stiffness and aching.

Top tips for protecting your back

- Keep mobile. Regular gentle exercise, such as walking, swimming, taking an aquanatal class or practising yoga will all help to keep your joints mobile, although this advice doesn't apply if you have weakened pelvic joints (see PGP, SPD and DSP, p. 116–17).
- Be careful when lifting. Because you're more at risk of injury from your relaxed joints and ligaments, it's important not to put your

back under any unnecessary strain. You can help avoid this by carrying your shopping in evenly spread loads rather than all in one bag; by lifting anything heavy with your knees bent, back straight and load held close to your chest (although preferably leave the lifting and shifting to someone who's not pregnant!); avoiding twisting whilst carrying anything; and bending at the knees to put your load down, too.

- Think about posture. The natural way to compensate for having a bigger belly is to lean slightly backwards, increasing the curvature of your spine. This will result in pain all along your spine, so try to think about your posture often. Tuck your bottom in, straighten your back and try to use your tummy muscles to support your bump. You'll probably find that standing with your legs slightly apart helps you to feel more centrally balanced than standing with your feet together.

- Get ergonomically checked. If your work involves you sitting down using a computer screen, ask your employer to get your workspace ergonomically checked. This means checking that your chair is suitably adjustable; that your screen is at the correct height; that you have any screen filters in place recommended for pregnant women and that you have a footrest and wrist support if necessary. If you work standing up, ask for a high stool or chair to sit on from time to time.

- Wear the right shoes. Experiment with heels of different heights. Some mums prefer to wear pumps; others find a slight heel more comfy for their backs. It's a good idea to keep both options handy so you can swap and change throughout the day depending on how your back feels.

Do-anywhere exercise for your back

Here's a quick exercise you can practise any time, any place, anywhere – although it'll help to try it out on the floor first so you can feel what you're doing better.
- Lie on the floor (not the bed – too bouncy) and bend your knees with your feet a few inches apart.
- Place the back of one hand at the top of your buttocks. Then,

keeping your lower stomach muscles tight, tilt your pelvis forwards until the small of your back flattens to the floor.

- Hold this position for a few seconds, then release and return your pelvis to its original position.
- Repeat slowly 10 times to relieve lower back pain.

Once you're proficient, you should be able to practise this exercise whilst sitting.

Pelvic girdle pain (PGP)

A specific type of back pain, known as Pelvic Girdle Pain (PGP) can occur at the back of your pelvis. It's also known as Sacro-Iliac Joint (SIJ) pain. Your sacro-iliac joints can be felt when you press into the dimples on either side of the spine at the bottom of your back. Although PGP is more likely to strike a bit later in pregnancy when you're a bit heavier, it's just as well to know what you're looking for now so you can act to get some help.

PGP is caused by the hormone relaxin increasing the mobility of your pubic symphysis (an important pelvic joint) and the sacro-iliac joints. This is in preparation for your baby's delivery, as looser joints mean more 'give', enabling your baby's head to pass through more easily. The downside is that this loosening can give you gyp with your pelvic joints throughout your pregnancy, making lifting, standing, walking and climbing stairs pretty uncomfortable!

Who'd have thought?

If you have a low-lying placenta in pregnancy, chances are it will lift away from your cervix as pregnancy progresses. Only 0.5–1 per cent of placentas remain low-lying at the end of pregnancy.

What are the symptoms of PGP?

The sorts of things you might notice include some or all of the following:

- pain in one or both buttocks
- low back pain around your pelvic region

- clicking in your pelvis
- a feeling of 'locking' in your pelvis
- lower back pain with pain in your legs.

SPD and DSP

If the pubic bone between your legs at the front of your pelvis feels very sore, you may be suffering from a condition known as Symphysis Pubis Dysfunction (SPD). This is a condition where the two halves of your pelvis that are normally held firmly together by strong ligaments separate slightly in pregnancy. Some degree of separation is normal, but if one side of the pelvis moves more than the other, or if the separation is too great, the result is severe pain and inflammation. There's another similar condition called Diastasis Symphysis Pubis (DSP) where the pubic joint loosens, leaving a wide gap between the two pelvic bones. It's very painful and thankfully very rare.

In both conditions, the pain is usually aggravated by any stance that means your legs are apart; by walking, going up and down stairs or turning over in bed.

What can help?

Once you've had either SPD or DSP diagnosed, your midwife, GP or obstetrician should refer you to a specially trained physiotherapist. You might be offered a pelvic support belt to help support the weight of your bump so that your pelvis doesn't come under so much stress, and be shown some exercises to strengthen your abdominal and pelvic floor muscles, but don't try to exercise these areas without being shown the proper techniques. A little gentle manipulation might also help.

Your mission this week: Go on a shopping trip

Either go shopping on the high street or online, just to research what kit you might want to buy for your new baby. Some items are essential, others aren't – but there's nothing to say you shouldn't buy what takes your fancy as long as you can finance it easily. Set yourself a budget and draw up a list of purchases that falls well within it; this will give you a bit of flexibility if you suddenly fall in love with something that's not on your list (and let's face it, you will!). Think about nursery furniture and decoration; bedding; first clothes (and spares!); a car seat; a crib or Moses basket (although this isn't strictly necessary); a cot or cotbed; a pram/pushchair or buggy suitable from birth; a jacket and hat; bibs and muslins for baby's possiting; nappies; a changing bag; a baby-listening monitor; a steriliser if you'll be using bottles at all; a set of bottles and bottle brushes; a blanket for daytime use; dummies if you'll be using them – factor everything in, however small.

Some items are OK to borrow or buy secondhand; others should really be bought from new for safety reasons. For a full rundown of baby essentials and frivolous luxuries, see p. 193.

Look no further

I'm too embarrassed to tell my dad face to face that I'm pregnant, but it seems unfair to leave it to Mum to tell him. How can I get over this?
There's nothing more guaranteed to make you feel like a naughty schoolgirl than telling your parents you're pregnant – and it's not uncommon for us girls to feel less inclined to tell our dads face to face. You might find it easier to say something like 'What kind of a granddad do you think you're going to be?', and let the news slip in a more oblique way, rather than announcing 'Dad, I'm pregnant', which does tend to conjure up images of how you got that way!

If you live near enough to tell your dad in person, don't be tempted to relay the news by phone, email or in a card. Depending on your degree of closeness, your dad will probably want to give you a hug, pat you on the back or shake your hand! But regardless of how he usually congratulates you, he'll appreciate you actually being there as he receives your news. Now that you're pregnant, remind yourself that you are, in fact, a grown-up – and also that your mum and dad not only had to have sex in order to conceive you; they also had to go through telling their own parents, so hopefully they'll appreciate how you feel.

Can I use ibuprofen gel on my back now I'm pregnant?
No, unless your doctor considers it essential. Even though it's not taken orally, the active ingredients are still absorbed into your bloodstream and can cross the placenta to your baby. In late pregnancy, ibuprofen gel can even delay the onset of labour, cause an overlong labour and cause complications in your newborn. See p. 115 for tips on minimising back pain.

Should I avoid using a VDU screen now I'm pregnant?
No, it's fine to carry on using your VDU. Although there used to be a lot of speculation about the risk of radiation from VDU monitors, there has been

loads of research done in recent years, and no evidence has been found to suggest they are harmful in any way.

Week 14 189 days to go!

Don't forget: Stretch marks do fade with time

Although this is the feelgood trimester for many mums, you won't escape all the niggles of pregnancy – or at least if you do it's only fair that you share your secret with the rest of us mere mortals! The sorts of things you can look forward to are stretch marks (which happen to most mums to some extent, depending on the natural elasticity of their skin, see p. 120); ill-fitting shoes as your feet swell and even seem to 'grow'; even bigger boobs (you may have mixed feelings about that one!) and more frequent peeing. None of these is likely to really cramp your style, although there are some more immediately obvious changes that can give rise to a crisis of confidence (see *You, your skin and other body bits* on p. 120).

Hey baby!

Your baby weighs around 25–30g this week (just under or just over an ounce) and has put on half his weight again! He's growing fast and measures around 7.5–8.5cm (3½ inches) now. From here on his growth rate will accelerate: previously all his energies were put into developing his human characteristics, features and organs; now all he has to do is grow and mature.

If your baby is a boy, he's already developed the structures that will produce sperm throughout his adulthood; if you're expecting a girl, she's already got ovaries, and by the time she's born they'll contain all the eggs she'll ever have – in fact she'll be born with at least two million, although lots of these will degenerate by the onset of puberty, leaving her with less than half a million (but still plenty!).

All about you

You, your skin and other body bits

We touched on the niggles that could plague you during this second trimester of pregnancy at the beginning of this section, more of which later – but this is also the time when lots of mums are described as 'blooming'. By now you'll hopefully be experiencing the beneficial effects of your pregnancy hormones rather than their less appealing side: lots of mums say that their hair feels thicker and more lustrous than ever before; that their nails are strong and healthy-looking; and that their skin is glowing. If this sounds like you, then you're probably enjoying yourself already. What with a nicely sized bump as well, you could be forgiven for thinking yourself the most beautiful creature alive! In fact, most of these changes are due to the fact that your skin is retaining more water and your heart is pumping more blood round your system.

If you're not reaping the rewards, however, and are still spotty (see p. 38–9), nauseous and grey-looking, don't despair. There's still time for you to start feeling better – and even if you don't you've still got your baby's arrival to look forward to, so try to console yourself with that if you can.

Now then: your Madonna-like looks aside (the Virgin Mother of God, not Mrs Ritchie!), as touched on previously, there could still be some problem areas for you to cope with. Here's a rundown of what to expect and what you can do.

Stretch marks

It's hardly surprising that once your skin gets over-stretched fairly rapidly it can begin to show a few signs of wear and tear, and this is exactly what stretch marks are: tears in the middle layer of skin (the dermis). Once you've got them, they are all yours for life, but you can take heart from the fact that they do become less visible with time, fading to a silvery colour. And it's also a little bit reassuring to know that somewhere between 75–90 per cent of mums get them during pregnancy.

Common places for stretch marks are across the belly; over the buttocks and upper thighs; on the breasts and under the upper arms (the parts often referred to, rather unkindly, as 'bingo wings'!). Happily most of these places tend to remain hidden under clothing unless you're on a beach holiday.

What you can do

Not an awful lot, to be honest. Although some body-cream manufacturers reckon their products help to prevent, minimise or cure stretch marks, there aren't enough scientifically controlled studies to back up this claim. Baby oil, cocoa butter and maternity massage creams might all help your skin to feel well conditioned, though – and using them on your bump means you'll have an opportunity for some quiet self-massage, when you can also make contact with your unborn baby.

Chloasma – the 'mask of pregnancy'

This condition, also known as 'melasma', is characterised by patches of pigmentation on the face. It's thought that up to 70 per cent of pregnant women develop these, although in the majority of cases it's pretty much unnoticeable. In extreme cases, though, a large butterfly-shaped 'stain' appears across the face, somewhat reminiscent of a cartoon burglar's mask. The condition is caused by the extra melanin produced in pregnancy. Melanin is the substance responsible for giving us a suntan, freckles and moles as well as dictating our skin, hair and eye colour, and is generated in increased quantities during pregnancy, triggered by pregnancy hormones. Chloasma/melasma is relatively rare, but can be traumatic if it's very pronounced as it's so startling to see – and because there's no hiding it.

What you can do

If it happens to you, you can minimise the effect by wearing sunblock and staying away from UV light – and take heart from the fact that in the majority of cases, the pigmentation fades and skin colour returns to normal within a few months of giving birth.

Linea negra

Also known as linea nigra, this is a line about 1cm wide that appears vertically from pubic bone to navel or sternum (breastbone) in some mums-to-be. Melanin is responsible again – just as it is responsible for chloasma/melasma. Again, it's the result of pregnancy hormones, which cause the body to produce more pigment.

What you can do

There's nothing you can do about this one – but it's something that doesn't affect all mums, and is most common amongst the dark-haired and dark-skinned. Lots of mums are more fascinated than disturbed by the development of a linea negra, and see it as another sign that pregnancy is moving on apace. The line fades away after pregnancy in most mums anyway, although it remains – albeit fainter – in some.

Thread veins

If you notice a mini roadmap appearing across your face or on your legs, don't be alarmed: the increased blood volume mums get in pregnancy means all the capillaries and veins become more engorged than normal, and this means that the tiny blood vessels that are usually hiding away far from the surface of the skin suddenly come to the fore. They're nothing to worry about, except from a cosmetic point of view.

What you can do
A good foundation should help to cover them if they bother you, and with luck they'll fade after the birth. If not, you can have them treated with laser therapy or injections after the birth – but definitely not beforehand!

Moles

Just as other areas of your skin will become darker because of an increased production of melanin, your moles and freckles might get darker in pregnancy, and you might even sprout new ones. Sometimes they fade after pregnancy, but in some mums they stay permanently darker.

What you can do
Keep an eye on any mole or freckle that changes substantially, alters in shape or size or bleeds. This could indicate a serious skin problem that's nothing to do with pregnancy, and must be referred to a doctor right away.

Your hair

If you are sporting a newly thick, lustrous mane and have put it down to glowing good health in pregnancy, you can be forgiven for thinking that's the cause. In fact, it's another of the more pleasant side effects attributable to those good old, bad old hormones. Most women notice some changes in the look and feel of their hair in pregnancy, and what's really happening is that your pregnancy hormones are preventing your usual rate of hair loss, and encouraging faster growth. Because your hair loss rate has been temporarily slowed, your hair really is thicker than usual – but the changes aren't usually permanent. Some mums also find that they grow hair in unwanted places, such as on their face or belly or around the nipples. Others find that their hair goes from straight to curly or changes colour – these changes are often permanent!

What you can do
Enjoy your brilliant new barnet while it lasts – but if you become disturbed

to find your hair apparently falling out in fistfuls after the birth or when you stop breastfeeding, don't be alarmed: you're simply shedding the hair you hung on to in pregnancy. It's just that you'll shed this at the same time as losing your usual quota of hair, so it can seem as if you're about to go bald! The fact that you shouldn't be able to find any hairless patches on your scalp ought to reassure you. In the case of growing excess hair, don't worry – this, too, should fall out eventually.

Your nails
Now this could go one of two ways for you, as some mums report having stronger, longer nails, whilst others find theirs becoming brittle, splitting and flaking. Fingers crossed you experience the former – but don't get too smug as these changes, too, are usually temporary.

What you can do
If you've got them, flaunt them, so go for a manicure and show 'em off! If you're one of the unlucky ones, however, avoid nail varnish as the chemicals will only worsen the condition of your nails. Instead, keep them trimmed short and apply nail and cuticle cream every day.

Your feet
Finding your shoes are a bit of a tight squeeze – or even that your feet appear to have elongated? Some mums develop flat feet as pregnancy progresses, and it's thought to be because of the extra weight bearing down on to the feet and flattening them out temporarily. This will, of course, have the effect of making your feet temporarily longer! Add to this the fact that extra fluid often accumulates in the feet and ankles, and you may find your normal shoes no longer fit properly. (For more on pregnancy footcare, see *Look after your feet*, p. 209, and *Be kind to your feet*, p. 264.)

What you can do
You might need to invest in a couple of pairs of shoes in a size bigger than usual, or in a different width fitting, to see you through pregnancy. In warmer weather, Birkenstock sandals, which have moulded inners to support your feet in all the right places, are a comfy option – and because the straps are adjustable you'll be able to wear them after pregnancy as well. Whatever you

choose, do try to buy leather as you're also likely to perspire lots more in pregnancy (nice!) and that could play havoc with your feet, leaving you with sore, smelly trotters. Don't turn into a modern-day Imelda Marcos, though, as this is another change that's likely to revert to normal after your baby's birth.

What the netmums say

'How pregnancy has affected my skin, hair and nails...'

My hair went really thick and shiny, and it seemed to grow so much! It's still looking good now! My nails were longer and stronger, and I never had any spots – so all in all, pregnancy suited me!
Georgina from Chester, mum to James, eight months

During my first trimester I was a bit of a fright! I had greasy hair, spots, the lot. But after about Week 16 I really bloomed. My hair was wonderfully glossy and so shiny, I only had to wash it once a week! I was feeling really good from then on. I loved being pregnant and I think it showed!
Mags from Lanarkshire, mum to Eve, two

I have suffered from psoriasis for the past 25 years and it has never been better than when I was pregnant. It really cleared up! Usually my nails are plagued by it and break easily, but they grew really strong and long, and so did my hair. I did suffer with a few spots breakouts, but I can't complain. My doctor suggested being pregnant all the time as a cure for my psoriasis as it has come back with a vengeance since!
Louise from Bury, mum to Lola Mae, 17 months

Sex in pregnancy

We looked at the issues of sex in early pregnancy in Chapter 1, but about now your thoughts might be returning to your love life, so let's have another look at some of the issues that can arise in this second trimester. Some couples love the added dimension pregnancy brings to their sex lives, but others find the idea off-putting, disconcerting or even downright worrying. There's no right or wrong about sex in pregnancy, but the important thing is that you and your partner talk about your feelings openly with each other; otherwise one or other of you may end up feeling rejected when it's actually the lovemaking itself that doesn't appeal, rather than your partner. In any case, lots of mums-to-be find that their libido rises and falls throughout pregnancy, and this is quite normal. Having said that, this middle trimester does tend to be the commonest time for mums to start feeling sexy.

If you're up for it, then go for it (as long as you haven't been advised not to); hopefully you're over the nauseous phase; you don't need to use contraception so can be spontaneous; you've got nine months clear of PMS and periods; and the long stretch of sleep deprivation that lies ahead of you might just spur you on to enjoy yourself while you may!

Some of the issues that might play on your mind – and which are common worries amongst pregnant couples – include:

- fear that having an orgasm could trigger premature labour
- fear that sex might harm your unborn baby
- discomfort about the thought of a 'third party' being involved in your sexual activity
- concerns that you are no longer attractive to your partner or that you no longer feel sexually attracted to him.

Fear of orgasm

Orgasms in pregnancy can feel very much like painless contractions – and there's a good reason for this as mild contractions do occur during a climax. No need to worry though, they won't be anywhere near strong enough to trigger premature labour. Near your due date, making love can help to induce labour, but it's the natural prostaglandin in sperm that's responsible rather than your own orgasm. Prostaglandin helps the cervix mature, and is used in the pessaries that are sometimes administered to induce labour in hospital. Don't worry that having sex will start labour prematurely, though: in a normal, low-risk pregnancy it only helps to trigger contractions once your body is ready to give birth.

Fear of harming the baby

Your baby is protected threefold: by the strong muscles of your uterus; by the cushioning sac of amniotic fluid; and by the mucus plug that covers the cervix until the onset of labour, so you have no need to worry that you'll harm him during sex. If, however, you've had recurrent miscarriages, a previous premature labour or other complications of pregnancy, you may be advised by your doctors to abstain from penetrative sex for a while. That's not to say you can't find other ways of pleasing each other though, so get inventive!

The 'third party' issue

For some couples, there's just no getting away from this one: the feeling that someone else is 'involved' in lovemaking is too strong to overcome and makes sex feel somehow wrong. In this case, as with the previous concern, you might find it easier to find non-penetrative ways of making love during pregnancy. Otherwise, it might help to realise that your baby is not lying close to your vagina – he's a long way further up inside you than that and quite remote from your lovemaking. In fact, the only way in which he is 'involved' is when your rush of feelings of wellbeing transmit to him, and that can only be a positive thing.

Concerns about attractiveness

Some mums-to-be feel wonderfully attractive; others couldn't feel less so. Some dads-to-be love the pregnant body; others don't. Sometimes you might feel like making love but your partner doesn't; sometimes he might fancy you when you're feeling anything but sexy. It's life, it happens – and some of it happens whether you're pregnant or not! Talk openly about your feelings along the way and reassure each other that not wanting sex has nothing to do with losing love for each other. Come together when you both feel sexy; accept those times when one of you doesn't. Discuss the fact that after the birth your love life will probably follow a different pattern from in your pre-pregnancy days and that it will most likely suffer a bit of a nosedive until your energy levels are restored and you're in a good routine with your baby. It's important to realise that most couples have to work hard at getting their sexual relationship back on any sort of track after the birth, but that with a bit of understanding on both sides things can come back together – albeit a bit differently from before.

Positions for sex in pregnancy

You have to become quite imaginative and inventive to find sexual positions that are comfortable in pregnancy. You probably won't want to take the full weight of your partner on your abdomen, and this will apply from now until the end of the 40 weeks. However:

- lots of couples find positions where the man is behind the woman easiest to accommodate – and they usually involve shallower penetration than face-to-face positions, which is often more comfortable for mums-to-be
- 'spoons', where you both lie on your sides with your partner's abdomen against your back and he penetrates from behind, is a popular position, especially if you both entwine your uppermost legs
- 'woman on top' positions are also worth a try: many mums like the fact that they are in control of the penetration and can keep it as deep or shallow as they feel comfortable with
- oral sex is an option if you fancy it, but a word of warning: your partner must on no account blow air into your vagina as this can cause an embolism that could have very serious consequences for you and your baby.

Your mission this week: Buy some maternity clothes

You'll need them in the next couple of weeks or so if you don't already, so you might as well spread the cost and get some now and some in another month's time. And anyway it's just *so* exciting to go into a maternity outlet and swan around legitimately. Before you buy, check the sizing policy – in most cases you buy clothes in your usual size. One thing to look out for is whether or not the clothes can 'grow' with you: maternity jeans are a good bet as most have a stretchy front panel and an expandable waistband. Other good choices would be roomy Empire-line tops, elasticated skirts, stretchy bootleg leggings and shaped kaftans. Go for slightly fitted styles if they're available: it's always better to look like an obviously pregnant woman than a wardrobe draped in dust covers!

Who'd have thought?

There is an old wives' tale associated with linea negra (see p. 121): if the line runs to the navel, you're carrying a girl, and if it goes all the way up to the sternum (breastbone), it's a boy. As with many old wives' tales, there's no scientific evidence to support this theory!

Look no further

Is it OK to use fake tan products in pregnancy?
Well, it depends to some extent on the product. Lotions, sprays and tissues impregnated with fake tan aren't toxic in any way but could trigger an allergy, so the British Medical Association's advice is to steer clear of them in pregnancy. The incidence of allergy is pretty low, but you might be more susceptible because of your pregnancy hormones. If you do decide to go ahead and use a fake tan, always do a patch skin test beforehand to check for a reaction. Remember, too, that you won't get any sun protection from a fake tanning product, so you must use a UV sunscreen in the sun.

Tanning tablets you sometimes see advertised in magazines do contain toxic ingredients that could be harmful to your baby, so don't take them under any circumstances.

I need an evening dress for a special occasion, but it seems such a waste of money. Is there an alternative to buying new?
Yes, there are companies that hire out pregnancy clothes, so you can find what you want and know you don't have to invest in it or squeeze yourself into what's basically the wrong size. Check out www.doesmytum lookbiginthis.com. Alternatively you could consider buying secondhand. There are websites specialising in this too: visit www.budget-bumps.com, www.bump2babe.co.uk or www.bumpsmart.co.uk.

I'm going to need a new bra soon. What's the best style for pregnancy?
A good support bra is your best bet at this stage of pregnancy. If you're not properly supported, the ligaments around your boobs will stretch and your breasts will become permanently saggy. You need to avoid underwiring, which can press against delicate breast tissue and become very uncomfortable. Choose a bra with an adjustable fastening so that you'll have some growing room; go for a natural fibre like cotton to absorb perspiration and keep you cool; look for wide straps and a deep panel of hooks at the back; choose a style with a wide band under the cups. Don't be tempted to buy more than two bras at this stage as they're unlikely to see you through your pregnancy and won't fit you afterwards either.

My boobs hurt in bed at night. Is there anything I can do?
Yes, you can buy yourself a special sleep bra, which is made from lightweight

cotton and available in maternity stores. This will give you a little much-needed support without feeling too cumbersome for bed. You'll find sleep bras online at www.mothernaturebras.co.uk and www.babiesrus.co.uk.

Week 15 182 days to go!

Don't forget: Try to do some moderate exercise

You could be forgiven, in early pregnancy, for putting exercise on the back burner – especially if you were feeling unwell – but now's the time to try to increase your fitness levels. This middle trimester is the time when you're likely to be feeling at your physical best, so you may as well capitalise on the fact and get a bit more active. Taking exercise will not only increase your general fitness, it will also help to improve your stamina, which will in turn enable you to cope better with labour. Exercise that demands some flexibility, such as yoga or swimming, will leave you more supple, and this will also help. Brisk walking is good exercise, too, and you can spend the time practising your breathing techniques for labour.

Hey baby!

Your baby is growing rapidly now and measures around 10cm (4in) from crown to rump, and weighs in at an impressive 50g – that's two ounces! His skin is beginning to sprout lanugo – fine, colourless hair that will help to regulate his temperature in the absence of much fat to keep him warm. The tiny bones in the middle ear (stirrup, anvil and hammer) have begun to harden so that, although the auditory centres in the brain are not yet fully developed, your baby's hearing capacity is increasing. His finger- and toenails continue to grow – most babies have overlong nails at birth – and the hair on his head is starting to sprout. His facial features are becoming more refined, giving him his own individual characteristics, and his ears are getting more defined.

Who'd have thought?

Your baby will play with his umbilical cord, flexing his fingers and gripping it quite hard for a moment at a time. Don't worry – this doesn't harm him.

All about you

Your uterus is creeping up stealthily towards your belly button and you might be able to feel the top of it about 10cm (4 in) below… which also means waving goodbye to your skinny jeans for a while, and enjoying the last couple of weeks of your boyfriend-cut or slouch pair. (Hey, wasn't it only last week you went shopping for all that new maternity gear? Might find some of it comes into its own next week or so!)

Some mums find themselves laid a bit low with coughs, colds and general snuffles. Guess what's responsible? The old enemy, your hormones (again!) interfering with your immune system, making it less effective – typical at a time when you're not supposed to take any drugs. If you're really suffering, ask your GP whether you can take paracetamol. It's usually considered safe in pregnancy, but you must always check first.

Are you considering amniocentesis?

If you've been offered amniocentesis – a diagnostic test of pregnancy – this could be the week you have it, but first you need to know all the implications the test can have. You don't have to agree to any test offered to you in pregnancy, so it's important you give it careful consideration before saying yes or no. To help you come to a decision, see *Your mission this week*, p. 135.

Circumstances under which you might be offered amniocentesis (or 'amnio') include the following:

- if you're over 35
- if there's a family history of birth disorders or defects
- if you have had an abnormal alpha-fetoprotein (AFP) blood test result
- if, for medical reasons, you want to find out your baby's sex – say, for example, if there's a family history of Duchenne Muscular Dystrophy (DMD), which is found almost exclusively among boys, and either parent is a carrier
- to check rhesus status: if your blood is rhesus negative and your baby's is rhesus positive, there's a risk of rhesus disease in any subsequent babies you may have, which can prove fatal. There's no risk in a first pregnancy, though. For a full explanation, see *Rhesus status* and *What if I'm rhesus negative?*, p. 140.

What happens during amniocentesis?

The test is usually performed between Weeks 15 and 20 of pregnancy – the sooner the better, really, as the results take around two weeks to come back. If you are considering terminating your pregnancy after a positive test result, it's better from all points of view that you are less far on.

Before you have the test, your doctor or midwife will explain everything to you in detail, from the procedure itself to the implications of the results. It's essential that you're fully informed before you decide whether or not to go ahead. If you do decide to have the test, the first thing that will happen on the day is that you'll have an ultrasound scan so that the doctor can find the best point at which to insert the needle to extract some amniotic fluid. You might be offered a local anaesthetic injection into your abdomen before the larger needle is inserted. A syringe draws a small sample of fluid out before the large needle is removed. All in all, the test can take between 10 and 30 minutes, depending on how clear a picture the ultrasound gives and how experienced the doctor performing the test is. It might be uncomfortable, but shouldn't be really painful.

After amniocentesis, you'll be told to rest for 24 hours to minimise the risk of miscarriage. You might experience some cramps in your bump afterwards, and this is normal. The sorts of things that sometimes (although rarely) go wrong include injuring the baby with the needle; introducing an infection into the amniotic sac or exposing the mum's blood to her baby's blood.

Results from standard amniocentesis take around two weeks to come through, but a new test called Amnio-PCR has been developed which can give results in 48 hours. Unfortunately you usually have to pay for this test. Ask your midwife, GP or obstetrician for details, or visit www.amniopcr.com/patients/summary/index.htm.

What the netmums say

'How I coped with amniocentesis'

When my triple test results* came back as high risk for Down's syndrome and I was offered an amnio, I was absolutely shell shocked,

* The triple test, offered by some NHS Trusts in the second trimester as a screen for Down's syndrome, is a blood test which measures the levels of three naturally occurring substances passed from baby to mother in pregnancy. Variations are the double and quadruple tests. Ask your medical team for details.

but there was no doubt in my mind that I needed to know for sure: forewarned is forearmed and all that. My main worry was that as I had had two miscarriages in the past I would be at a higher risk of losing the baby. The midwife and consultant assured me that previous miscarriage didn't affect my risk and I felt slightly more confident. Luckily our baby was lying in a perfect position to be out of the way. They took half a dozen scan pictures beforehand to be as sure as possible. The test itself was a little uncomfortable and within an hour I was starting to feel the period-like cramps they'd told me about. I took the rest of the week off work – I wasn't taking any chances at all – and just rested. The hospital told me that if the results were clear they would phone me, but if they were bad then I would get a home visit. I was at work when I got the call, and as soon as the voice announced that she was a midwife from the hospital I just burst into tears of relief: she didn't even get as far as telling me the results were clear. The wait was the longest period of my life, as I constantly went through different scenarios in my head, preparing myself for the worst – but it was totally the right decision for me. Due to my age and the fact I was high-risk with Nathan too, I'll probably ask to have one done automatically should I be lucky enough to fall pregnant again.
Sam from Hampshire, mum to Nathan, 13 and Lucy, 21 months

We didn't have the screening test for Down's syndrome at first as we had decided that we wouldn't terminate in any case. We had done exactly the same with our first baby. However, our 20-week scan showed cysts on her brain, and more tests at a specialist hospital showed a problem with the bowel, and clenched hands, so we had the screening and got a high-risk result. After weeks of tests, scans and a foetal MRI scan we were recommended to have amnio. We decided that if we knew ahead of the birth we could either prepare ourselves for her arrival – or relax knowing she was OK. We had the test 30 minutes after it was offered and it was pretty scary for me as I'd developed a bit of a needle phobia when pregnant with my first daughter. We had to wait a week for the results and it was a very long week. Meanwhile I researched into Down's, including looking at childcare possibilities. I hardly slept the night before I was due to ring for the result, and was up at about 5 a.m. waiting for 8 a.m. to come round. When we got the result we were so happy and rang all our relatives to give them the good news. Further scans showed the cysts gradually disappearing and everything else normalising. We never did find out what had been wrong with Paris – not because the hospital didn't bother trying to give us a diagnosis, but because there wasn't one. She's just special!

Rachel from Buckinghamshire, mum to Leila, three and Paris, five months

Your mission this week: To amnio or not to amnio?

Sit down with your partner and have a proper chat about whether or not you want to go ahead with amniocentesis. Things to consider are:

- what you would do if you got a positive test result for any of the conditions the test detects
- whether or not termination would be an option for you
- whether you would feel better able to cope with an affected baby by getting advance warning
- whether you're prepared to undergo the test despite a slight risk of miscarriage, which could mean you lose a perfectly healthy baby.

There is an organisation called Antenatal Results and Choices (ARC) which offers counselling to help you come to a decision before, during and after the antenatal testing process. Visit the website at www.arc-uk.org or call the helpline on 0207 631 0285 (Mon–Fri, 10 a.m.–5.30 p.m.). Your medical team should also be able to offer you support and advice.

Urinary tract infections (UTIs)

Sometimes just referred to as urine infections, UTIs are common in pregnancy because of those same old culprits, your hormones. Progesterone relaxes the muscles of your ureters (the drainage pipes leading down from your kidneys to your bladder), slowing down the flow of your pee. The fact that your uterus is growing all the time and constricting your bladder doesn't help either. The result is that your bladder becomes the perfect home for bacteria, because they've got more time to grow and spread before they are peed out.

This is another reason for frequent urine testing during pregnancy. Some UTIs have no symptoms, but just show up as bacteria in your pee. Others let you know in no uncertain terms that they've taken up residence in your bladder by giving you some or all of the following symptoms:

- pain or a burning sensation on peeing
- pain in your pelvis, lower abdomen, small of your back, or in your sides
- high temperature
- hot and cold flushes
- nausea and vomiting
- tremors
- frequent urge to pee
- passing much more or less urine than usual
- incontinence
- strong-smelling pee
- dark-coloured pee (which could indicate the presence of blood)
- pain during sex.

If the infection has spread to your kidneys, which is more unusual, you might have a very high temperature and constant kidney pain in your back and sides, or on one side only.

If you're found to have a UTI, you'll almost certainly be put on a short course of antibiotics, then have your pee re-tested afterwards to ensure it's clear of bacteria. Sometimes drinking lots of water can help to flush the bacteria out of your system, speeding up the recovery process. In the case of cystitis, however, there is no evidence that this is helpful, although drinking at least two litres of water per day is generally good for your health.

Why the damp pants?

You might notice about now that you appear to be producing rather a lot of your usually scanty vaginal secretion. No need to worry about this – it's perfectly normal and caused by – all together now – HORMONES! To be honest, it's probably going to keep on increasing throughout pregnancy, so it's worth making sure you always line your underwear with a panty liner and keep a supply in your handbag, too. On the plus side, if you're into the idea of a spot of nookie, it will help things to go more smoothly, as long as your other half isn't put off by it. Just to let you know, it should be either clear or milky white and inoffensive in odour – not yellow, blood-stained or smelly, in which case you have probably got an infection.

Look no further

I've heard about other NHS tests for detecting your risk factor for Down's syndrome without amniocentesis. How do these work?
The 'combined test', which involves nuchal translucency (NT) measurement by ultrasound (see p. 69) plus blood tests, is offered in the first trimester to detect your risk factor. The 'quadruple test' measures four markers for Down's syndrome in a mum's blood during the second trimester, and should be offered to all mums who come for screening tests in the second trimester. The 'serum integrated' test involves blood tests at Week 10 or 11 and then again at Week 15 or 16 of pregnancy, and is thought to be the best alternative to NT measurement where it's not available. The 'integrated test' is even more accurate if good quality NT measurement is available and the mum is prepared to wait until the second trimester for the results. Detection rates of Down's syndrome from these tests vary from 81–85 per cent.

How soon do I have to decide whether or not to have amniocentesis?
The latest that amnio is usually performed is during Week 18 of pregnancy, and given that the results take around two weeks to come through, you can understand why. You could potentially be 20 weeks pregnant and trying to make decisions about whether or not to continue with your pregnancy, and you might need another week or so to decide finally. This does mean, though, that at 15 weeks you still have a little time before you have to commit to the test. Take your time to think things over and, if you think it will help, contact ARC (see p. 135) for support.

Week 16 175 days to go!

Don't forget: Get your partner involved with your pregnancy too

Maybe your other half is something of a natural Earth Daddy and can tell you exactly what's happening at each stage of pregnancy before you've even had a chance to pick this book up! Maybe he's as disinterested in what's going on inside you as he is in how many programmes there are on the washing machine. He's probably something in between these two extremes. Either way, it's harder for him to feel properly engaged in something that's not happening directly to him – especially when there's not a lot of physical evidence to remind him of what's going on day to day. But now that you have probably sprouted a little bump and changed in other noticeable ways, too, you might just be able to get him on board with a bit more enthusiasm.

Don't talk pregnancy all the time (what a turn-off!) but leave your book open at the right page for him to read about what's happening each week; get him involved in massaging your bump, your back, your feet – whatever feels good for both of you; and give him some 'alpha male' tasks to do, like building a changing table or checking out which baby car seats fit your model of motor.

Hey baby!

You're fairly unlikely to feel it yet, but your baby often gets bouts of the hiccups, which is a precursor to breathing. Later on, when you're able to feel his movements distinctly, this will feel like a series of little twitches or 'jumps'. Of course, your baby can't make a hiccuppy noise because his windpipe is full of amniotic fluid, not air. This week he'll weigh almost 80g (nearly 3oz) and measure 11.5cm (4½ inches). His legs are elongating and his body is growing faster than his head at last, to bring things into proportion. From time to time he sucks his thumb, makes a fist and prepares for when he tries to 'punch his way out' in late pregnancy!

All about you

Are you up to reading other mums' birth stories yet? It's actually a good idea to get used to the sorts of things that might happen during labour, both good and not so good. You can always focus on the more positive things you've heard (in fact, that's a really good thing to do, along with self-hypnosis techniques like visualisation, to up your chances of having a better experience yourself), but it would be foolhardy to ignore all the less encouraging stories. Supposing you headed off to the labour suite without any inkling of the sorts of hurdles you could potentially face: what sort of a shock would it be if something actually didn't go quite according to plan?

For starters, read the Netmums' experiences of preparing for labour (p. 311, 359). They talk about how what other people told them influenced their attitudes to birth, and how similar their actual experiences were compared with their expectations (p. 373). Then turn to p. 252 for an in-depth look at the whole process of labour in its three stages.

Who'd have thought?

About 80-90 per cent of urinary tract infections are caused by *E. coli* bacteria, which are normally present in the rectum. Women are eight times more likely than men to get a UTI, partly because of how close the anus is to the urethra.

You and your nose!

In the same way that your gums are more liable to bleed in pregnancy because of the increased blood volume you've generated, your nose might bleed from time to time too. As if that isn't enough, your pregnancy hormones (yes, them again!) can make your nasal lining and sinuses swell a bit so that you feel congested and stuffy. And nature's final trick in the nose department is to combine stuffiness and nosebleeds with running mucus, also due to your increased blood volume! So whilst you're trying to catch the drips, you'd be ill-advised to actually blow your nose in case of a nosebleed, and in any case you'll still be left unable to breathe properly. So no good news, then? Well, yes: these niggles, like so many others in pregnancy, will soon resolve after the birth of your baby – and by then they'll be a dim and distant memory. Oh yes, and there are things you can do to relieve your symptoms, too.

What you can do
- First of all, be careful when you blow your nose: proceed with caution and go gently
- If you do get a nosebleed, sit leaning slightly forward and pinch the sides of your nose together, just below the bone. You'll probably need to continue squeezing your nose like this for up to 10 minutes
- Try inhaling steam: add a decongestant capsule or a few drops of tea tree oil to a bowl of very hot water and lean over it with a towel over your head.

It makes a great facial treatment too!

- Don't pick at your nose
- Steer clear of ingestible decongestant medications and over-the-counter remedies unless prescribed by your doctor
- If you get lots of minor nosebleeds or have more than two bad ones, tell your doctor, as you may become anaemic, or there may be some other underlying problem.

Who'd have thought?

Your amniotic fluid can pick up the aroma of different things you've been eating, especially stronger flavours such as curry, garlic and onion. Some studies have shown that this can influence a baby's preferences when it comes to weaning on to solids!

What the netmums say

'Dealing with nasal congestion'

I did antenatal yoga and we were shown an exercise to alleviate nasal congestion, which really helps if done regularly: place your thumb and index finger on either side of your nose, then cover one nostril with your index finger and breathe in through the open nostril. Close this nostril with the thumb and breathe out through the other nostril. Breathe in through this same nostril, cover with your index finger and breathe out through the other nostril, and so on. Gradually your nose should clear.

Lisa from Eastcote, mum to Ellie, five months

I got this in my second pregnancy and it became a problem quite late on when I got really bad sinus pains. The midwife sent me to see a doctor, but he said they don't like to give any medication to pregnant women, and suggested steam inhalation with a few drops of decongestant oil. This did help relieve it, and I used to do it just before bedtime as I suffered most at night.

Samantha from Ipswich, mum to Shaun, three-and-a-half and Jasmine, eight months

Rhesus status

Your rhesus status means whether you have rhesus positive or rhesus negative blood. People with rhesus positive blood have a protein called 'D antigen' on the surface of their red blood cells, and they are said to be 'RhD positive'. People without D antigen are known as 'RhD negative'. Most mums – around 90 per cent – are RhD positive.

Rhesus positive cells contain a substance which can stimulate rhesus negative blood to produce harmful antibodies that destroy red cells; this can occur where a mum is rhesus negative but her baby is rhesus positive (known as rhesus incompatibility), but only if their two blood supplies become intermingled. Happily, there isn't a problem with a first pregnancy, because the antibodies aren't already present in the mum. If there's rhesus incompatibility in a subsequent pregnancy, though, there's a serious risk that the antibodies that might have been produced meanwhile will recognise the baby as a 'foreign' body and try to break his or her blood down.

What if I'm rhesus negative?

In the UK an injection of anti-D is given as routine to all rhesus negative mums at 28 weeks and sometimes also at 34 weeks of pregnancy, to stop the possible production of the harmful antibody. After delivery, your baby's rhesus status will be checked from an umbilical cord blood sample. If he's rhesus positive, you will be given another injection within 72 hours. This will stop you building up antibodies between the delivery and any subsequent pregnancy with another rhesus positive baby.

Eczema in pregnancy

Around 60–80 per cent of mums who develop eczema in pregnancy have never suffered from it before, so if you suddenly find yourself with dry, itchy patches of skin – commonly on the nipples in pregnancy as well as elsewhere – then do get it checked out by your doctor. For most mums, the symptoms appear some time during the first two trimesters of pregnancy. Itchy skin in pregnancy can be a symptom of other underlying problems (see p. 244), so you need a proper diagnosis; also a lot of the treatments for eczema (including over-the-counter remedies) are not recommended for use in pregnancy as the effects on a developing baby haven't been established, so you do need to take advice on what you can and can't use to alleviate symptoms.

What can be done?

Usually the first line of attack is to use a non-greasy daily emollient, such as E45, which comes as cream, lotion and bath additive. Emollients are thick, water-based moisturisers that keep the skin hydrated. You should avoid using creams that contain even a tiny percentage of steroid such as hydrocortisone unless it's on the advice of your doctor. If you have a bad case of eczema you may well be prescribed a steroid cream, but it needs to be used under medical supervision.

If the eczema gets bad enough to become infected, there are some antibiotics that are considered safe to take whilst pregnant, so it's certainly worth going back to your doctor if this happens to you. Some mums find that cutting wheat and/or gluten and/or dairy products out of their diet relieves the symptoms of eczema, so this might be worth a try, but only in consultation with your doctor or hospital dietitian. You can find gluten-free, wheat-free breads, pastas and other products in most supermarkets these days, as well as dairy-free milk, yoghurts, cheese and spreads, so you won't have to go hunting through health-food shops to find alternatives. If you do go dairy-free, though, it's important that you get enough calcium in your diet so step up your intake of green vegetables, sesame seeds or tahini, cow's milk, tofu, cheese, yoghurt, wholegrain cereals and pulses. Your doctor may prescribe a calcium supplement.

What the netmums say

'Tips for relieving eczema in pregnancy'

At 12 weeks pregnant with my third baby I suddenly had an eczema flare-up. I hadn't had an attack for a good 10 years and was so surprised to be told it was linked to the pregnancy as I didn't suffer with the other two. It was at its worst on my hands, so I couldn't even cover it up, and although the doctor prescribed 1 per cent Diprobase, it didn't help. It was sore, itchy and flaky. All I could do was keep slathering on aqueous cream loads of times a day. I washed with it instead of soap or shower gel, too, and kept a small tube in every handbag! It cleared up about a month after Jonah was born.
Celine from Leicester, mum to Kieran, six, Luca, three and Jonah, one

I found aloe vera gel cooling and soothing when my eczema worsened in pregnancy. Usually I use a steroid cream, but I didn't want to use it whilst pregnant, even though my GP said it should be safe. The gel didn't reduce or improve the appearance of the eczema, but it certainly helped to relieve the itch, which in turn helped prevent it from becoming infected. Now I've had Cassie, I'm back on the steroid cream and it's more under control again now.
Gaynor from Truro, mum to Cassie, six months

Who'd have thought?

Continuing the theme of comparing your baby to a tasty snack, he's currently about the size of an orange!

Your mission this week: Consider the future

Start to have a think about whether or not you'll be returning to work after you've had your baby (assuming that you're working now). You may think you already know your decision, or that you have no choice in any case – but once you've done your research and really thought about how you and your partner might be able to make changes to accommodate a new way of working, you might just see possibilities you hadn't otherwise considered. There's no need at all to make decisions yet – and in any case you may change your mind again after your baby's born – but it's a good idea to get the old cogs turning in your brains and let ideas come and go.

Things you might want to consider include: looking at your partner's work situation as well as yours – perhaps he could work closer to home to cut down on his journey time, or agree with his employer to work from home one day a week; going back to work part-time yourself or on flexible hours; approaching a family member or friend to be your child's main carer; changing your own career further down the line – becoming a childminder, for instance – so that you stay home and still earn money. There's plenty of food for thought when you get started, and if you start thinking about your options from around now you won't have the same sense of panic as if you leave it until you're largely preoccupied with the birth itself.

If you already know that you will be returning to work and are not planning to use a friend or family member as a baby minder, it's worth starting to think about formal childcare. You'll need to weigh up the pros and cons of the different types, which are:

- a registered childminder
- a day nursery
- a workplace nursery or crèche
- a nanny or au pair

You can find out about their services, costs and other important information by visiting Daycare Trust at www.daycaretrust.org.uk or the National Childminding Association at www.ncma.org.uk.

For lots of information and advice on what you're entitled to in terms of maternity leave and pay, see p. 225.

Look no further

Someone at work has just told me she has chickenpox, and I don't think I had it as a child. Is my baby at risk if I get it?
The chances are that even if you don't recall getting chickenpox as a child, you have developed antibodies through a 'silent' (symptomless) mild infection with it at some point during your life. In fact, 80 per cent of pregnant mums who are checked for these antibodies do have them – and one of the blood tests taken at booking can be analysed by the lab at any time during pregnancy to check your immunity status. If you're immune, there's no risk to you or your baby. If you're found not to have these antibodies, however, there are a couple of times when your baby could be at risk. These are:

- before 20 weeks of pregnancy. If you develop the infection before this time, there's a risk of chickenpox syndrome, although this is rare (up to 14 weeks, the risk is around 0.4 per cent; between Weeks 14–20 it rises to 2 per cent)
- if you develop a rash within a week before your baby is born or up until a month afterwards, when he could be at risk of overwhelming infection.

In any case, you should contact your GP or midwife if you've come into contact with chickenpox: either you or you and your baby will be given manmade antibodies within 10 days of exposure to lessen the severity of the infection and avert disaster. It's worth knowing that the incubation period for chickenpox is about two weeks before symptoms appear, and a person is infectious from two days before the rash appears until after the blisters crust over.

Who'd have thought?

Although you will still probably not be experiencing the same sleep quality that you did before you were pregnant, slowly rising progesterone levels in the middle months mean you'll get your best sleep in your second trimester.

Do my parents have to become registered childminders before they can care for my baby?
No, they don't, although there might be financial benefits all round if they do. If your parents or in-laws do agree to become your main childcarers – and are forward-thinking enough – they might decide to attend a special parenting course for grandparents if there's one running locally. These should be considered as refresher courses, and this is a good way of suggesting them to your parents, who will probably take umbrage (understandably so!) if you cast aspersions on their ability to care for your baby. The fact is, though, that much changes from generation to generation in terms of the thinking around baby- and childcare. When you were a baby, for example, your parents might have thought nothing of keeping you waiting for a feed because it was less than four hours since your previous bottle or breastfeed, whereas feeding on demand is more widely accepted now as being better for a newborn baby.

Is dancing good exercise in pregnancy?
Much depends on what you mean by dancing: a gentle dance class that doesn't put undue stress on your back or pelvis, and doesn't involve you flinging yourself around or leaping high in the air (with the possibility of falling) should be fine – but do let your teacher know you're pregnant so she can keep an eye on what you're doing. Over-stretching can cause a ligament injury, so take it easy and don't do any moves you find difficult. The other thing, as with all exercise, is to ensure you drink plenty during breaks, and don't allow yourself to overheat as this can be dangerous for your baby.

I've found a really nice body cream that soothes my eczema, but it contains chamomile. Is it safe to use in pregnancy?

Yes, when used topically, chamomile is one of the recommended essential oils for pregnancy, so a body cream that contains it is absolutely fine to use. Herbal medicines to be taken internally should never be used in pregnancy unless prescribed by a reputable, professional herbalist with a special interest in pregnancy as some can be powerful uterus stimulants, which could trigger premature labour.

Who'd have thought?

Sleeping on your back as you get bigger in pregnancy puts pressure from your uterus on important blood vessels that run down the back of your abdomen. This can restrict blood flow to your baby and parts of your body. Because there's a major blood vessel on your right side, lying on your left helps to optimise blood flow.

How are you feeling?

Tick the box that most closely represents how you feel about the given statements, then look back to the charts in previous chapters to see how you've changed over the months.

Physically	Emotionally
I still feel sick Strongly agree ☐ Agree ☐ Neither agree nor disagree ☐ Disagree ☐ Strongly disagree ☐	I'm worried about diagnostic tests Strongly agree ☐ Agree ☐ Neither agree nor disagree ☐ Disagree ☐ Strongly disagree ☐
I feel better than in previous weeks Strongly agree ☐ Agree ☐ Neither agree nor disagree ☐ Disagree ☐ Strongly disagree ☐	I'm comfortable with the idea of being pregnant Strongly agree ☐ Agree ☐ Neither agree nor disagree ☐ Disagree ☐ Strongly disagree ☐
My back aches Strongly agree ☐ Agree ☐ Neither agree nor disagree ☐ Disagree ☐ Strongly disagree ☐	I don't know what to do about returning to work Strongly agree ☐ Agree ☐ Neither agree nor disagree ☐ Disagree ☐ Strongly disagree ☐

I've noticed more vaginal discharge than usual	I feel closer to my parents
Strongly agree ☐ Agree ☐ Neither agree nor disagree ☐ Disagree ☐ Strongly disagree ☐	Strongly agree ☐ Agree ☐ Neither agree nor disagree ☐ Disagree ☐ Strongly disagree ☐
My nose is driving me nuts!	I'm happy with my partner's level of involvement
Strongly agree ☐ Agree ☐ Neither agree nor disagree ☐ Disagree ☐ Strongly disagree ☐	Strongly agree ☐ Agree ☐ Neither agree nor disagree ☐ Disagree ☐ Strongly disagree ☐
My bump's getting more noticeable	I'm keen to hear other mums' birth stories
Strongly agree ☐ Agree ☐ Neither agree nor disagree ☐ Disagree ☐ Strongly disagree ☐	Strongly agree ☐ Agree ☐ Neither agree nor disagree ☐ Disagree ☐ Strongly disagree ☐

Who'd have thought?

Boys still outnumber girls in the UK. In 2006, there were 1,047 baby boys born for every 1,000 baby girls*.

*Source: National Statistics

Quick quiz

What's behind all the physical changes?

1 What causes spidery thread veins?

a. Staying in the sun too long

b. Leaking blood vessels due to increased blood volume

c. Not eating enough fruit and vegetables

2 Why is your hair thicker in pregnancy?

a. Because hormones make it grow more

b. Because hormones stop it falling out as it usually would

c. Because of a more balanced diet

3 How can you stop stretch marks happening?

a. By massaging a special cream into your belly

b. You can't – they're genetic

c. By not putting on weight too quickly

4 What is a linea negra?

a. A Latin term for an epidural

b. A dark line of pigmentation that runs vertically down your bump

c. A mole that gets darker in pregnancy

5 Why might your shoes feel too tight in pregnancy?

a. Hormones make your feet start growing again

b. The weight of pregnancy can make you flatter footed, elongating your feet

c. You accidentally put them in with a hot wash because your brain's gone to mush

Answers: The answers to this quiz are all 'b'.

Mostly a: Some of your answers sound like reasonable enough guesses, but they won't get you very far if you act on them. Have another read through this chapter when you get a chance – the better informed you are, the more in control of your pregnancy you'll feel.

Mostly b: You're obviously very interested in all the changes that have been happening, as well as those that are still to come. Keep absorbing information at this rate and you'll be writing your own book on pregnancy!

Mostly c: Pardon me for waking you, but you can't really read this book with your eyes shut... Seriously, though, it's worth trying to inform yourself as much as possible – not to show off to doctors and other mums, but so that you'll have a good idea of what's normal and what needs checking out with your medical team as you go through pregnancy.

Chapter 4
Weeks 17–20

By the end of this chapter you'll have completed half your pregnancy! Isn't it going quickly! No? Oh well, from here on in, it should feel like full steam ahead as you teeter at the crest of the mountain and hurtle down the other side. (Although it has to be said that approaching your due date towards the other end of pregnancy can feel interminable... No matter – we'll address that when we get there, OK?)

These next months will see opportunities for you and your partner to connect with your baby in new, more intimate ways. This is the month most mums get to see their babies in much greater detail at the anomaly scan (around Week 20) and you may be among the lucky mums who feel their babies move this month – at around 18 weeks or so. (It's not unusual, though, not to feel anything until Week 22 or, in some cases, even later. Don't panic!)

Week 17 *168 days to go!*

Don't forget: Your amnio results could come back this week

We've talked already about what you would do with the results of an amniocentesis test if it proved positive, and this could be the week that important decisions have to be made about the future of your pregnancy. Chances are that all is fine – and we mums have everything crossed for you that it is – but it's just as well to have another good chat with your partner about what the results will mean for you both. You might want to consult with ARC again (see p. 135) to help you to see things as objectively as possible – and this might be particularly applicable if you and your partner can't agree on your next course of action. Remember, though (and this is vitally important), that this is your body carrying your baby, and no one – not even your partner – can force you into any decision to which you don't feel reconciled.

Hey baby!

The length of your baby is roughly equivalent to the short side of a DL envelope (go on, raid the stationery cupboard) at 11–12cm (around 4½ inches). He's made another good effort at piling on the ounces and has doubled in weight from Week 15 to around 100g (4oz). This week sees him laying down fat – a very important part of his growth. This will fill out all the wrinkles in his skin and will play a vital role in regulating his body temperature and metabolism. At the moment, your baby's make-up is still largely water (almost 90 per cent!) but this will change as he plumps himself up so that fat is responsible for two-thirds of his weight at birth.

All about you

Around now, you might start to feel a bit of pain or discomfort down one or both sides of your uterus if you bend or stretch suddenly, which is commonly known as a 'round ligament' pain. Don't worry – it doesn't mean there is anything wrong, just that your uterus is continuing to grow and expand. Your baby will remain blissfully unaware of any discomfort you might be feeling – just as he will be when he seemingly tries to kick his way out of you in the coming weeks! Don't ignore the pain if it's severe or persists after a little rest, though – it could be symptomatic of some other problem. Consult your GP or obstetrician for a quick check-up to make sure. Chances are there's nothing seriously wrong in any case.

Puffy fingers, ankles, feet...

Now whilst it's quite normal to get swollen digits and extremities – and sometimes even a slightly swollen face – in pregnancy, it's important you keep an eye on the extent of it (and that your midwives or GP do) as excessive water retention can be a symptom of pre-eclampsia, a serious condition of pregnancy which, if allowed to progress to eclampsia, can be life-threatening for both mum and baby (see p. 274). You might be unaffected as yet, but it's as well to be forewarned so you'll know what to look out for and what action to take.

The medical term for swelling of the extremities in pregnancy is oedema. Here comes the yukky bit now: it's caused by some of your capillaries (tiny blood vessels) leaking because of the extra blood volume that's circulating round your body. Also, as pregnancy continues, the weight of your uterus compresses some of the veins in your pelvis, making the blood pool rather than flow freely – and this in turn causes the water normally contained in other body tissue to be squeezed into the tissue in your hands and feet.

If all of that sounds hideous, it might help to know that it's not at all uncommon, with around half of all mums noticing some oedema, if only in the latter stages of pregnancy – and it's almost unheard of for a mum carrying twins not to get it to an extent. You might notice more water pooling around your ankles and across your feet after you've been standing or walking for a while – in fact it can almost feel as if your feet are sloshing about in water! It's not a problem, though, unless it's accompanied by headache, visual disturbances, pain under the ribs, vomiting, a decrease in urine output and/or high blood pressure, which are all additional signs of pre-eclampsia. If you do notice any combination of these symptoms, get yourself seen by a doctor straightaway.

What you can do
Given that you haven't got pre-eclampsia symptoms, the best remedy for oedema is to rest with your feet slightly higher than hip height. You can also benefit by:

- drinking plenty of water – and if this sounds like crazy advice, take our word for it: you're less likely to retain water the more you drink
- trying to keep mobile when you're not resting with your feet up
- staying off your back in bed
- removing your rings before the swelling means they have to be cut off
- raising the foot end of your bed slightly so that your legs are elevated while you sleep.

What the netmums say

'Swelling up!'

I had such excessive swelling in my feet towards the end of pregnancy I went up two shoe sizes. As I normally take a size eight in shoes, this meant I was having to buy men's sandals in a size 10! It was purely uncomplicated oedema, nothing more sinister, and about three days after Zak was born my feet went back to normal.
Niki from Liverpool, mum to Zak, 23 months

I had terrible swelling in my ankles, feet, hands and fingers. I could only wear flip-flops, and I had to leave my wedding and engagement rings off for months. When I got home from work in the evenings I used to lie on the settee and put my feet up on the back of it until my feet and ankles went down. They were very painful, but I was told it was nothing serious. The swelling took a couple of weeks after the birth to go down fully. It was lovely to finally be able to put on a pair of high heels and my rings again!
Ruth from County Durham, mum to Ben, four

My feet swelled so badly during pregnancy that I actually felt the skin might tear, it was stretched so tight! I spent most of my time barefoot and the rest of the time in crocs – which was unfortunate as it was winter so I had to wear them with socks, not the fashion statement of the moment! My face swelled up, too, which only added to the feeling that I was turning inflatable! Everything went back to normal a few days after I delivered my lovely little daughter, though – thank goodness!
Jackie from Liverpool, mum to Sophie-Rose, eight months

Thrush

You may be interested to learn that the fungus that causes thrush is commonly found in your vagina. You could also be forgiven for being not remotely interested in this information – but you may become interested as pregnancy goes on, because thrush is quite a common problem for mums-to-be.

The fungus responsible for thrush is called *Candida albicans*, and it usually resides in our privates benignly enough without making its presence felt. The problem arises in the absence of the normal bacteria that stem its growth. The balance of these bacteria can be upset by a number of factors, all to do with the workings of the immune system. If you're on antibiotics, for instance, or very stressed out, you might notice persistent and troublesome itching, soreness and a thick, creamy discharge in your underwear. We talked about your immune system being compromised by pregnancy when we were discussing snuffles and colds, and similarly those mischievous hormones can give rise to a bout or two of thrush, especially in the third trimester, but sometimes before.

So what next?

Luckily, there's no evidence to suggest that thrush can harm an unborn baby and there is an antifungal treatment available in pessary form that your GP can prescribe for you in pregnancy. Don't use any over-the-counter treatments, though, as most antifungals contain an ingredient that can be harmful in pregnancy. You might get some relief by eating live natural yoghurt, which helps to restore the balance of bacteria in your vagina, but it will take a bit of time to work.

Sometimes babies catch thrush during delivery if Mum has it at the time of the birth, but it's not a worry and is easily treated.

Your mission this week: Look after yourself

- If you work, reassess your working conditions. If you've told your employer you're pregnant, make sure you get an ergonomic check to ensure you've got all the comforts you need to keep you safe in the workplace. Try to rest as much as possible – and if this means trying to renegotiate your working hours so you start and finish a bit later to miss the rush hour, then try. It could also mean a valuable extra hour in bed every morning. Don't offer to give up your lunch break – or any other breaks – and work through, though, as you need these as much as you need the extra time.
- Get into the habit of cooking simple meals now so that you're not trying to think up new, speedy ideas once your baby has arrived, and so that you get used to shopping a bit differently.
- Don't forget that exercise actually energises us, so build a good brisk walk, an evening swim or an antenatal exercise class into your regular routine.

Look no further

Despite me pushing my now-visible bump out in front of me, no one ever offers me a seat on public transport. What can I do?

Don't be shy to ask someone to get up for you, man or woman. The feminist movement has taken off so much in recent decades – and the PC 'police' have become so ardent – that men are usually only reluctant to offer seats to mums-to-be and the elderly in case of rejection. (Also, unless you're heavily, indisputably pregnant, people can be fearful of offering a seat to someone who turns out to be just a bit too fond of the high life!) If you ask politely whether anyone feels able to give up their seat because you're pregnant (without even a hint of confrontation, as that would make you as bad as the PC extremists themselves!), you'll probably get lucky. Don't assume, though, that just because your fellow passengers appear to be able-bodied and as fit as a flea, they're not also in need of a seat: they may have an invisible but debilitating complaint. However, there's no harm in asking, and the more you practise, the more confident you'll become, despite a few people ignoring you or just staring at their shoes...

When does pre-eclampsia turn into eclampsia?

This happens relatively rarely these days now that pre-eclampsia is screened for closely, but it can happen if symptoms aren't picked up on and addressed immediately. This is one reason why it's so important for you to keep all your antenatal appointments and to report any interim symptoms (see p. 274) to your medical team. In eclampsia, a mum may have fits and lose consciousness, and the condition can be fatal for baby and/or mum. If eclampsia does happen, it is usually in late pregnancy or shortly after delivery.

How does pre-eclampsia affect unborn babies?

The main problem is that the placenta stops working properly, restricting the amount of oxygen and nutrients getting to the baby – this is termed 'placental insufficiency'. This in turn can cause severe growth impairment and may mean a baby has to be delivered prematurely. For more on pre-eclampsia see p. 274.

Week 18 161 days to go!

Don't forget: Get your eyesight checked

Some mums find their eyesight changes during pregnancy – and even, in rare cases, that they need a new prescription for glasses or contact lenses. Three guesses what might be causing such a disruption? Right first time – hormones! Other changes you might notice include dry eyes, blurred or distorted vision, spots before the eyes and floaters (those little black specks that can hover around your line of vision). It's important to get yourself checked out by an opthalmologist or your GP to rule out any other underlying problem. Normal or near-normal vision usually returns a few weeks after the birth, or once you've finished breastfeeding – so don't chuck out your old specs or lenses! And to make the most of any 'two for one' offers in the event that you do need to get new specs, why not update your look by choosing a new pair of frames with your old prescription, or see if you can get prescription sunglasses in your old prescription. These will come into their own once your eyesight has normalised.

Hey baby!

Your baby will have gained half his body weight again by the end of this week, and will end up a whopping 150g (well OK, not whopping, but it's still the equivalent of 6oz). His crown-to-rump length is somewhere between 12.5–14cm (5–5½ inches). Roughly speaking (and depending on the size of your hands) this is about the same as the distance between the middle of your wrist where it joins your palm and the tip of your thumb. Your baby is looking more and more human now. Although his hearing won't mature fully until the third trimester, he's able to hear you, so sing and chat to him throughout the day. Not only will it soothe him and help him recognise your voice at birth – it will be company for you too! From this week, your baby's growth rate will slow a little, but he'll still continue to gain weight all the time.

Who'd have thought?

Toxaemia, hypertension of pregnancy, proteinuric pregnancy-induced hypertension, gestosis and pre-eclamptic toxaemia (PET) are all terms for pre-eclampsia.

All about you

It could be another milestone for you this week, as lots of mums feel their babies move for the first time at about Week 18 (see *Was that you, baby?*, below). This week your uterus takes on the size and shape of one of the smaller melon varieties – say a galia or cantaloupe! You'll probably find that you can feel the top of it about two finger widths below your belly button. Several other developments we discussed earlier might happen for you this week as well: you could develop a linea negra (dark line) vertically down your bump; you might notice the onset of the 'blooming' period with your hair going all thick and glossy and your nails taking on a new invincibility. On the minus side, you might find that backache creeps up on you (if it hasn't done so already) because your centre of gravity is beginning to change. Re-read the advice in *Top tips for protecting your back*, p. 115, to try to minimise the discomfort.

Was that you, baby?

This week – or some time over the next four or so – you'll feel your baby move for the very first time, and this is known as 'quickening'. In fact, according to the *Oxford English Dictionary*, to 'quicken' means 'to reach the stage of pregnancy at which the child shows signs of life'. This is obviously rather an outdated idea, as modern technology means that signs of life can be detected very early in pregnancy via ultrasound scan – but it can't harm to get of a bit of history under your belt, so hey.

Some mums describe quickening as feeling like a series of tiny bubbles bursting in their tums; you might feel it more as a fluttering sensation – as if a butterfly has somehow made its way into your uterus and would like to come out again now please-and-thank-you-very-much!

There's no need to worry if you don't feel your baby move this week. As long as your scans have been normal and your baby's heartbeat has been heard recently, that's all you need to know. First-time mums, in any case, tend to notice movements a bit later than mums who've done it all before because they don't really know what they're expecting to feel. If you're a bit overweight and have more fat than most laid down across your belly, you might not feel movements this early either. Or you might well have felt something but thought it was a bit of wind brewing! And if you've been rushing from A to B and not really had much quiet time, you might simply have missed the movements.

'Earth receiving baby!'

From this point in pregnancy you can focus on your baby's movements, whether or not you've felt them yet, because feel them you will – and soon. It can help if you build some quiet time into your daily schedule when you can lie down, concentrate on your bump and wait patiently. A warm bath sometimes provokes some movement, especially at night when you're ready to collapse into bed, as this is often the time an unborn baby is at his most active! (Well, to be fair, it's often the time a newly born baby is at his most active, too…) Don't expect your partner to be able to feel anything yet if he lays his hands on your bump: what you'll feel first are internal sensations. What he'll feel are the stronger kicks that resonate through to the outside world!

What the netmums say

'Feeling my baby move for the first time!'

I felt my baby move at 17 weeks. I was sitting at the PC and kept feeling a fluttering in my tummy like I had butterflies: it felt like the sensation you get when you drive over a hump-backed bridge. As the pregnancy progressed I felt more definite kicks and flips, and little feet and hands pushing out, plus feet nicely jammed up under my ribs. Some of the movements took my breath away – especially when he'd turn right over to face the other way, which he used to do right up until he was born!
Nicola from Norwich, mum to Jacob, three-and-a-half

I was just over 20 weeks when I felt funny flutterings down below. I thought, 'Oh my God, was that my baby?' His timing was perfect as I was due to have my 20-week scan two days later, and had been worried that I hadn't felt him move yet. As the pregnancy progressed, the movements grew stronger, and at 28 weeks my partner got a kick in the ear when he had his head on my bump, which he's never got over to this day! It was really amazing for him to feel the movements I'd been feeling and be able to share that with me.
Charlotte from Derby, mum to Joshua, three

I first felt my baby move between Weeks 16 and 17, and it felt like butterflies – in fact, I wasn't sure if it was a touch of wind. But the first real big movement was at around 19 weeks and I was so chuffed I lay in bed all night with my hands covering my tummy, just in case I felt it again. But then, of course, I thought I'd imagined it all along until the next time!

Mags from Lanarkshire, mum to Eve, two

You and your pelvic floor

Now we don't want to be indelicate, but how're things down below? You could ask your partner, but just in case you hear something you'd rather not concerning the various large objects that could fit inside your lady parts – with each new description accompanied by loud guffawing – there are other ways of assessing how toned your vagina is. You'll know if your vaginal muscles need strengthening if, for example, you can't cough, laugh loudly or sneeze without the comfort of knowing you are wearing a panty liner. This is known as 'stress incontinence'. You can test the muscles out, too, by trying to stop yourself from peeing mid-stream. If you find it a bit of a challenge, there's room for some toning-up there.

Strengthening the vaginal walls is important on several levels: firstly, it'll help to prevent stress incontinence, which often starts or worsens in pregnancy (so if you passed the peeing test, you can wipe the smug grin off your face – you're not home and dry yet. Forgive the pun.) Another reason for working out 'downstairs' is that the pelvic floor muscles support your uterus and bowel as well and your bladder, configured as they are in a sort of pelvic sling. Lastly, your vagina is likely to come in for a bit of a hammering if you give birth through it, and not only will strengthened muscles help you push your baby out, they will give you a head start to getting back into pelvic shape afterwards!

Secret exercise (no one need ever know...)

The basic exercise for strengthening the pelvic floor muscles should really be practised by all mums – pregnant or not – every day of our lives. And you don't have to be a mum to benefit either. No, no, we don't mean dads should do them as well! We mean that all women can benefit, not just those who have given birth.

Try to repeat this exercise three or four times a day and remember to do it. It's very discreet, can be done sitting, lying or standing and – as long as you don't pull 'concentrating' faces – no one need ever know you're doing it:

- pretend you're trying to hold your pee, then gradually pull these same muscles up and squeeze them hard. You'll feel your anus automatically tighten at the same time
- you'll know you're pulling the muscles up gradually enough if you envisage yourself travelling upwards in a lift from basement to top floor: with each passing floor, tighten a bit more and feel a slightly wider area responding
- hold the squeeze for a slow count of five, breathing freely, then 'take the lift back down' through every floor until your muscles are fully relaxed
- repeat as many times as you can.

What the netmums say

'Me and my pelvic floor'

Never, never neglect to do your pelvic floor exercises! For me it sorted out the slight postnatal stress incontinence problem, reduced the swelling and numbness after being stitched up and gave me quite pert buttocks for a while, too!
Sam from Hampshire, mum to Nathan, 13 and Lucy, 21 months

I loved doing my pelvic floors even before I fell pregnant with my first baby – but now, after two babies, it doesn't feel like I have the strong 'grip' I had before. At least I can still enjoy sex – and my partner sure isn't complaining! – but I'll be doing a lot more now I'm in my third pregnancy!
Alicia from London, mum to Kyrus, two, Demiyah, one, and 14 weeks pregnant

Who'd have thought?

Over the coming weeks your breasts will begin producing colostrum – the nutrient-rich first food that will nourish your baby in the first few days after birth, before you get breastmilk.

That giddy feeling

Dizziness is to the second trimester of pregnancy as nausea and tiredness are to the first. There are a few reasons why you might feel you're going to go into a silent-movie swoon while you're expecting:

Reason: You haven't eaten for a couple of hours and your blood-sugar levels have plummeted.
Remedy: Keep a supply of easily portable snacks in your handbag, desk drawer or coat pocket. A cereal bar, an apple or a few rough oatcakes will give you a lasting blood-sugar boost. As a rule, try to eat five small meals a day rather than three substantial ones.

Reason: You've let yourself get too hot.
Remedy: It's not uncommon to get 'flushes' in pregnancy, so whatever the season make sure you dress in layers that you can adjust according to your temperature. It's dangerous to get really hot, as there's some evidence that over-heating during pregnancy may cause damage to the baby's developing nervous system, so don't exercise to the point of overheating.

Reason: You've stood up too quickly.
Remedy: It's difficult to remember to get up gradually each time you want to leave your seat, but do try to come to standing slowly. This is to avoid 'postural hypotension' where your blood pressure suddenly drops and blood doesn't reach your brain quickly enough.

Reason: Your growing uterus brings pressure to bear on your blood vessels, constricting the flow.
Remedy: Hmmm… there isn't one. You'll just have to sit this one out!

Whatever the reason for your dizziness, lying on your left side or sitting with your head between your knees will help to increase the blood flow to your brain. If you get persistent dizziness or fainting spells, get medical help straightaway as this could be a symptom of anaemia or another underlying condition.

Your mission this week: Girl or Boy?

Chat with your partner about whether or not you want to find out the sex of your baby: your anomaly scan will ideally have happened by Week 20 (although in some areas this may happen a week or so later), and you may well get an opportunity to find out, depending on how your baby is lying and the clarity of the image.

How you decide whether or not to ask about your baby's sex – if indeed your hospital's policy is to tell, and it isn't in all cases (see *Look no further*, p. 163) – will depend on a few factors. Firstly, does your partner feel the same way as you do? If so, the decision will be easier. If not, it's probably better for neither of you to know the sex than for just one of you to have the information. (It would be very easy, for example, to blurt it out in anger: 'Is this the way you'd like *your daughter* to learn about relationships?' Just imagine…)

Secondly, how will you cope if you don't hear what you want to hear? Say you've been longing for a girl and find out you're carrying a boy: will this knowledge spoil pregnancy for you or give you time to adjust to the news? If, of course, it's confirmed that you're expecting a girl, you can't lose! (Unless your partner was hoping for a boy…) Some couples prefer to wait until the birth, knowing that they'll be equally happy either way.

Finally, if you decide that neither of you wants to find out the sex of your baby, make sure you say so to your sonographer: so many couples do want to know that he or she may just mention it during your scan unless you request not to be told.

What the netmums say

'Deciding whether to find out the sex of my baby'

I really wanted to know – and was sure I was having a boy – because I thought if I could imagine a boy or a girl, it would help me bond with the baby in pregnancy. When I was told I was having a boy I was really happy, and we decided on the name Thomas at about 30 weeks. It really helped me think of him as a little person, and I used to talk to him and say his name. When Thomas was finally born, I felt like I already knew him.
Jennifer from Chesterfield, mum to Thomas, two years

We found out in my first pregnancy that we were expecting a boy, but after he was born we wished that we hadn't known – it felt a bit of an anti-climax. I think we only asked in the first place because everyone expected us to. With my second baby we kept it as a surprise and I'm so glad that we did – it was lovely for my husband to be the one to tell me 'it's a girl' rather than a sonographer! Our third baby is due in four weeks, and again we've chosen not to know. I think we're in the minority, though, as there were eight of us from my son's year at school having babies this year, and I'm the only one who hasn't found out the sex. I also think it is a bit of an obsession with other people, because whenever I say I don't know whether I'm having a boy or a girl, they usually start trying desperately to guess from the shape of my bump! My husband and I don't feel our lives will be greatly different whether we have another boy or another girl, and I have carried all three babies in exactly the same way.

Susan from Northants, mum to James, five, Grace, four, and 36 weeks pregnant

I didn't find out with my first baby as I wanted a surprise, but I felt very strongly it was a boy, which it was. My second pregnancy was a happy surprise and we decided to find out what we were having as the two babies would be so close in age. I really wanted a girl and it was a second boy, but once I knew, those longings disappeared. My third pregnancy was much planned, and I'd bought a book on how to try and conceive the gender of your choice naturally in case I could swing the odds in favour of having a girl. However, I must stress it was a baby I wanted – boy or girl. I followed the book's suggestions about temperature, diet and timing of sex so when we conceived we felt sure it would be a girl, especially as the pregnancy was very different. At the 20-week scan we were told it was another boy, and initially I was a little disappointed, but we booked a 3D scan and it was amazing: I absolutely fell in love with my third little man. Maybe it's natural for a mum to want a girl, but I can truly say I feel like the proudest mother in the world when I look at my three boys.

Nadia from Hadfield, mum to Ethan, four, Jacob, three and Theo, five months

With our first child it really made no odds to us what the sex was: we were just so pleased to have a little one on the way. I thought at first that I'd want to find out in subsequent pregnancies, but I've changed my mind. I think it's because I've got a preference now, and I really feel it would be better to wait until the birth to find out, as I would then love the baby whatever, rather than finding out early and 'coming to terms' with the idea. Another point is that it's a bit of an anti-climax for other people waiting to be told about the birth. Rather than asking, 'What did they have?', because they already know the sex they're just told, 'They've had him/her' and that's that.
Jenny from east Sussex, mum to Laura, three

Look no further

Why won't my hospital divulge the sex of my baby? I'm uncomfortable with the medical team knowing the sex when I don't.

It's not uncommon to feel as you do, and it can feel like a bit of an intimate intrusion for a complete stranger to know more about your unborn baby than you do, but it may help to know that the reasons are usually ethical. In some cultures where either gender is more highly prized, couples may terminate a perfectly healthy baby purely on the grounds of it being the 'wrong' sex. This is not only ethically indefensible, but can also upset the natural order of things, bringing about an imbalance in the sexes. Because hospitals can't discriminate between cultures, some make a blanket rule for everyone.

The other reason some hospitals choose not to divulge the sex of a baby is that they may get it wrong and they don't want any reprisals. Sometimes the decision lies with the sonographer. Someone very experienced and highly skilled might be more prepared to be put on the spot than a less experienced technician.

Who'd have thought?

In the UK, 90 per cent of mums stop breastfeeding before they want to because of a lack of support and preventable breastfeeding problems.*

*UK Infant Feeding Survey 2000

I've heard you can get special 'cones' to help exercise your pelvic floor. What are they and can they be used in pregnancy?

Vaginal cones are small conical weights, similar in shape and size to a tampon, that you can place in your vagina to help you train your pelvic floor muscles. They were originally devised to help women to overcome stress incontinence but are also suitable for improving the tone of the vaginal muscles generally. There are two types:

- a set of cones of increasing weight
- a single cone of adjustable weight.

The cones are probably safe to use in pregnancy – but only on the advice of your GP, obstetrician or midwife. However, for most mums-to-be, practising regular pelvic floor exercises (see p. 158) should be perfectly sufficient. There are some circumstances in which it's not considered safe to use vaginal cones, such as if you have a history of miscarriage or if you have been advised to avoid sex in pregnancy. Of course, scrupulous hygiene is important as you don't want to introduce germs into your vagina. You can find Aquaflex vaginal cones at larger branches of Boots.

Is it safe for me to continue wearing contact lenses in pregnancy?

Yes, as long as you're not suffering from dry eyes or distorted vision, which are both common side-effects of pregnancy, so it's as well to have a pair of specs you can wear in the correct prescription, even if you have to get a new pair due to temporary changes in your eyesight. Wearing the wrong prescription will leave you prone to accidents; wearing contact lenses with dry eyes will aggravate the problem. If comfort drops don't ease your eyes whilst wearing contact lenses, stop wearing them altogether until the problem resolves itself. If in any doubt, consult your opthalmologist. See *Don't forget: Get your eyesight checked*, p. 155.

Who'd have thought?

Some people believe that you can tell a baby's gender by its heart rate in the uterus: that if you're having a girl it will be above 140 beats per minute, and a boy's will be below 140. However, there's no scientific evidence to support this pregnancy myth.

Week 19 154 days to go!

Don't forget: Think about names for your baby

It might seem a bit early, but there's no time like the present for starting to consider names for your baby. It can be a bit more involved than you might imagine. There are plenty of considerations:

- how many syllables will best complement your surname? A long surname might go better with a short first name (eg Mark Ramprakash); a two-syllable surname can take an equivalent or longer first name (Lourdes Ritchie; Romeo Beckham); a short surname can take a more elaborate first name (Arabella Weir); a long first and surname can be a bit of a mouthful (Natasha Kaplinsky)
- how 'trendy' do you want to go – and will your child thank you for it later? Fifi Trixibelle, Peaches Honeyblossom and Pixie Geldof are all relatively high-profile, eccentric media types (and who knows what will become of little half-sister Heavenly Hiraani Tiger Lily?), but if you name your shrinking violet Zowie Bowie or something along those lines (you see where we're going with this?), chances are he or she will change it later in any case. (Zowie renamed himself Joey at first, but is now known as Duncan Jones!)
- are there any family names you want to include? Will they be first or middle names? And whose family takes priority?
- how do the initials look when written down? Christopher Robin Andrew Pearson, for instance, would not make a great combination; neither would Philippa India Grayson…
- Does the first name sound good with the surname from the point of view of sense? Russell would not be the best choice for a son of Mr and Mrs Sprout; Mr and Mrs Thyme may want to re-think their choice of Justin…

Make a long list, then a shortlist, with contributions from both you and your partner. You might think you've found the perfect name now, but you may well go off it later – or you might prefer to wait and see whether your newborn seems to suit a particular name. Either way, there's no harm in thinking now – and it's one of the more pleasurable tasks of pregnancy.

Hey baby!

Your baby nows weighs around 200g (almost 8oz). Although he still looks rather scrawny in relation to his crown-to-rump length – which is around 14.5cm (just under 6 inches) – fat is continuing to fill out his wrinkly skin and plump him up all over. He can now nod his head backwards and forwards since the muscles in his neck have strengthened. These muscles will continue to grow stronger throughout pregnancy, but they won't be strong enough to hold his head steady until he's around six months old – although some babies do manage this sooner.

A thick, creamy-white substance called vernix is starting to coat your baby's skin. This protects his skin from its watery environment. After all, if you can turn all prune-like after a soak in the bath, imagine what nine months spent in a watery amniotic sac could do to your skin!

All about you

If you're suffering from any of the niggles we've already discussed, from skin irritation to swollen ankles, make sure you're doing all you can to alleviate them – and don't be afraid to bring them up with your medical team if you're really suffering and not getting any relief. Keeping yourself hydrated can help with lots of things – dry skin; oedema (swelling); urinary tract infections – so keep a bottle of water handy and try to drink around two litres a day.

Allergies in pregnancy

In order for your body to accept your baby as a 'non foreign' entity, your immune system dampens down during pregnancy. This can be a double-edged sword: on the one hand, you'll find yourself more prone to viruses and bacterial infections; on the other hand, you'll be less likely to react as strongly to allergens as you would do normally – unless you're one of the unlucky few for whom allergies actually get worse in pregnancy. Autoimmune conditions also tend to improve, although it's a bit arbitrary who will feel better and who will feel worse.

Let's hope you're one of the fortunates who does feel the benefit of reduced allergic reaction, because lots of the medications you may have been taking before you were pregnant won't be compatible with pregnancy, and you'll have been advised to stop using them. If you are really suffering, though, speak to your doctor, as there may be an alternative medication you can take.

Don't use over-the-counter antihistamines or any nasal sprays without your doctor's advice, as they could contain potentially harmful ingredients.

Heartburn

Heartburn is, in fact, nothing to do with your heart, but is a term used to describe a burning feeling in your chest, usually after eating. It's caused by acid juices from your stomach leaking back up into your gullet and is very common in pregnancy, affecting two-thirds of mums-to-be. The reason is that the pregnancy hormones responsible for just about every other ill and happy event in pregnancy cause the valve at the entrance of your stomach to relax so that it isn't fully closed.

If you're already suffering from heartburn, much as we'd like to be the bearers of good news, the truth is it'll probably get worse as your bump grows because your uterus will put pressure on your stomach, forcing some of the acid back up. Because of the laws of gravity, the problem tends to worsen at night or any other time you're lying down. Just as with lots of the other niggles in pregnancy, though, it should resolve immediately with the delivery of your baby.

Help with heartburn

- Some mums find relief from sitting astride a chair, back to front, and leaning their arms on the chair back. This tips you forward slightly, making it hard for acid to come back up, and helps to create a bit of space around your stomach.
- Keep your diet simple, avoiding rich, fatty, tomatoey or spicy foods, coffee and fizzy drinks, which are all thought to make things worse. Alcohol is another culprit, so if you're still enjoying a glass of wine every now and then it might be best just to give it up for now.
- Try to sleep in a semi-upright position by propping yourself up with an extra pillow or putting a V-shaped pillow behind your usual one. This will help to defy gravity and prevent your stomach from being squeezed!
- Avoid big meals: indigestion is another reason why it's a good idea to eat small, regular meals rather than three main meals a day.
- Try not to eat close to bedtime.
- Some mums have found that eating a small amount of acid-neutralising

food, such as apple or raw carrot, or sucking a peppermint, can help to ease symptoms. Others find that chewing on a raw piece of root ginger prevents an attack in the first place. Not scientifically proven, but worth a try...

- Milk can have an antacid effect, so drinking half a glass might help alleviate symptoms.
- If things get really uncomfortable, consult your pharmacist, who may be able to recommend an antacid over-the-counter treatment that's OK to use in pregnancy.

Indigestion

Another uncomfortable tummy complaint in pregnancy is indigestion, but the discomfort is lower down than in heartburn and likely to feel more like bloating, rumblings and unpleasant sensations. Things are invariably worse after a big blow-out meal, so perhaps it's time to put the weekend fry-up or three-course Sunday lunch on hold for now. (The cries of 'What else are you expecting me to give up?' are deafening at this point, we know. But it's for your own good...)

You'd be forgiven for assuming that indigestion is also caused by your hormones – because you'd be right! Yes, it's all down to the general relaxation of muscles throughout your body that makes your digestion sluggish.

Help with indigestion

- Best advice is to avoid the foods and drinks that make indigestion worse. They're similar to the heartburn triggers – rich, fatty, spicy foods, alcohol and fizzy drinks. (Bah, humbug!)
- Keep your meals small and frequent – five snack meals a day rather than three large ones might suit you better.
- Try not to bolt that little meal of yours, however hungry you are. (But then if you're eating little and often, you shouldn't be hungry anyway.)
- Don't eat close to bedtime.
- Prop yourself up in bed (see *Help with heartburn,* p. 167).
- Eat a peppermint or drink a small cup of peppermint tea after eating.
- Avoid restrictive clothing and tight waistbands.

What the netmums say

'How I coped with indigestion and heartburn'

The only thing that worked for me was home-made milkshake. I used to put loads of ice, milk and ice cream (chocolate or vanilla) in the blender with a chopped-up banana and whizz it together. During the last three weeks it was the only thing I could drink!
Niki from Liverpool, mum to Zak, 23 months

For me, heartburn was the worst part of being pregnant. I suffered really badly right the way through both pregnancies and the only thing that would ease it was drinking a glass of cold milk. I found I couldn't sleep lying flat or on my sides, so I had to prop myself up with about three pillows and sleep like that.
Kelly from Ashford, Kent, mum to Reese, four and Riley, seven months

Every time I went to lie down, the heartburn was unbearable. I bought lots of extra pillows to try and prop myself up a bit, but I even had the scary feeling I was going to be sick lying down. I tried eating little but often and not eating after 5 p.m., but all to no avail. In the end I ate whatever I fancied and carried a large box of indigestion tablets around with me. My sister-in-law said to me, 'Don't worry: as soon as that baby comes out, the heartburn will stop' – and she was right!
Mags from Lanarkshire, mum to Eve, two

I had terrible heartburn, but I didn't do much to help myself as I just couldn't stop eating the stuff that caused it: I couldn't resist takeaways! I did find that the chewy indigestion tablets you can buy over the counter were a great help, though.
Amanda from Bristol, mum to Ruby, one

I slept propped up on four or five pillows and kept a bottle of liquid indigestion remedy by the bed at all times towards the end of both pregnancies, which I would just take swigs from! I also found that drinking cold water helped slightly if I didn't have the indigestion remedy to hand.
Lisa from Liverpool, mum to Joshua, five and Rose, three

Who'd have thought?

Your weight gain at this point in pregnancy should be around 4.5–6kg (10–13lb), although this can vary a lot depending on your frame, pre-pregnancy weight, age, race and height. By the end of pregnancy, the average weight gain for mums at the recommended weight for their height at the outset is 10–12.5 kg (22–28lb), although lots of mums whose weight gain falls outside these guidelines go on to have healthy babies. Consult your midwife, GP or obstetrician if your gain is far outside of the parameters, as you might need to see a dietitian.

Breathlessness

Another of the many marvels of pregnancy is that your body does try to adapt to work more efficiently. For example, your respiratory system changes the way it works so that it can process oxygen and carbon dioxide more efficiently. In pregnancy you tend to breathe more deeply as you have greater lung capacity than before. This is because there's more space around your lungs as a result of your ribcage expanding.

Later on in your pregnancy, when your baby is large enough to compress your diaphragm, you'll probably experience breathlessness again, and it can feel as if your baby couldn't possibly get any higher in your belly! Some mums know their baby has dropped down in readiness for birth when they experience a sudden relief from this rather overstuffed feeling. (The pay-off in this case, though, is a less-than-alluring waddling gait and the feeling that you're carrying a sack of spuds around in your pelvis!)

'I need to pee – again!'

About now you might find that, as in the early days of pregnancy, you need to rekindle your love affair with the loo. The urgent need to pee doesn't have the same cause at this stage: in early pregnancy it's a response to hormones, but as your uterus grows it's more to do with the fact that your bladder is being compressed and can't hold as much urine before you feel the need to go. So really it's ongoing until your baby is delivered – probably peaking in the last month, when your baby's head engages and presses on your bladder even more – and even after the birth you'll need to go frequently for up to another week, until all the excess fluid you've been carrying in your body tissues is expelled. (It's marvellous fun, this pregnancy caper, isn't it?)

Your mission this week: Beg, borrow or swap maternity clothes

Chances are your pregnancy wardrobe is still somewhat limited, and if your only other option is slopping about in your partner's tracky bottoms and a big, baggy T-shirt, it's time to reinject some pizzazz into your look. See if you can borrow a friend's old maternity gear – she'll probably have things in different sizes to accommodate you as you grow. Shop for tops in larger sizes in budget outlets like supermarkets and cut-price clothing stores. The A-line, Empire line and kaftan styles will flatter you as well as feeling comfy. If you have made some friends at your antenatal group or have an existing friend who's pregnant at the same time as you, swap clothing items to ring the changes.

As you buy more clothes, try to keep to colours and styles that will mix and match with each other so you create a sort of 'capsule' wardrobe. You can make up several different looks by wearing the same top over trousers or under a dress; by wearing a shirt done up under a cardigan or open over a vest; by accessorising with chunky or delicate jewellery, depending on your mood and the occasion. Swapping flat shoes for a low wedge or modest heel can totally alter the 'feel' of an outfit, too.

Look no further

How can I get total strangers to stop touching my bump without asking?
Isn't it funny (well, perhaps not) how people who would usually sit at least two empty seats away from you on a train, would clamp their knees tightly together when seated next to you on a bus for fear of making contact, and will say 'Sorry' if they so much as pass by you too closely in the street will suddenly think nothing of laying hands on your pregnant belly! There are a few ways of getting around this, some of them more comfortable for you than others:

- try carrying a long-handled shoulder bag slung across your bump, making it harder to access
- fold your own hands over your bump as you walk or stand still, again making it harder for a stranger to touch

- if a hand comes towards your bump and you're quick enough, shake it warmly and say 'How do you do?'!
- simply say 'I'd rather you didn't touch, thanks' (a bit uncomfortable, we know, but completely acceptable nonetheless)
- in extreme circumstances, or in the case of a persistent offender, rub their tummy back and say 'Gosh, you've got a bigger belly than mine! Are you sure you aren't expecting?' This will certainly stop most women in their tracks, and should make your point loud and clear to a man.

My partner has offered to massage my sore back. What essential oils can we use and which should be avoided?

There's a good choice of essential oils you can use, mixed with a base carrier oil, for pregnancy massage. They include chamomile, citrus oils, geranium, lavender, neroli, rose and sandalwood. Those to avoid – mostly because they have been associated with triggering premature labour – are basil, clary sage, hyssop, juniper berry, marjoram, myrrh, pine, rosemary, sage, thyme and bay, although some aromatherapists believe that they are safe to use. If you're in any doubt at all, consult with a qualified aromatherapist who has a special interest in pregnancy.

Your partner should mix only two drops of essential oil per teaspoon of carrier oil and massage very gently, concentrating on stroking rather than rubbing vigorously, chopping or kneading. At this stage of pregnancy, it's best if you lie on your left side (which encourages good circulation) rather than on your tummy.

Sometimes I get so tired at work I don't know how I'm going to cope until my maternity leave. Any suggestions?

Well your employer is obliged, if it's at all possible, to provide you with somewhere to rest – and this includes somewhere you can lie down – so do make enquiries to see what can be done. Try to have naps during your breaks and at lunchtime. Just remember to set your mobile phone alarm to wake you up again, and don't sleep for longer than about 20 minutes as you'll feel more exhausted than ever when you wake up if you do. You might find it easier to sleep if you keep a small pillow and lightweight blanket at work: lying down isn't necessarily conducive to a nap unless you're comfy and warm.

Week 20 147 days to go!

Don't forget: Celebrate the halfway mark this week!

So you've got the first half of your pregnancy under your belt (although for your baby, halfway was last week as his gestation, from conception to birth is actually 38, not 40 weeks). Having climbed a steep hill in terms of adapting to this life-changing new experience, the remaining 20 weeks of pregnancy could feel like the downward hurtle of a rollercoaster ride as you get ever nearer to the birth. For lots of mums, the next three months pass by in a flurry of preparation for the baby's arrival, but the last few weeks tend to drag as they tire of dragging around a huge belly like a modern-day Mr Pickwick, have less energy than ever and become increasingly impatient to get the birth over with and meet their new babies. You can afford to pat yourself on the back this week, then take stock and start to plan for the rest of your pregnancy so that by the time your baby arrives, you'll have thought of everything!

What the netmums say

'Reaching the halfway mark'

I felt relieved once I got to 20 weeks, although I suddenly realised I'd have to get through the same amount of time again to even get to my due date! I really enjoyed feeling my baby move, though – and finding out whether we were having a boy or girl was priceless.
Alicia from London, mum to Kyrus, two, Demiyah, one, and 14 weeks pregnant

Getting to the halfway point this time around was great for me as I'd been sick almost all the way through the first part of pregnancy and by around Week 20 I started to really bloom: it made me look forward to a happier, healthier second half. Plus I loved my growing bump, and it took until almost 20 weeks to start showing properly!
Lucy from Devon, mum to Leo, three and Alicia, one

Who'd have thought?

Your uterus needs five times the blood supply it usually does when you're not pregnant.

Hey baby!

This week your baby is developing his own unique fingerprints! His growth rate has slowed to allow his lungs, digestive system and immune system to mature. Having said that, he now weighs about 260g (9oz) and has grown to a crown-to-rump length of around 15cm (6in). For reference, that's about the same as the height of a standard can of lager! Other developments include your baby's digestive system becoming developed enough to begin to absorb amniotic fluid as well as some of the nutrients and enzymes it contains. This can give rise to more hiccups – and this time you might even feel them!

All about you

The top of your uterus has reached your navel now, and you might find you want to wear looser clothes again. Your medical team will be watching to see the upward curve of your belly increasing until the last month of pregnancy, as this is a good indication that your baby is growing well. Lots of mums notice their bums and thighs getting bigger around now, and their nipples darkening. Although other changes in pigment usually reverse after pregnancy when hormones normalise, your nipples will probably always remain darker than before.

Your anomaly scan

For most mums, this is the week of the much-anticipated anomaly scan, at which the baby's major organs are all looked at and any major physical abnormalities can usually be spotted. You might have mixed emotions about seeing your baby in such detail for the first time: joyful anticipation, but also anxiety in case there's anything wrong. After all, the whole reason for the scan is not to allow you to have a good old look into your own uterus and wave hello to your baby – it's to look for any potential problems that might need treatment in utero (while your baby's still inside you) or shortly after delivery, or to detect any abnormalities you might want to know about in advance of your baby's birth. Don't forget that you are not obliged to have any tests in pregnancy –

including scans – so if you think the results might throw up unwanted implications, or if you know that you would never consider terminating a pregnancy no matter what, don't feel pressurised into having them.

If you choose to go ahead, your sonographer will be looking at the development of your baby's head, spine, limbs and organs, as well as measuring the circumference of his head and his thigh bone, which are both good indicators of his growth rate as well as providing confirmation of how many weeks' pregnant you are. Problems that can be detected during an anomaly scan include spina bifida; hydrocephalus (water on the brain); serious heart and kidney abnormalities; abnormalities of the digestive system; and cleft lip/palate, although the rate of detection is never 100 per cent and depends partly on the type of anomaly. Abnormalities of the central nervous system, for instance, have a high rate of detection at around 76 per cent, whilst only around 17 per cent of heart defects are spotted at an anomaly scan. Any problems with the placenta can also usually be found at your anomaly scan.

Most hospitals will give you a printed picture of your baby to take home with you; some Trusts make a small charge for this, and you will almost certainly have to pay if you want more than one image.

What the netmums say

'Having a 20-week scan'

Going for my scan was a weird and wonderful experience – weird because I felt more anxious than excited, and wonderful because everything appeared to be fine once the scan was underway. My heart leapt when I saw my baby quietly resting inside me: those tiny fingers and toes took my breath away. I definitely felt much closer to him once I'd seen him – although I didn't know he was a 'he' until the birth as we chose not to know the sex.
Jen from Cheshire, mum to Jordan, one

It was fantastic to see our daughter on the screen and find out that we were having a girl – it meant we could focus on names, and within hours we were calling her Rosie-May. The downside was that my placenta was found to be low-lying, which could have been a worry and played on my mind all throughout the rest of pregnancy.

I had a few extra scans to check whether or not it had moved up, but in the end I had to have a planned Caesarean. She's worth all the anxiety though, without a doubt. This time I've got my fingers crossed that I don't have placenta problems again.
Lindsay from Hereford, mum to Rosie-May, two, and 11 weeks pregnant

Extra scans

Some mums are offered extra scans in pregnancy if they have a particular complication or are expecting more than one baby. If you've suffered a previous stillbirth, you may also be offered more scans for your own reassurance, especially late in pregnancy when your baby's movements diminish because of a lack of space in your uterus.

The sorts of complications that might mean you have extra scans include gestational diabetes (to check on the size of your baby, as babies of diabetic mums tend to overgrow); carrying a small-for-dates baby; fibroids; placenta praevia (where your placenta lies low down, obstructing your cervix); and other problems with the placenta.

Cordocentesis

Also known as foetal blood sampling or cord blood sampling, cordocentesis offers another test for Down's syndrome or Edward's syndrome (a severe chromosomal disorder with a very low survival rate) if your anomaly scan suggests that your baby may have either of these. There are, however, other reasons why cordocentesis might be suggested to you. They include:

- if there's a risk you might have caught toxoplasmosis, which could cause severe abnormalities in your baby
- if you have started producing rhesus antibodies, which would threaten your baby's survival
- if your baby is anaemic and needs a blood transfusion while he's still inside you
- if your baby's not growing well.

The procedure is similar to amnio and CVS (see p. 60) in that it involves a needle being passed through your abdomen and into your uterus where the umbilical cord meets the placenta. A small sample of blood is extracted from this point and sent for analysis. The results usually come through within a few days. The procedure is complex and usually has to be carried out at a specialist centre. As with amniocentesis and CVS, there's a slight risk of miscarriage: in the case of cordocentesis it's around 1 per cent.

Who'd have thought?

By now your breasts may have increased in weight by around 180g (almost 7oz).

Headaches in pregnancy

Perhaps it's another of nature's little jokes that some mums-to-be seem to suffer from pregnancy-induced headaches – just at a time when they're not supposed to take painkillers! Conversely, those mums who are migraine sufferers often report an improvement throughout pregnancy, which is a real blessing. Although lots of mums report that their headaches have worn off by the second trimester of pregnancy, lots more find that they persist throughout the 40 weeks, albeit on and off. No one really knows for sure what causes these headaches, but we think we can make an educated guess – can you? You've got it: hormones! It's also thought to be associated with the increased blood flow that goes on throughout pregnancy, putting your body under extra, unaccustomed stress.

Another possible cause is if you've recently decided to go caffeine-free for the duration of your pregnancy: this can give rise to the most searing headaches as your body adjusts, even if you considered yourself a fairly moderate caffeine fiend before. Things should improve after a few days. If not, consult your doctor as there might be some other underlying cause.

Who'd have thought?

The number of women who become pregnant each year in Britain is around 700,000.

Self-help for headaches

- Next time you get a headache, write down all the circumstances you can think of: whether you were particularly stressed at the time; whether you had missed out on sleep or skipped a meal; what you had eaten and drunk within the previous six hours; and so on. If you do this for the next four or five times you have a headache, you might be able to discover a trigger.

- Paracetamol is considered safe to take, in moderation, in pregnancy, but do talk to your GP before taking it, to get advice on how much is too much.
- Try to relax as much and as often as you can. Practise a relaxation technique, such as deep breathing, visualisation (see p. 324) or yoga.
- Don't go too long at a time without food, as low blood-sugar levels can cause headaches. Have small, regular, nutritious snacks.
- Take a cool shower (not shockingly cold though!).
- Rest in a darkened room with a cool compress on your head and neck.
- Take some regular, moderate exercise: brisk walking and swimming are particularly good – but avoid breaststroke, which can put a strain on your lower back.
- Some mums find acupuncture helpful.
- Talk to your GP or midwife to see if they can shed light on your headaches. It may be, for example, that you have altered your posture since becoming pregnant and this is having a knock-on effect. Regular headaches in pregnancy need medical attention in any case, as they can be a symptom of pre-eclampsia, especially if accompanied by other symptoms (see p. 274).
- If you suffer from migraines, take advice from your doctor, as there may be a treatment you can take in pregnancy. Never self-medicate with over-the-counter drugs, though, as many migraine treatments contain ingredients that could be harmful in pregnancy.

Who'd have thought?

A recent US research study conducted over 60 years* found that women in their forties give birth to more girls than boys, whilst late-teenage mums are more likely to have boys than girls.

*Source: National Center for Health Statistics

Your mission this week: Create some memories

Now that you're sporting a bump, why not start a pregnancy album to go alongside the video diary you may have started earlier. You could include your positive pregnancy test, your scan picture and lots of photos of each other: if you've seen pictures of your own mum pregnant, you'll appreciate how fascinating it can be to look back at this special time in your parents' lives. And after all, pregnancy is a big part of your baby's life, too!

If your camera is digital and you keep your photos on your computer hard drive, do print some off, and do back up your photo files by copying them on to a disk in case they get lost. Organise the photos into chronological files and type a little caption underneath each plus the date.

Look no further

Can I pay to have extra scans if I want them but don't need them?
You could always pay to go private to have extra scans, but you might want to ask yourself why you would want to undergo tests you don't need, especially as most major abnormalities will have been seen or ruled out at your anomaly scan (although ultrasound screening can never carry a 100 per cent detection rate). It might be helpful to discuss your feelings with your midwife or doctor before spending on expensive private scanning. A single private scan can cost £100–£200.

Can acupuncture help with headaches?
Yes, and it's a safe therapy to try in pregnancy as long as you find an experienced, qualified acupuncturist with a special interest in pregnancy. Some mums also find that acupuncture helps with other complaints including backache, stress, nausea and tiredness; others use it throughout pregnancy for the feeling of general wellbeing it can give; and some mums even take their acupuncturist into the labour suite with them for pain relief during the birth. If you're planning to do this, you should mention it to your midwives and doctors beforehand.

Why do I keep getting cramp?
Cramp is especially common in pregnancy, particularly in the second and third trimesters, and often happens in the night, especially if you flex your calf muscle. There are several reasons why you might get cramp: muscle fatigue due

to the extra weight you're carrying can cause your legs to protest by cramping, and too much phosphorus – a chemical element found in processed meats, crisps and snacks – and a lack of potassium and calcium can result in cramp.

Try to rest your legs as often as possible and massage the muscles, especially before bedtime. Cut out as many processed foods and snacks as you can. Have a glass of milk and a potassium-rich snack such as a banana, kiwi fruit, half an avocado, a slice of cantaloupe melon or a banana before bed. If you do get cramp, stretch your leg out and flex your foot backwards so your toes are pointing towards the ceiling. This effectively lengthens your calf muscle, which has shortened and gone into spasm. Gently massage the muscle until you release the spasm. (For more on cramp, see *Leg cramps*, p. 233.)

Who'd have thought?

Those little bumps that have sprouted on your nipples are called Montgomery's tubercles. They secrete an oily fluid that helps keep your nipples supple and moisturised, and were named after nineteenth-century Irish obstetrician William Fetherstone Montgomery. They usually get smaller after pregnancy or when you stop breastfeeding, but are unlikely to disappear altogether.

How are you feeling?

Tick the box that most closely represents how you feel about the given statements, then look back to the charts in previous chapters to see how you've changed over the months.

Physically	Emotionally
I feel better than I've felt up till now Strongly agree ☐ Agree ☐ Neither agree nor disagree ☐ Disagree ☐ Strongly disagree ☐	I was/am anxious about the anomaly scan Strongly agree ☐ Agree ☐ Neither agree nor disagree ☐ Disagree ☐ Strongly disagree ☐
I've felt my baby move Strongly agree ☐ Agree ☐ Neither agree nor disagree ☐ Disagree ☐ Strongly disagree ☐	I feel sensitive and am easily upset Strongly agree ☐ Agree ☐ Neither agree nor disagree ☐ Disagree ☐ Strongly disagree ☐

My boobs are 'pimply' Strongly agree ☐ Agree ☐ Neither agree nor disagree ☐ Disagree ☐ Strongly disagree ☐	I feel elated most of the time Strongly agree ☐ Agree ☐ Neither agree nor disagree ☐ Disagree ☐ Strongly disagree ☐
I'm doing my pelvic floor exercises regularly Strongly agree ☐ Agree ☐ Neither agree nor disagree ☐ Disagree ☐ Strongly disagree ☐	I'm anxious about the birth Strongly agree ☐ Agree ☐ Neither agree nor disagree ☐ Disagree ☐ Strongly disagree ☐
I fancy eating non-edible substances! Strongly agree ☐ Agree ☐ Neither agree nor disagree ☐ Disagree ☐ Strongly disagree ☐	I really want a boy/girl Strongly agree ☐ Agree ☐ Neither agree nor disagree ☐ Disagree ☐ Strongly disagree ☐
I've noticed pigment changes in my skin Strongly agree ☐ Agree ☐ Neither agree nor disagree ☐ Disagree ☐ Strongly disagree ☐	I really want to know the sex of my baby Strongly agree ☐ Agree ☐ Neither agree nor disagree ☐ Disagree ☐ Strongly disagree ☐

Who'd have thought?

The cheesy white vernix that coats your baby's skin in the uterus is made from fat and dead skin cells. (Yummy!)

Quick quiz

Your pregnancy health

1 Can you take any painkillers while you're pregnant?

a. Yes, anything you like

b. No, nothing at all

c. Paracetamol, on your doctor's advice

2 Why is it dangerous to get very overheated in pregnancy?

a. Because you could faint and have a fall

b. Because you'll sweat too much

c. Because too high a core body temperature can be harmful to your baby

3 What causes thrush in pregnancy?

a. Eating too much yoghurt

b. You catch it from your partner during sex

c. There aren't enough bacteria in the vagina to keep it at bay

4 What's the correct term for swelling due to water retention?

a. Edina

b. Chloasma

c. Oedema

5 What dangerous illness can swelling be a symptom of?

a. Diabetes

b. Hydrocephalus

c. Pre-eclampsia

Answers: The answers to this quiz are all 'c'.

Mostly a: You're not really taking this seriously, are you! Either that or your brain really has gone to mush and you're struggling to recall information. Have another read about the health issues covered in the mini quiz so you'll feel more in control of your pregnancy health.

Mostly b: You've been trying to absorb health information all right, but in doing so you've got a bit muddled! It's worth you reading some sections again as forewarned is forearmed when it comes to your pregnancy health.

Mostly c: Well done, you've taken some important health messages on board. By doing so you've put yourself one step ahead of the game and will probably be aware of any potential problems before they take hold. That's a great situation to be in.

Who'd have thought?

Breastmilk doesn't come out of the pointy bit of your nipple, but out of lots of little holes around it, so your nipples are really just like a watering-can rose!

Chapter 5

Weeks 21–24

My goodness, we're hurtling through this pregnancy, aren't we? No? Some mums find the time passes quickly; others find it drags a bit – and the second half of pregnancy can seem like a longer haul than the first. There's a reason for that: remember at the outset we explained how for the first two weeks of pregnancy you weren't even pregnant? So really your pregnancy has only lasted 18 weeks so far and there are 20 more to go!

The second 'half' is largely about enjoying your last months as a childless couple, getting your home organised for your new arrival, maybe having a last holiday and – last, but by no means least – preparing for the birth. Yes, it's time to give some serious thought to how you envisage things going on the big day; what you'll do if your birth plan doesn't work out for you; how you'll cope if you end up having a Caesarean or other assisted delivery; who you're asking into the labour suite with you; whether you want to bring any special practitioners; whether you want a water birth – and all those other decisions that up until now have probably seemed so far off you haven't been dwelling on them. Of course, you might be the sort of mum who's had it all sorted in your head for weeks on end, in which case apologies for casting aspersions!

Who'd have thought?

Braxton Hicks contractions, which you may experience from around now, don't have any kind of adverse effect on your baby.

Week 21 140 days to go!

Don't forget: Build some 'feet up' rest into each day

You might feel yourself getting heavier from this point on, and it's quite common for mums to find their feet or legs swelling around now, especially in warmer weather. You might also get the dreaded varicose veins as your uterus starts to compress other blood vessels. What better excuse, then, to put your feet up and let your partner fetch and carry for you? In fact, you may as well do so even if you haven't got any symptoms – you'll certainly be doing the lion's share of babycare in a few months' time!

Try to ensure that whenever you're sitting and relaxing, you elevate your legs to just above hip height; this will allow excess fluid to drain away from your feet. Lying down on your left side with your feet up on a pillow will also help prevent or minimise varicose veins: because the inferior vena cava (a major blood vessel) is on the right side, left-sided rest takes the weight of your uterus off this blood vessel and reduces pressure in your legs.

Hey baby!

Although his growth rate has slowed down a bit now, your baby is still gradually piling on the grams and now weighs around 300g (10½oz). His crown-to-rump length is about 18cm (7in) and this takes him to around the same size as a large banana! Now that he can swallow amniotic fluid and his digestive system is maturing and beginning to work as it will once he's born, your baby is ingesting more and more fluid all the time. It's thought that by full term, a baby can be swallowing as much as 500ml of amniotic fluid a day!

All about you

By now most mums will have noticed big changes happening: try hiding the fact that you're pregnant now! Around the same time, you might find your libido creeping back up on you – or roaring round your system like a tiger in your tank! With a manageable bump, more fulsome boobs and that much-talked-about 'glow', you'll (hopefully) be. feeling attractive and womanly. Proven fertility can have this effect on mums- and dads-to-be alike: your partner might be at his randy best about now, too, seeing the evidence of his own fertility right before his eyes. There's nothing more guaranteed to make a bloke feel all macho than the thought that he's got plenty of lead in his pencil! For more on sex in pregnancy, see p. 125.

Blood clots

Blood clots, whilst not specific to pregnancy, can be a serious problem for mums-to-be due to more sluggish circulation, with symptoms including a rapidly swelling, painful leg, often with a red, warm patch over the affected area. Some unfortunate mums even get blood clots in the groin. The danger is when the clot is deep-seated, as in a deep-vein thrombosis (DVT), as a piece of the clot could break off and travel to the lungs causing a pulmonary embolism. In the worst case, this can prove fatal. Thankfully, DVT is a rare complication, reported in around one in 1000 pregnancies, and prompt, appropriate treatment can stave off disaster. Other types of blood clot which are less threatening, known as superficial thromboses, can also occur. A superficial thrombosis, as the names suggests, is usually close to the surface of the skin and can be felt as a lumpy or swollen vein.

What you can do about it

Diagnosis and treatment of DVT usually involves an ultrasound scan to locate the clot, followed by injections of heparin (a blood-thinning drug), which will prevent it from getting bigger, and give the body a chance to reabsorb it. Mums with DVT usually need to stay in hospital for treatment, which can take between a week and 10 days. After the crisis has passed, heparin is usually given until the birth and for a few weeks afterwards. Treatment of a superficial thrombosis is often with a support stocking to help compress the vein and frequent elevation of the leg to encourage blood flow back towards the heart.

Varicose veins

You'll know when you've got a varicose vein or veins as they're quite distinctive (if not to say somewhat ugly) in appearance. They come in a range of hues, from blue-black to purply red (not that you can choose) and can be lumpy or twisted to look at – another of the great joys of pregnancy. Some mums are more prone to getting them than others (see *Look no further*, p. 19. Varicose veins can develop when the small valves inside the veins which prevent blood from flowing backwards stop working efficiently, allowing blood to pool in the veins. In pregnancy, although you have a greater volume of blood in your body, your actual rate of circulation slows and becomes sluggish (yes, because of hormones!) so the valves can't open and close properly.

Who'd have thought?

You'll put on more weight in your second trimester than in the first or third because these are the weeks when your baby gains weight most rapidly.

What you can do about it

Varicose veins are unlikely to be treated in pregnancy unless they're severe and are causing you discomfort. Compression stockings, which squeeze the legs gently and steadily to help circulation, may bring some relief – although these can't cure your veins or prevent others from occurring. It's important to get the fit right or the stockings won't work properly, so you'll need to consult your doctor about the size and type for you. If your veins are severe, they may be treated by injection or surgery, but this is usually deferred until a few months after delivery, as your veins will probably shrink to a certain extent by this time.

Self-help for varicose veins

- Try to keep as mobile as possible so that your circulation is on the go. Avoid standing still for long periods, and if you must stand up, exercise your legs and feet.
- Elevate your legs as often as possible, ideally to just above hip height.
- Don't sit with your legs crossed, as this further restricts blood flow.
- Avoid shoes with more than a low heel.
- Don't wear restrictive tights or socks, but do wear maternity support tights.
- Talk to your doctor about taking vitamin C with bioflavonoids and vitamin E supplements, both of which are thought to be helpful in strengthening and protecting the walls of blood vessels.
- Step up your intake of berries, especially the dark ones such as blueberries, blackberries and cherries, as these are all rich in bioflavonoids.

What the netmums say

'Coping with varicose veins'

I developed quite prominent veins in both lower legs, which would really ache if I was on my feet for any length of time. I was advised by my midwife to try to lie down on my left side when resting as this takes pressure off a big blood vessel. I also rested with my legs up as much as possible and wore some light support tights. I think I could have done with heavier support, but it was so warm when I was pregnant that I couldn't bear the thought! I used to put my clean pants and support tights on while I was still in bed in the mornings before I stood up and the blood had pooled in the veins (yuk!). Happily the veins subsided quite a bit in the months after the birth and I can live with them now.

Georgie from New Malden, mum to Matthew, 14 months

Before I was pregnant I never knew you could develop varicose veins in your vulva! I had a large, throbbing one on my right labia, which was made much more painful by the leg of my pants. Then a friend suggested wearing a thick sanitary pad, and this not only applied a bit of helpful pressure to the vein, it also stopped the rubbing. I can't say it wasn't still uncomfortable, but I did find some relief from applying a bag of frozen peas whenever I could find the privacy!

Leanna from Gateshead, mum to Alfie, two

Your mission this week: Get your entitlements sorted

Now's the time to think about applying for Statutory Maternity Pay (SMP), and this week or next you should get a special form called MATB1 from your doctor or midwife that entitles you to claim it. By law you need to let your employer know you're intending to claim SMP at least 28 days before you plan to take maternity leave. The MATB1 form provides medical evidence of your pregnancy; you can't obtain it any earlier than this week. You might need to ask for the form, so make a note to yourself to bring the subject up at your next antenatal appointment. For more about your maternity package see p. 225.

Look no further

Who is most at risk of getting varicose veins in pregnancy?
Varicose veins tend to run in families, so ask your mum if she suffered from them in pregnancy – or if she does now – as this is the main predisposing factor. They tend to be more common in mums who stand for long periods, too, as well as those who gain excessive weight in pregnancy. Whilst you may not be able to prevent varicose veins appearing altogether, you can reduce your risk of them or minimise their severity by taking the self-help measures outlined on p. 188.

I'm still getting migraines despite hearing that they tend to stop in pregnancy. Can I take my usual medication?
Poor you, that's really unlucky. Some of the drugs for migraine, especially those which contain triptans designed to stop the attack in its tracks, are not recommended for use in pregnancy because the effects on the unborn baby are unknown, but do talk to your GP as there may be alternatives to paracetamol that you can take with medical supervision to help you over migraine. For more on headaches in pregnancy, see p. 177.

I want to start drafting a birth plan. Is there an actual form I need to fill in?
Some hospitals do have a pre-printed tick-box list of things for you to fill in, and whilst this might help you to cover everything that might happen on the day, it's by no means necessary for you to use it as your final plan. You can write or type your ideas out any way you like, although it's best to try to keep things in chronological order so that whoever is referring to it on the big day doesn't have to do too much hard work! Well done for getting started now – it'll put you one step ahead of the game when it comes to honing your ideas (see p. 294), which might change in the meantime in any case. You might want to talk your ideas through with your medical team as your pregnancy progresses, and it'll make a good talking point for you and your birth partner, too. It's important you realise, however, that many mums have to abandon their birth plans on the day: as with all the best-laid plans, things can happen that are out of your control, so whilst it's well worth having an 'ideal world' running order, try to keep your expectations realistic.

Week 22 133 days to go!

Don't forget: Make a habit of sleeping on your side from now on

We've touched before on how lying on your left side can encourage better blood flow to your baby and better circulation for you as it helps prevent the uterus compressing major blood vessels (the aorta and the inferior vena cava that runs down the back of your abdomen). From around now, it's a good idea to try to adopt a side sleeping position in bed, too. It'll probably be your natural inclination: sleeping on your back might make you breathless and put a strain on your lower back; lying on your tummy puts your uterus under pressure and is probably pretty uncomfortable by now. Some mums find sleeping on their side also pulls the lower back, but this is easily rectified with a couple of well-placed pillows. Place one pillow between your two knees and another behind your back to stop you from rolling fully on to your back while you sleep. You might find putting a pillow under your bump for support is good, too. There are special wedge-shaped pillows you can buy for your bump and back, but they'll have limited use after pregnancy. You can even buy full-length 'body pillows', which you can throw one leg over and use to get really comfy, but you might find it takes up rather a lot of space in your bed unless you've got a king-size or bigger (or are prepared to chuck your partner out of bed for the duration of your pregnancy! What do you mean 'That sounds appealing…'?

Hey baby!

This week your baby weighs about 350g (12oz) and measures around 19cm (7.5in) crown to rump. His inner ear is now the size of an adult's and he's sporting not only a pair of eyebrows but also some hair on his head. Your baby's two layers of skin begin to perform their different functions at this stage: the outer layer or epidermis is a protective coat for your baby; the dermis, which is underneath the epidermis, develops a network of tiny blood vessels and nerve endings. This is what gives your baby's skin its sensitivity: at birth, your newborn's skin will be around five times more sensitive than your own. His lungs are producing a substance called 'surfactant', which helps to keep them open as he breathes. Very premature babies often spend time on ventilators which perform the function of the surfactant they lack.

Who'd have thought?

Your baby can hear and identify your voice clearly: if you sing to him during a quiet, restful moment, you might notice that he responds by moving about a bit or, if he was already moving about, pausing to listen!

All about you

Sweats

Because your thyroid gland becomes more active when you're pregnant, it's not unusual to find that you sweat more than usual. Some mums worry that this is a sign of dangerous overheating, and that their babies might suffer, but it's more uncomfortable than serious.

To keep your cool during the day, try the following tips:

- dress in natural fibres such as 100 per cent cotton, linen or pure wool
- keep a can of cooling facial spray with you
- carry a mini fan in your handbag
- dress in light layers so you can take one or more off
- wear your hair off your face and wear a brimmed hat in the sun
- keep hydrated by drinking around two litres of water a day
- keep a gel eye mask in the fridge and lie down with it over your eyes
- hold your wrists under cool running water.

You might find that you're sweating more at night, especially in warmer weather when the heat rises to the top of the house. Here are some tips for a more comfortable night:

- run a fan in your room with windows and doors closed for an hour or so before bedtime
- choose nightwear in 100 per cent cotton
- have a cool bath or shower just before bed
- reduce the number of covers on the bed, and choose layers of cotton sheets rather than blankets
- keep a cooling body spray next to the bed
- you can buy chilled pillows (no refrigeration or power required) from www.chillowpillow.co.uk.

Newborn essentials and frivolous luxuries

Now's the time to start actually buying the essentials you'll need to care for your newborn. It's worth shopping ahead, not only so you can spread the cost, but also because you may find that the exact cotbed you'd wanted is out of stock and needs to be re-ordered. It's also helpful to start feeling organised during your second trimester because by the time you hit your third, you're likely to be feeling less energetic and more cumbersome.

So what do you really need and what can you do without? (That's not to say that you shouldn't splash out on some luxuries if you can afford to!)

Essentials

- **A good supply of nappies** Bear in mind that your newborn may get through up to 12 every 24 hours. If you're buying washable nappies, buy at least 24 so that you always have a day's supply, even while the others are being washed. You'll also need a supply of liners and a nappy bucket. If you're using disposables, you'll also need nappy bags for wrapping the nappies in before throwing them away. Do consider washable nappies from an environmental point of view: many are completely machine washable now, and although you'll have to lay out a fair chunk of cash to buy them in the first place, it's an awful lot cheaper in the long run than buying disposables.
- **At least half a dozen clean vests and stretchsuits** Choose vests with an 'envelope' neckline and poppers that fasten at the crotch, as these are easiest to put on and take off. You can get long- and short-sleeved vests, so be guided by the season. The stretchsuits will have long arms, so bear this in mind. There's no need to buy sleepsuits – stretchsuits can double as day- and nightwear at first. It's best to avoid 'newborn' sizes, unless your baby is premature, and go for 0–3 months as it's more cost effective – and it won't matter if they're a little roomy at first. Your baby will grow so rapidly you'll be into 3–6 months before you know it! Unless you know your baby's sex for sure, avoid blues and pinks and go for the more unisex colours and patterns – there are loads around. For bargain buys, check out supermarkets and branches of George, Primark and H&M.
- **Two cardigans** These are always useful and easy to get on and off. In the summer, a cardigan can replace a jacket; in the winter it's a convenient extra layer.

- **Bottles, bottlebrushes and steriliser** These are essential if you're going to express breastmilk, if you're planning to mix bottles with breastfeeding or if you're bottlefeeding exclusively. Buy at least six bottles if you're planning to bottlefeed exclusively so that you can be sterilising four at a time whilst keeping two fresh ones ready for use as and when. (It's no longer recommended that you make up a day's feeds in advance as some fridges don't keep formula at the correct temperature, and incorrect storage can cause gastroenteritis in a baby.) You can find different shaped bottles and teats, as well as different types of steriliser, from cold-water types which have soluble tablets added to the water to microwave and electric steam sterilisers. Do some homework by researching online or asking other mums' opinions before you buy.

- **Formula milk (if you're bottlefeeding exclusively)** All infant milks contain all the nutrients, including proteins, a baby needs from birth to six months. Your midwife or health visitor can advise you on which infant formula to use, but most bottlefed babies are started on a whey-based milk, such as SMA Gold.

- **A baby car seat** You'll need this to bring your baby home in. It's really important that you either buy this item brand-new or borrow one from a friend because if you buy secondhand you can't be sure whether the seat has ever been involved in an impact, and so you won't be 100 per cent certain of its safety. Check that it is compatible with whatever car you'll be using to transport your baby: most outlets that sell baby car seats will check the fit for free.

- **A crib, carrycot or cot** Bear in mind that a crib will have a limited lifespan of about six months. If you are buying a pram/pushchair rather than a stroller style, you can use the carrycot part as a crib until your baby outgrows it, although you might need to buy a firmer mattress to add to it for nighttime sleep (check with the manufacturer). A cot is safe to use from birth as long as you follow the safety guidelines of making the bedding up so that your baby sleeps with his feet to the foot of the cot (and so can't wriggle down under the covers). Some parents like the idea of a Moses basket, but although these have the advantage of being easily portable, they're expensive to buy from new and will only last for up to three months. If you manage to borrow one from someone or buy secondhand, it's best to buy a new mattress for the sake of hygiene, unless the one that comes with the cot is completely waterproof and the cover has no cracks or holes in it. A cotbed is a great idea as it converts from a cot into a toddler's first bed.

- **Bedding** Choose brushed or plain cotton sheets and two or three cellular blankets, as these will allow air to circulate as well as keeping your baby warm. You should never use a pillow, duvet or hot-water bottle with a baby under one year old. When the room where your baby is sleeping is at the optimum temperature (see below), a sheet and one or two blankets is all he needs to be comfortable. In colder conditions, he might need three layers of blankets. In summer, if it's very warm, he might not need anything more than a sheet. Remember that a folded blanket counts as two layers.
- **A room thermometer** The optimum temperature for your baby's nursery is between 16°C (61°F) and 20°C (68°F).
- **Baby-listening device** Not strictly an essential, but lots of parents find these so reassuring that they're starting to feature on just about everyone's list. One unit plugs in in the room where your baby is; the other is a carry-around unit that allows you to listen in on your baby from elsewhere in the home.
- **Pram, pushchair or stroller** There's a wide choice of styles, so you'll need to do some homework to work out the best product for you. You can buy a pram/pushchair/car seat combination; a pram/pushchair or a stroller (some are suitable from birth, but you'll need to check this out). Racing-style, three-wheeled 'jogger' pushchairs are popular and manoeuvrable; umbrella-folding styles are useful if you use public transport a lot or have a small car. A raincover is also essential.
- **A hat, coat and blanket** When you're out and about you'll need to be prepared for all weathers, so keep a hat, coat (lightweight jacket in warm weather; warmer coat for winter) and blanket with your pram or pushchair. In summer, a cotton sunhat and parasol will also be needed (on the offchance that we get any sun, that is!).

Who'd have thought?

Sex selection in the UK is illegal unless for proven medical reasons such as the avoidance of having a baby with a major inherited disorder such as Duchenne Muscular Dystrophy (DMD), which occurs almost exclusively in boys.

Luxuries

- **A changing bag and mat** You might think these are essential, but really any largeish rucksack will do as a changing bag and a towel will serve just as well as a changing mat.

- **A baby changing station** This is a piece of furniture that houses all your baby changing essentials and incorporates a changing mat into the tabletop. It's sheer luxury and you'll need a surfeit of space as well as spare cash in order to justify it!

- **A nappy disposal system** Although it's handy to be able to pop your nappies into a special bin that seals them in plastic and stores up to 28 nappies at once before it needs emptying, it's unnecessary and does tend to become a bit smelly! And unless you have one downstairs as well as upstairs it will have limited value in any case.

- **Baby wipes** In the first month baby wipes can cause nappy rash on a baby's delicate skin, no matter how hypoallergenic they claim to be. Warm water is much kinder than a cold wipe!

- **Top-and-tail bowl** In the first few days or weeks your baby can be kept clean by wiping him over with cotton wool balls and cool water, and you can buy special bowls with one compartment for the water and another for the cotton wool. In reality any two plastic bowls will do! It's just important to use separate bowls for the water and the used cotton wool so that the water doesn't become contaminated.

- **A baby bath** Some mums do find it's easier to use a baby bath than a big bath as it's more manageable – and those that sit on top of the big bath do bring a baby up to a more comfortable height. You can manage just as well bathing your baby in a basin in the early days, though: just make sure you wrap the taps with a face flannel to prevent scalds.

- **Dummies** Whether or not these are essential depends on your own personal viewpoint, but a baby can comfort himself just as well with his thumb as with a dummy, and some experts would say you're making a rod for your back by offering a dummy in the first place as they can be hard to get rid of. The same is true, of course, of thumb-sucking – and both practices are frowned upon by orthodontists! Up to you, really…

- **A baby sling** A sling, which allows you to carry your baby around with your hands free, is undoubtedly a useful piece of kit, especially when your baby is young, but probably can't be classified as essential. There are different types to choose from, including some that carry your baby facing either inwards or outwards, and others that tie or clip around your body, more like the ones used by African tribal mums. Best thing is to try some out in the shops and see which are easiest to use, or ask a mum who's used them.

- Cot mobile This is a nice-to-have item, but your baby won't gain much benefit from it in the early days. Maybe you could ask for this as a present if anyone asks you for ideas?
- Cot activity centre Frankly, this is a waste of money for a newborn, although these toys can come into their own once a baby is able to focus, aim and kick, and becomes interested in 'cause and effect'. This is the point at which it might just buy you an extra 10 minutes in bed if your baby amuses himself with it on waking.
- Cot bumper This is a cushioned border that ties around the inside edge of a cot. They're unnecessary and may prove hazardous as the strings could become untied and put your baby at risk of strangulation, or the bumper could suffocate your baby. If you're keen to use a cot bumper, look for the type that Velcroes on to the bars or cut any strings short and tie them outside the bars.
- Baby toiletries They might make your baby smell all soapy and fresh, but there's nothing as appealing as a newborn's natural smell, and he doesn't need the chemical additives that are in most toiletries.

Who'd have thought?

Most Caucasian babies have dark-blue eyes at birth, even though this can change in the first few weeks or months of life. So your blue-eyed newborn might well turn out to have brown or green eyes as time goes on. Most babies from African or Asian parents are born with dark-brown or grey eyes, and these will get darker in the coming weeks or months.

What the netmums say

'Our best and worst baby buys'

My best buy was a baby sleeping bag – I couldn't have imagined life without it! My worst, moneywise, was a big combination pram with all the bits (car seat, carrycot, accessories). I hardly ever used it as we used the car a lot and didn't need anything so heavy-duty. It did look lovely, and the feeling when I put my baby in it was amazing, but after about two months it wasn't the same, so that was £600 wasted! With my second, I chose a lightweight buggy for about £100. I could use it from birth, fold it easily into the boot and am still using it now.
Rachel from Blyth, Northumberland, mum to Hollie, seven and Lewis, two

My baby carrier has been used for all three of my children and was invaluable once I had a toddler and a baby to contend with. My baby bath was a brilliant buy too – it's quite a large one and is moulded inside so that basically your newborn is supported, leaving you both hands free to wash and play with your baby. I bought it for my first and have just stopped using it with my third. My travel cot was a brilliant buy, even though I mainly used it at home for the children to nap and play in. One of my worst buys was one of those moulded seats designed to allow your baby to sit upright from about three months onwards: our little boy hated it, and actually worked out how to tip himself over and get out of it!
Fiona from Doncaster, mum to Emma, five, Samuel, three and Holly, seven months

My worst buy was a baby bath set: it was a complete waste of money as within weeks both of my children had outgrown it, and I ended up using the normal bath. My best buys include my baby monitor with breathing pad underneath, which means complete peace of mind for me throughout the day and night. I also love the digital children's 'in ear' thermometer, which is so quick and easy to use with a built-in alarm for fever temperature, and is perfect from babyhood to toddlerhood and beyond.
Lindsay from Chester, mum to Jasmyn, three and Logan, seven months

What I thought was my best buy soon became my worst: I chose to give my baby a dummy and it turned into the bane of all our lives. Nita was three before I could get it off her and it was so embarrassing turning up everywhere with it jammed in her mouth. Eventually I took it off her without discussion and she resorted to thumb-sucking for the next two years! I think if I'd done without in the first place she'd have found her thumb for a short while and not depended so heavily on having a comforter. With Sajiv I've left him to his own devices and he usually falls asleep rubbing his blanket under his nose.

Alisha from Bolton, mum to Nita, six and Sajiv, eight months

Your mission this week: Buy yourself some maternity underwear

If you haven't done so already, you'll probably want to get some pregnancy knickers as your ordinary ones have probably developed an embarrassing tendency to slide over your bump and fall down to your upper thighs! Pregnancy pants come in two styles, and you'll have to experiment to see which suits you best: you can either find 'big knickers' that stretch over your bump and accommodate it snugly whilst still fitting on your 'waist'; or you can buy tanga-style briefs which are designed to go under your bump. Either way, it'll pay to get 100 per cent cotton underwear as this will be more comfy if you have a tendency to sweat or if you are prone to thrush. Buy underwear in your pre-pregnancy size – perhaps just a pair of each to start with until you're sure which style you prefer.

In all likelihood you'll need another bra soon, too. Go for a professional fitting – which is offered by most department stores – and choose natural fibres.

Who'd have thought?

There's a plus side to your skin retaining more fluid in pregnancy: it plumps up and smooths out any fine lines and wrinkles you may have had before! (Obviously this is a temporary effect which will be lost once your baby's been born, but hey! Enjoy it while it lasts.)

Look no further

Is it safe for me to continue driving, even with my bump getting bigger?
As long as you adjust your seatbelt so that it still fits snugly but without being constricting, and as long as you alter the seat back and position so that you are quite comfortable, there's no reason to stop driving. You might have to find new ways to manoeuvre yourself in and out of your car later in pregnancy – especially if yours is low to the ground – but this shouldn't stop you.

What can I do to help relieve my piles?
Haemorrhoids (piles) often get increasingly worse in pregnancy as the weight of the uterus compresses important blood vessels and your circulation continues to be sluggish. There are several things you can do to help:

- drink plenty of water and eat plenty of fibre to keep your stools as soft as possible. This will help prevent you from straining on the loo and making matters worse
- try to keep moving. Sitting or standing in one place for a long time can compound the problem – you need to give your circulation a boost by keeping mobile
- dabbing a little witch hazel on to your piles with a ball of cotton wool can help soothe them
- sitting on a bag of frozen peas can bring instant relief
- using a glycerine suppository can help ease the passage of a hard stool
- sitting in a warm, salty bath may help
- lying down for an hour a day with your legs elevated above hip height can take the pressure off piles.

I recently had a fall and bumped my bump, although not that hard. It was painful for me, but do you think I've hurt my baby?
The cushioning effect of your amniotic sac will protect your baby from most minor bumps and bangs throughout pregnancy, so it's very unlikely he's come to any harm. You'll find it reassuring if you feel him moving around normally, too. It's best to check things out with your medical team, though, just in case, and to put your own mind at rest. Had you suffered a more major fall, even though your baby would probably have been fine, there might have been implications (see p. 241).

Week 23 126 days to go!

Don't forget: Disregard other people's comments

One of the common cries of mums-to-be is that they are sick of people sharing their pregnancy horror stories, old wives' tales and opinions on bump size without being asked! It does seem that expectant mums are regarded as fair game for busybodies and scaremongers alike – all of which is just so unfair that we'd forgive you for stamping your feet like a petulant toddler or doing a Princess Anne and telling the lot of 'em to 'naff off'! Probably the best way to deal with unwelcome advice is to smile benignly, nod sagely and reserve comment yourself – then disregard everything you find unhelpful. That's not to say that you won't hear good stories and useful nuggets along with the dross – it's just filtering one from another that can prove tricky.

Just for the record, though:

- there's no scientific evidence whatsoever to support the idea that the size, height or shape of your bump is related to the gender of your baby
- you can't get the umbilical cord wrapped around your baby's neck by sleeping with your arms above your head (although it will put a greater strain on your circulation so is best avoided from this point of view)
- you can't accurately 'divine' the sex of your baby by dangling a crystal, a ring or a garibaldi biscuit over your bump and watching to see whether it'll make clockwise or anticlockwise circles
- taking iron supplements in pregnancy won't give you a dark-eyed, dark-haired baby any more than drinking saffron-flavoured milk will make your baby fair!
- there's nothing to say that if your mum had a Caesarean, you will too. Your own birth experience will depend on several factors including the lie of your baby and your own body type.

Who'd have thought?

You'll know you're drinking enough fluids in pregnancy when your pee consistently looks almost clear in colour – or the colour of weak jasmine tea!

Stop press!

At the time of writing, a new research study, which is the result of a collaboration between Exeter and Oxford Universities, suggests that a diet high in calories – and including breakfast cereals – at around the time of conception can predispose hopeful mums to having a boy. Researchers discovered that 59 per cent of mums who ate at least one bowl of cereal per day had boys, compared to only 43 per cent of women who ate less than one bowl per week. It seems that mums who eat a high-energy diet of around 2,200 calories a day are one-and-a-half times more likely to have a boy than those who eat less than 1,850 calories a day. It's already known from IVF studies that high levels of glucose encourage the growth of male embryos whilst discouraging females, and skipping breakfast lowers glucose levels because the body thinks there is not going to be much food around that day.

What the netmums say

'The stupid things people say!'

I was six months gone and I was in the local chip shop when the woman in front said (in a thick Brummie accent), 'Bl**dy hell, you're massive!' I said, 'I'm only six months gone!' and she said, 'Well, that's a Caesarean for sure!' I just laughed it off at the time, but I was really worried for ages! Actually I was 3cm smaller than I should have been for my dates and I didn't end up having a Caesarean. Ruby was eventually delivered by ventouse.
Amanda from Bristol, mum to Ruby, one

I was pretty overweight whilst pregnant and I had my family constantly asking me, right to the end, 'Are you sure you're pregnant, and not just fatter?' Nice! The only thing anyone ever needs to say to a pregnant woman is, 'You're looking beautiful.'
Erin from Leeds, mum to Connor, 11 months

I had a huge bump in pregnancy, and goodness knows enough people made the remark, 'Are you sure you're not having twins or triplets?' with the usual casual laugh. That hurt in itself as I just wanted to look and feel 'normal', especially as it was my first pregnancy. Then an elderly woman at church – who claimed she'd been a midwife in her younger life – said, 'Good luck getting that out!' I was only six months pregnant at the time and was mortified. It made me anxious all the way up to the birth – which, by the way, went beautifully with just gas & air for pain relief. It did make me wonder which poor women had been attended by this terrible old crone!

Alison from Humberside, mum to Charlie, three

While I was pregnant one of my mum's friends said, 'Your Gail's put on weight since she got married.' Mum pointed out that that's what happens when you're pregnant but she was really mad with her. Then four days after I had my daughter I met one of my mum's friends in the supermarket and she said, 'I thought you'd have had your baby by now.' I somehow managed to hold the tears in and say, 'I have. She's in the car with her daddy.' She apologised, but I just left my shopping basket and went out crying to my husband in the car! I was gutted. She must have felt very bad because she phoned my mum and asked her to pass on her apologies to me.

Gail from Glasgow, mum to Brodie, six and Zoe, four

A girl I worked with when I was pregnant was always saying, 'Your bump is really small, I'd get that checked out and make sure everything is OK.' As it was my first pregnancy, I didn't know about these things and would go to my midwife appointments all worried. I'm 5' 10" and the midwife said, 'Look, you're tall and slim and the perfect size for your dates, so stop worrying.' I later heard the same workmate had been telling another girl that she was huge and it could be twins, making her panic too. Incidentally, this girl had never been pregnant and was just a know-it-all – who knew nothing as it turned out!

Mags from Lanarkshire, mum to Eve, two

Who'd have thought?

Although your baby is inside your uterus, his world is far from silent, and has been compared to being underwater in a swimming pool! All sorts of sounds from your blood flow, your digestive system and outside noises like music and your voice will all make their way through to your baby!

Hey baby!

At 450g, your baby is only just shy of 1lb in weight – that's almost half a standard bag of sugar! He's around 20cm (8in) long from crown to rump, and is plumping up nicely. His facial features are similar to those of a newborn now, and his pancreatic function is increasing. The pancreas produces the naturally occurring hormone insulin – an important hormone for controlling levels of glucose in the blood.

All about you

Don't be surprised to find yourself getting all emotional again around now. You might have had a reprieve from the dreaded (well, by everyone around you anyway!) mood swings, but lots and lots of mums report suddenly feeling overwhelmed by pregnancy and the fact that they're embarking on the home strait. Don't run away from your feelings: talk everything through with someone sympathetic, whether it's your partner, a close friend, a relative or your midwife. Bear in mind that your partner might be having a few wobbles and misgivings, too, so it's up to you to judge whether now is a good time to share, or whether it might be more helpful all round to go to an outside source for an outpouring. Be reassured, though, that you're not alone in feeling like a confused teenager again. It's quite normal (even if it feels like the exact opposite!).

On the positive side, you're likely to be more and more aware of your baby's movements with every passing day now, and might already have pinned down his most active and restful times. Feeling your baby move can be absolutely thrilling, especially as often you're the only person who knows it's happening. It can feel like a secret communication going on between the two of you. For some mums, the bonding process begins in earnest around now.

What the netmums say

'When my partner first felt our baby move'

My husband was terrified – he wouldn't touch my bump at all. I made him do it once or twice and he actually squirmed! I think he was just scared of becoming attached to the baby and then something bad happening.
Jen from Hertfordshire, mum to Jack, four and Theo, 17 months

My hubby was fascinated to know what it felt like to me when our baby moved. The only way I could think to give him an idea was to have him hold his hand out flat, palm down, then I scraped my knuckle hard along his palm and asked him to imagine that sensation pushing against his abdomen. He used to chat to my bump, and he loved it if he got a reaction.
Lisa from Liverpool, mum to Joshua, five and Rose, three

My other half felt our baby move only a couple of days after I first felt it! It wasn't just movements – it was kicks! The first time for him was amazing: he was so quiet and the look on his face said everything! He said that it was the moment my pregnancy actually felt 'real' to him. It took more than a movement for me to realise it!
Amanda from Bristol, mum to Ruby, one

My hubby was feeling for movement from very early on in the pregnancy, yet he was still freaked when he finally did feel Owain. From then on, every night he'd put his hand on my bump and talk and sing to him. Now, as a two-year-old, Owain sings and chats all day long!
Lynette from Aberdare, south Wales, mum to Owain, two

Who'd have thought?

Breast milk contains the Omega-3 fatty acid DHA, which is important for brain and eye development. It's a complete food for your baby in the first six months of life, and his eyesight, speech and jaw development will all be boosted by breastfeeding.

Braxton Hicks contractions

Sooner or later you're likely to feel your uterus going into involuntary spasms in what are known as 'Braxton Hicks' contractions – first described by nineteenth-century British gynaecologist John Braxton Hicks – and they can, in fact, start from quite early in pregnancy. These are a sign that your uterus is limbering up and practising for labour, and are nothing at all to worry about. Having said that, not having them is nothing to worry about either, as some mums either don't experience them or don't notice them. If you do, it'll feel like your abdominal muscles are tightening and relaxing all on their own.

The difference between how Braxton Hicks contractions feel and how labour contractions feel is significant: Braxton Hickses are painless in most cases, if sometimes a little weird-feeling, and kind of random; labour contractions are most definitely uncomfortable (to say the least) and will be evenly timed and become stronger and more frequent on a pretty relentless basis. An exception to this can occur late in pregnancy, just before true labour. 'False labour', as it's known, happens when a mum experiences a series of painful contractions before her amniotic sac ruptures (or 'waters break') and real labour starts. In false labour, contractions usually last for less than a minute at a time, and are irregular. (For more on false labour see pp. 206–7.)

Braxton Hicks contractions are nothing to worry about and you don't have to take any action if you feel them happening. Mention them to your midwife if you like, just so you can be sure that the tightenings you're feeling are indeed Braxton Hickses.

Who'd have thought?

It seems that left- or right-handedness is decided in the uterus. Ultrasound studies show that the same proportion of babies are right-handed (90 per cent) as adults, and that the preference for using the left or right hand predominantly emerges from around 10 weeks' gestation when independent arm movement is first observed.

What the netmums say

'How Braxton Hicks contractions felt'

I didn't really get Braxton Hicks with my first two pregnancies, but with this one, I've been getting them on and off for the past few weeks. They're quite nasty pains – a bit like bad period pains – and they've actually had me doubled over.

Gillian from Preston, mum to Brendan, four, Nicole, 18 months, and 22 weeks pregnant

My Braxton Hicks were a lot more painful than actual labour pains! With my first daughter, I was in hospital due to a fall, and was getting what I thought were Braxton Hicks. However the contractions measured so strong on the monitor that the midwives were certain I was in labour. As it happens I went another 10 days before giving birth. With my second pregnancy, the Braxton Hicks were about the same strength as my labour pains.

Sara from Swaffham, Norfolk, mum to Georgie, four and Hollie, one

I didn't get any Braxton Hicks contractions that I noticed, and I actually felt quite left out when all my pregnant mates were having them! My midwife said it was probably because I was on the go a lot and was too distracted to notice. Some people apparently feel them much more strongly than others, and it's not so unusual to miss them. It did mean that when I started labour at 38 weeks I assumed the early contractions were Braxton Hicks – but they weren't! By the time I realised and went into hospital, I was already 5cm dilated!

Hollie from Kingston, Surrey, mum to Cory, four months

Carpal tunnel syndrome

You might be one of the unlucky 30 per cent or so of mums who get the annoying affliction that is carpal tunnel syndrome. It's a condition that affects the hand and wrist, although occasionally symptoms can spread up the arm. Symptoms are numbness or tingling in the hand and/or fingers, with the notable exception of the little finger! This is because it's caused by pressure on the 'median' nerve in the hand, which serves the thumb, index and middle fingers and part of the ring finger. In pregnancy the pressure is usually due to fluid retention, which causes a bit of swelling in the hand and wrist and compresses the median nerve. Usually symptoms disappear within a week or so of the birth. While you've got it, though, you might find your symptoms are worse at night or first thing in the morning.

Self-help for carpal tunnel syndrome

Some mums find all or some of the following suggestions helpful:

- hold your hand up in a 'high five' and stretch your fingers as hard as possible for a few seconds, then relax them. Repeat this 10 times
- ball your hand into a tight first, then relax. Repeat this 10 times
- make circular movements from the wrist, then shake your hand vigorously downwards as if trying to flick glue off your fingers
- plunge your hand alternately into ice-cold then hand-hot water
- raise your hands and arms with pillows while you sleep (but avoid sleeping on your back at this stage of pregnancy)
- consider acupuncture or acupressure – but only with a fully qualified practitioner with experience of working with pregnant women
- talk to your doctor or midwife about providing you with a wrist support.
- consult your doctor if your symptoms don't improve at all or get worse. A short course of ultrasound treatment might help.

What the netmums say

'Having carpal tunnel syndrome'

I had it in my second pregnancy and it was awful – I couldn't grip anything at all, and as I worked in a kitchen that made it very tricky and a bit dangerous. My doctor advised me to go and buy hand splints, and said that it would go after the birth – and it did.
Maresa from Buckinghamshire, mum to Charlotte, 15 and Olivia, 19 weeks

I've recently had surgery for this condition as mine never really got better after the birth: it was done under local anaesthetic and the relief is fantastic! In pregnancy it was a constant distraction and I'm sure I burnt up loads of calories just through rubbing and shaking my hands! I wouldn't wish carpal tunnel syndrome on anyone really, but if you do get it, I understand that it usually goes away after pregnancy: I was just a bit unlucky.

Dana from County Antrim, mum to Jamie, two

Your mission this week: Look after your feet!

You might have found that the old trotters are playing you up a bit lately – and even if they're still relatively comfy, you might find you become rather footsore as you get bigger. This is because your arches can become somewhat flattened by the extra weight they're carting around (medically known as 'over-pronation') and, as a result, your feet can start to roll inwards when you walk. This can cause inflammation of the fibrous band of tissue (the 'plantar fascia') that runs from your heel to your forefoot. There are several things you can do to relieve the discomfort. It's worth trying to get your feet measured several times in pregnancy so you can buy new shoes as and when you need them. You could also ask your doctor to refer you to a podiatrist, who may prescribe orthotic foot supports for you to wear in your shoes to support your feet. Soaking your feet in cool water for half an hour at the end of the day can bring some relief, as can wearing cotton socks or shoe liners rather than putting shoes over bare feet. Finally, get your partner to massage your feet using a specially formulated foot cream: look for a cream containing peppermint or citrus oil for a really revitalising result.

Look no further

I keep secretly wishing I wasn't pregnant any more, then feeling terribly guilty. How can I get over this?

You might be reassured to know that, along with the mood swings that often recur at around this time, it's really common to get 'cold feet' as pregnancy continues, and there's absolutely no need to feel guilty. Loads of mums admit to feeling they'd like to turn back the clock, stop lovingly eyeing up everything with an elasticated waist and start partying again – and it's a perfectly natural response to the idea of giving up that extra degree of freedom enjoyed by non-parents.

The best way to deal with these feelings is simply to go with them. OK, so you might be waving goodbye to nipping down the pub for a quick few on the way home from work or inviting three other couples at short notice for a weekend drinks party, but your life is heading for enrichment like you've never known before – and believe us, there are very, very few mums who'd want to turn the clock back once their precious babies are born. (Having said that, you can fully expect to be revisiting feelings of 'I don't want to do this any more' once you're in labour. Ask any midwife: it's one of the commonest cries they hear from labouring mums!)

Why is my bump so much smaller than other mums' at the same stage?
When it comes to bump size, a lot has to do with your pre-pregnancy size and weight, the strength of your abdominal muscles and the size of your baby as well as with genetics – and, for all these reasons, there can be vast differences in the rate at which mums expand! As long as your baby is growing normally, which your midwife or doctor will confirm at each antenatal appointment, you have no cause for worry. You'll probably find that you grow more quickly in future pregnancies because your abs might not be quite so toned second time around. This is also normal.

How come my friend's baby is more active than mine?
Some babies just seem to be more lively in the uterus, just as some children are livelier newborns and toddlers than others. Perhaps you are generally more active yourself than your friend, and don't have as many opportunities to slow down and feel your baby's activity. Another explanation is that your friend could be more physically sensitive to her baby's movements than you are or that your baby's sleepy and wakeful patterns are opposite to your own so that he's moving about more when you're asleep than when you're awake: this is quite common and is one cause of sleeplessness in pregnant mums. As long as you're feeling movements consistently every day, however faintly, and the pattern is more or less the same, everything should be fine. If things deviate a lot from what has become your baby's norm, contact your midwife straightaway so she can monitor your baby and check on his wellbeing. Finally, you might end up thankful that your baby is a little less rumbustious than your friend's: one US study conducted in the nineties discovered that foetuses who were very active in the uterus tended to make more irritable babies!

Week 24 119 days to go!

Don't forget: Buy a supply of breast pads

Hey, as if you didn't have enough physical symptoms to deal with, now you could very well find that your boobs start leaking – and it'll probably happen on a day when you're wearing a dark-blue shirt and attending an important meeting or event... OK, so it doesn't happen to all mums-to-be, but it's well worth being prepared just in case. The stuff that might come oozing through is colostrum, the first nutrient-dense substance that's a forerunner of full-on breastmilk. It might seem a bit previous of your boobs to start manufacturing baby food at this early stage, but you know there's a lot about pregnancy that seems to be unrelated to rhyme or reason! Get yourself a pack of breast pads just in case, then just slip one inside each bra cup; avoid wearing tight, clingy tops that will reveal your secret; choose light-coloured shirts just in case the colostrum takes you by surprise – and breathe easy again.

What the netmums say

'Me and my leaky boobs'

I was on my honeymoon at 22 weeks pregnant and I had the shock of my life to wake up in the morning to find a wet patch on the sheets and all over me. I was leaking! I had no idea if it was normal or not and was so embarrassed that I didn't want my husband to see. I later found out it was perfectly normal.
Erin from Leeds, mum to Connor, 11 months

From 19 weeks of pregnancy I had to wear breast pads, and I've tried them all: the throwaway ones, the washable ones, and so on. I first noticed the leakage in bed; then I was aware of the possibility everywhere I went just in case it showed. The really embarrassing moment came when I leaked whilst on a night out: the only totally sober person in the room, leaking around the chest area, walking around with arms folded, wishing the band would sing more quickly so I could go home!
Louise from Newcastle-under-Lyme, mum to Grace, five

The first time it happened to me was just before I was singing in a concert! We all had to wear red T-shirts and I didn't have a spare one! It was really early in pregnancy so I wasn't prepared and I was absolutely mortified. All I could think of to do was pretend I'd spilt something: I think the men fell for it but not the ladies! Also, I went into early labour at 32 weeks and was put in a bed on the maternity ward with all the mums who had just had their babies: every time one cried I was leaking milk everywhere! Luckily they managed to stop the premature labour with drugs.

Joanna from west Sussex, mum to Isabella, 21 months

Hey baby!

Weighing in at just over 1lb – 540g – your baby now has some chance of survival if he were to be born this prematurely, although he would still be facing a major uphill struggle and there are no guarantees he'd be able to pull through. He now measures around 21cm (8.5in) crown to rump – or roughly the length of the short side of a sheet of A4! This is the week when your pregnancy is rather charmingly referred to as 'viable' – as if it wasn't to you beforehand. Used in this way, though, the word 'viable' means that your baby is deemed capable of living outside the uterus, and termination is no longer lawful after this week.

All about you

Gestational diabetes

Gestational diabetes is a temporary condition that affects around 2–5 per cent of all mums-to-be. It's usually detected in the second or third trimester of pregnancy and is triggered in susceptible mums by the growing demands of the unborn baby and the impact of pregnancy hormones on the pancreas. You're more at risk of developing gestational diabetes if you have a family history of diabetes, or if you were very overweight when you became pregnant.

What's going on?

Every time we eat, the food we consume turns into glucose. When the pancreas is functioning properly it produces insulin – a hormone that transfers glucose from the blood into the body's cells for energy. In diabetics, the pancreas fails to produce enough insulin to cope with the extra demands of pregnancy, so glucose remains in the bloodstream.

The main problem with having too much glucose in your blood when you're pregnant is that it crosses the placenta and makes your baby grow too large. Having a big baby can lead to a complicated labour and delivery, and you're more likely to have a Caesarean if you have gestational diabetes. You'll probably be offered more scans throughout pregnancy, too, so that your medical team can monitor your baby's growth. You're unlikely to be allowed to go overdue with gestational diabetes and might even be induced a bit earlier than your EDD.

Signs and symptoms

Gestational diabetes is often without symptoms because it's picked up very quickly before any effects are felt. It's one of the things your midwife is looking for when she tests your urine, so the first sign will probably be a positive test for glucose in your pee. If glucose is found you'll be referred for a random blood test to get a more accurate idea of how much glucose is in your blood. If the result is high, you'll be sent for a glucose tolerance test (GTT). You'll be asked to fast the night before the test, then given a glucose solution to drink. You'll have two blood tests – one at the start of the GTT and one at the end – to measure how quickly your body is dealing with the glucose. The results will be sent to your GP or midwife.

If you do have gestational diabetes, you'll be referred to a hospital dietitian who'll prescribe a strict low-fat, low-sugar diet and advise you to increase your activity levels. This is usually all you need to control your diabetes. Very few mums need insulin, but if you do it will ensure your blood-glucose levels stay within a range that's safe for you and your baby. Either way you'll be given a blood-glucose monitor for self-testing at home, and a record book for keeping a note of your test results. The self-test involves pricking your fingertip and collecting a drop of blood on a testing strip, which slots into a battery-operated monitor. The monitor analyses the blood sample for glucose content and displays the result digitally.

What about my baby?

Because your baby makes extra insulin in pregnancy to combat the high blood-glucose levels crossing the placenta, he might continue to do so during the delivery and then have a low blood-glucose level (hypoglycaemia) at birth. If so, he might need to spend a little time in special care. Regular normal feeding may be enough to correct his blood-glucose levels, but sometimes babies are given a sugary solution (dextrose) via an intravenous drip. Your newborn baby is also at risk of jaundice, but this isn't serious and usually disappears without treatment.

What next?

In most cases, gestational diabetes disappears shortly after the birth, although some mums remain diabetic; these mums may well have had undiagnosed diabetes before they became pregnant. If you do get gestational diabetes but it goes away after your baby's born, you have an increased risk of developing type 2 diabetes later in life, but you can prevent or delay the onset by keeping your weight down, exercising regularly and continuing to eat a low-fat, low-sugar diet.

What the netmums say

'Having diabetes in pregnancy'

I had sugar in my urine at about 22 weeks and was sent for a glucose tolerance test (GTT) at 28 weeks which showed I had diabetes. I was shocked and upset, as no one in my family is diabetic: apparently I was just unlucky. I was given a little monitor for checking my blood-sugar levels, which I then had to record in a book several times a day. I was told to cut down on sugar and carbohydrates, and this was enough to regulate my blood-sugar levels. I even lost weight after I combined my new diet with light exercise – which was good as I'd been overweight before. I was also given extra scans every four weeks to check on my baby's growth. I made it to 38 weeks, when I was offered a sweep to start labour. I was told that if that didn't work I'd be induced on my due date, but it did work and my little boy was born the following day weighing a healthy 7lb 10oz. His blood sugars were tested and were fine. I had another GTT six weeks after the birth and was given the all-clear, but I've been told I'll be monitored for

gestational diabetes from the outset in any future pregnancies.
Kerry from Surrey, mum to Rhys, 10 months, and 14 weeks pregnant

I had gestational diabetes with all three of my pregnancies: it was discovered during a routine antenatal test. I had to monitor my blood-sugar levels several times a day, and had to use insulin from about five to six months onwards in each case. I had scans every four weeks and had to attend a special clinic at the hospital frequently. My babies' weights were 8lb 3½oz, 8lb 15oz and twins (six weeks premature) at 4lb 2oz and 5lb 5oz. My first two pregnancies were induced on the due date, but the girls couldn't wait that long! In all cases, my diabetes disappeared after the delivery.
Kathleen from South Shields, mum to Arran, 12, Luke, five, and Kate and Natalie, three

Thinking about breast- or bottlefeeding

The decision about how you're going to feed your baby is a very personal one and you shouldn't feel pressurised or judged when you come to make it. For some mums it's a no-brainer – the message that 'breast is best' couldn't be any more prominent, and even baby-milk manufacturers agree that there's no better food for a baby than his mum's own breastmilk. That's because it's formulated uniquely for your own baby and contains antibodies which protect against infections including gastroenteritis, respiratory illness, urinary infections and ear infections. It also reduces the risk of childhood diabetes and leukaemia, as well as allergic conditions like asthma and eczema.

The vast majority of mums are physiologically able to breastfeed: the secret is getting your baby latched on to your breast properly, and your midwife should be able to help you with this. (The key is to make sure your baby gets a good mouthful of boob as well as nipple.) If you feel any pain or discomfort during a feed, it's almost certainly because you've got the positioning wrong. A breastfeeding counsellor can also offer lots of great practical advice and support, either in person or by phone. Contact your local National Childbirth Trust (NCT) branch to find one.

Who'd have thought?

Wilhelm Preyer, a nineteenth-century German physiologist, first detected foetal movements when he placed a stethoscope on a mum's bump and 'heard' the baby move at around 12 weeks' gestation. We now know, through ultrasounds research, that babies can be seen to move from as early as eight weeks.

If you know you'll want to share the feeding with your partner you'll need to explore the options for 'expressing' your milk, which basically means milking yourself! Feeding your baby breastmilk from bottles as well as from the breast is known as 'mixed feeding'. It's not as difficult as you might think to express your milk: you can buy manual or electric pumps or express by hand (although this last option tends to be rather hard work), then store your milk in the fridge or freezer until it's needed. You can find guidelines on expressing and storing breastmilk on the Association of Breastfeeding Mothers website at www.abm.me.uk.

If you decide, as some mums do, that there's no way you want to breastfeed, or if you're in the tiny minority of mums for whom it's an impossibility (because of prior breast surgery, for example), then bottlefeeding will give your baby all the nutrients and calories he needs to thrive as long as you follow the formula manufacturer's instructions to the letter and are scrupulous about hygiene. There's a range of different bottles and teats you can try until you find ones that suit your baby best, and you'll also need to buy bottle brushes and a sterilising system (see *Newborn essentials*, p. 193).

Think about your options, do your research and try to come to a decision that you're happy with.

Who'd have thought?

If you're going on holiday, it's worth checking with your insurance company whether or not you need a written 'pre-travel health statement' from your GP, as travel insurance companies differ in what they need in order to cover you in pregnancy.

What the netmums say

'Deciding how to feed my baby'

I knew from the moment I fell pregnant that I wanted to breastfeed. Unfortunately with my first baby my milk didn't come in, so after two weeks of just colostrum and with a baby rapidly losing weight I had to give up and formula feed. My second baby was an absolute dream to feed, and I continued breastfeeding him until he was nine months old. My third was born with tongue tie [where the membrane connecting the underside of the tongue to the floor of the mouth is abnormally short, making the tip of the tongue partially or wholly immobile] and couldn't latch on. They don't snip them where we live, so for six months I expressed and fed her my milk in a bottle. If I had another baby I would still plan to breastfeed, but I've learnt that things don't always go to plan!

Delyth from Wales, mum to Rhys, five, Siôn, three and Carys, two

I knew with both pregnancies that I wanted to breastfeed. Luckily for me I was in hospital for a week on the Transitional Care Unit after having Morgan, and if it wasn't for them I think I would have quickly given up, as I found it hard to get him to latch on for the first few days. I breastfed him successfully right up until a month before my daughter was born. Unfortunately I haven't been as successful in breastfeeding my daughter: we managed up until 12 weeks, but then for some reason she stopped latching on properly and didn't want to take the breast, so I ended up combination feeding. Now she only has her first morning feed from the breast and will only occasionally take it at other times of day. I'm still trying, though, as I believe it's better for her.

Julie from Leeds, mum to Morgan, 17 months and Paige, three months

I knew I was going to bottlefeed long before I was pregnant. I don't mind other people breastfeeding, but it's not for me. My mum bottle fed my brother (now grown up) and he's fine. I had some not-so-nice looks from other mums for bottlefeeding, but I didn't really care.

I was lucky to have a midwife who didn't try to push me to breastfeed. I'm due my second next month and I have my bottles and formula ready in the kitchen. One big downside is that formula is really expensive, and it's really gone up over the past two years.
Carmen, Catterick Garrison, mum to Charlotte, 22 months, and eight months pregnant

When I was pregnant with my first I knew I'd always give breastfeeding a go, and I started the day he was born. Yes, it took me a while to get a good latch, but I was lucky to get it established before I went home. I breastfed for five weeks, but then I found that my near-10lb-born baby was just too hungry. I was exhausted by the constant feeding demands, so I switched to bottles and I felt better instantly: my stitches began to heal properly and I felt so much healthier instead of drained. My son thrived and settled to become a fantastic sleeper, which has lasted! When I had my daughter a year later I decided breast was best and she took to breastfeeding fantastically. I breastfed for seven months and found it more convenient and less tiring at night to be able just to scoop her up in the dark and put her on the breast. She was an excellent feeder, never lost an ounce of weight and to this day has never been ill. Persevering with breastfeeding is worth the benefits for your baby and is an ultimate bonding experience.
Alicia from London, mum to Kyrus, two, Demiyah, one, and 14 weeks pregnant

Your mission this week: Find an antenatal class

Make sure you book yourself into an antenatal class if you haven't done so already (see p. 19): you don't want to miss the boat. However much you might think you can go it alone and you don't need a class, you can only benefit – and so can your birth partner – by getting yourself enrolled in one. It'll also give you a fantastic opportunity to meet lots of other parents who are due about the same time as you. You might only want to stay in touch in the early days of new parenthood to compare notes, empathise and indulge in lots of baby talk; but on the other hand, you might make a friend – or group of friends – for life! Antenatal groups often form babysitting circles as well, which beats trying to find someone from cold. Go on – you won't regret it.

Look no further

Could my baby's kicking damage the amniotic sac?
No – along with the amniotic fluid it contains, it's actually there to take all the impact your baby can give it and to protect him from external impact at the same time. Athough a 'bag of waters' might sound pretty fragile, the sac is, in fact, made from two very tough membranes – the amnion and the chorion.

Is it safe to colour my hair in pregnancy?
Although there hasn't been much investigation into the subject, studies have found that the chemicals in permanent and semi-permanent hair dyes are not highly toxic. The chemicals in hair colourants would be dangerous if you were exposed to very high levels, but the amount found in these products is comparatively tiny. What you do need to consider, though, is that your hair might not react the same as it would if you weren't pregnant. Lots of mums report their hair changing colour, texture and condition in pregnancy, and this can make the results of using hair products unpredictable. Semi-permanent pure vegetable dyes, such as henna, are a good non-chemical alternative.

My friend, who's in her twenty-fourth week of pregnancy, has been told she needs a pelvic X-ray, but isn't it dangerous to have X-rays in pregnancy?
There used to be a lot of near-hysterical outcry about X-rays in pregnancy, but latest research suggests that almost all types are safe after the first 12 weeks of pregnancy when the cell-division phase of development is over, and that they don't involve enough radiation to affect your baby adversely after this time. Having said that, research is ongoing and this view could alter again, so as a precaution it's best to avoid any unnecessary X-rays until you've had your baby and are no longer breastfeeding.

Sometimes X-rays are deemed necessary in later pregnancy, as in your friend's case, and especially in mums who've suffered a pelvic or spinal injury or have a bone disease. In these cases X-rays can help to determine whether or not a straightforward delivery is likely to run into further complications.

The doctor and radiologist who carry out an X-ray will only go ahead if the benefits will outweigh any risk.

How are you feeling?

Tick the box that most closely represents how you feel about the given statements, then look back to the charts in previous chapters to see how you've changed over the months.

Physically	Emotionally
I'm proud of my new figure Strongly agree ☐ Agree ☐ Neither agree nor disagree ☐ Disagree ☐ Strongly disagree ☐	I'm bored with being pregnant Strongly agree ☐ Agree ☐ Neither agree nor disagree ☐ Disagree ☐ Strongly disagree ☐
I'm familiar with my baby's sleepy and wakeful times of day Strongly agree ☐ Agree ☐ Neither agree nor disagree ☐ Disagree ☐ Strongly disagree ☐	I love it that strangers comment on my bump Strongly agree ☐ Agree ☐ Neither agree nor disagree ☐ Disagree ☐ Strongly disagree ☐
My boobs are leaking colostrum Strongly agree ☐ Agree ☐ Neither agree nor disagree ☐ Disagree ☐ Strongly disagree ☐	I'm looking forward to maternity leave Strongly agree ☐ Agree ☐ Neither agree nor disagree ☐ Disagree ☐ Strongly disagree ☐
I'm finding it harder to sleep comfortably Strongly agree ☐ Agree ☐ Neither agree nor disagree ☐ Disagree ☐ Strongly disagree ☐	I feel closer to my partner than before I was pregnant Strongly agree ☐ Agree ☐ Neither agree nor disagree ☐ Disagree ☐ Strongly disagree ☐
I'm hungrier than I've been for weeks Strongly agree ☐ Agree ☐ Neither agree nor disagree ☐ Disagree ☐ Strongly disagree ☐	I feel my friends are treating me differently Strongly agree ☐ Agree ☐ Neither agree nor disagree ☐ Disagree ☐ Strongly disagree ☐
My feet seem to have grown Strongly agree ☐ Agree ☐ Neither agree nor disagree ☐ Disagree ☐ Strongly disagree ☐	My mood swings are back with a vengeance Strongly agree ☐ Agree ☐ Neither agree nor disagree ☐ Disagree ☐ Strongly disagree ☐

Quick quiz

How do you cope with pregnancy niggles?

1 What's the best way to deal with varicose veins?
a. Keep moving to promote better circulation
b. Sit down as often as possible
c. Hide them under trousers or a long skirt

2 How can you stop a pregnancy nosebleed?
a. Lean slightly forward and pinch the bridge of your nose
b. Lie back and wait for it to dry up
c. Bung a lump of cotton wool up each nostril

3 What can you do to ease carpal tunnel syndrome?
a. Stretch and relax your hands and fingers repeatedly
b. Raise your arms above your head when sitting
c. Sorry, carpal *what*?

4 What's a good strategy for combating the sweats?
a. Drinking plenty of water
b. Drinking less so you don't produce so much sweat
c. Spraying yourself all over with anti-perspirant

5 What's a good self-help measure when you have piles?
a. Sitting on a bag of frozen peas
b. Sitting on a hot-water bottle
c. Sitting on a stone wall

Answers: The answers to this quiz are all 'a'.
Mostly a: Top marks go to you for paying attention. OK, so you might not be lucky enough to escape all the niggles of pregnancy, but you'll know what to do to make yourself more comfy. Nice one.
Mostly b: Yes, well it seems you may have absorbed some of the information in this book back-to-front or upside-down. A little knowledge can be a more dangerous thing than none at all, so

have another browse at the correct answers then take the quiz again in a week or so's time.

Mostly c: Are you missing the point here or having a laugh with your answers? If it's the former, we mums really recommend you have another look at the correct answers (which were all 'a', in case you skipped over that bit!). And keep this book with you at all times in case you need to refer to it suddenly!

Chapter 6

Weeks 25–28

So 24 weeks down, 16 to go – give or take a week or so! When you think of it in these terms, it does start to feel like you're getting somewhere, doesn't it? Try to continue making the most of your energy (if you've still got any!). Your baby's about to embark on another rapid growth spurt, so you'll probably notice yourself getting bigger more rapidly from around now. Once you're into your third trimester, you'll need to rest more, exert yourself less and generally get yourself into the best frame of mind for the birth.

Use this time to go out and buy whatever you still need to get (see p. 193), and perhaps make a list of stuff you'd like but don't need, for when friends, family and colleagues start asking what they can treat you to. It's hard to think exactly what would be useful when you're caught on the hop, so indulge yourself in another spot of catalogue shopping/internet browsing so you've got lots of ideas. At this stage it's best to think about practical things (which doesn't mean they can't be attractive) rather than baby toys. People will buy these anyway once the new arrival has made an entrance – and even if you don't get many baby toys, it doesn't matter: your baby won't show much interest in anything specially bought for him for the first few months, and even then is likely to be just as fascinated by a set of car keys as a cuddly, fluffy duck!

Finish up any abandoned decorating or reorganising projects: have you set aside some room for your baby's stuff, for instance? Do you have a nursery organised? (Not necessary for at least the first six months, but probably easier to think about now than it will be when you're in the thick of babycare!) You'd be amazed how 'back seat' these things can become, the longer they're left. And the severely sleep-deprived don't tend to be the most active home-improvers either!

Week 25 112 days to go!

Don't forget: Book a visit to the maternity suite

If you're attending NHS antenatal classes you'll probably be told when you can have a tour of the maternity suite, but if you haven't enrolled you'll have to make your own arrangements. You might have mixed feelings about setting foot in the very place where you'll be labouring and giving birth, but believe us mums, in this case a known quantity is always better than the unknown! Hopefully you'll come away from your visit reassured that you know where things are, that the suite is comfortable (even cosy, in some hospitals) and that you'll be able to picture yourself giving birth – which is particularly useful when you're practising visualisation techniques (see p. 324). See *Visiting the delivery suite*, p. 227, for a list of questions to ask when you get there.

Hey baby!

Those fat stores are building up under your baby's skin and he now weighs around 700g (1.5lb) and measures 22cm (nearly 9in). Your baby's kicks will probably feel quite vigorous now as he gets bigger and stronger. It's a good sign that he's exercising his muscles and using his motor skills. You might find he objects to you putting things on your own belly! There have been reports of grumpy babies kicking books off their mums' bumps as if they object to their style being cramped! On the plus side, your partner should be able to feel the movements more strongly now. Don't freak out if he doesn't seem as interested as you'd hoped, though: some blokes just find the whole concept hard to get their heads round because they're not the ones having the experience directly. (Do you think you could imagine the wonder of feeling your baby moving inside you if you weren't the one who was pregnant?)

All about you

Just look at you, with your uterus the same sort of size as a football – which is appropriate enough as your baby will be kicking an imaginary football around inside you by about now! You may feel that you're about as big as you'd like to get, sporting a still fairly neat and manageable bump, but your baby will have other ideas as he still has lots of fat stores to lay down and a good deal of growing to do. You'll probably be expanding widthways as well as upwards and outwards. The top of your uterus has risen by around 4cm (1½ inches) in the last four weeks so that it's now around 25cm (10in) above your pubic bone, and approximately halfway between your belly button and the bottom of your sternum (breastbone).

Qualifying for maternity leave and pay

You've got to have been in continuous employment with the same boss for 26 weeks up to and including this week in order to get Statutory Maternity Pay (SMP), so if this applies to you, you'll officially qualify for maternity leave and all your allowances at the end of this week. It's also the latest you can leave it to let your employer know that you're intending to take maternity leave. Make quite sure that you've planned the right split of maternity leave for you – before and after the birth –and that you're not jumping ship earlier than you really need to. If you want to change the start date of your leave – even by putting it back – you'll officially have to give your employer 28 days' written notice unless you have medical reasons. Most employers are likely to be sympathetic, though, if you have to start your maternity leave early for any reason.

You may feel that you want as much time as possible on your own at home before your baby's born to make up for the lack of 'me' time you'll get after the birth: perhaps this bit of your pregnancy has fallen during a spell of really hot weather and you're tempted by the idea of relaxing in the garden rather than commuting to work. However, it really is best to save up as much leave as possible for after the birth, unless you're really unwell. Hard as it may be, do try to project yourself forward to when you have your baby home with you: although you might be feeling quite blasé now about the prospect of eventually leaving your baby with someone else (especially if you know you'll have to return to work fairly soon after the birth anyway), once you've held that newborn in your arms you might well feel that no one but you could possibly look after him well enough, or that you can't bear the idea of separation too soon. So do plan to give yourself as much time as possible with your new baby.

Who'd have thought?

The amniotic fluid surrounding your baby is warmer than your own body temperature – no wonder your baby is so cosy in there!

How long is maternity leave?

Compulsory Maternity Leave

By law, you can't work for an employer straightaway after the birth of your baby. The rules are that you have to take Compulsory Maternity Leave (CML) for at least two weeks from the birth, or four weeks if you're a factory worker. In some cases, there might be a statutory reason why CML has to be longer still.

Statutory Maternity Leave

As long as you were in employment when you became pregnant, you're entitled to 52 weeks' maternity leave, no matter how short a time you've worked for your employer – so right from day one of your employment. This is made up of 26 weeks Ordinary Maternity Leave (OML), during which time you'll enjoy all your contractual rights except your full wages or salary (see *What is Statutory Maternity Pay?*, below), and an optional further 26 weeks Additional Maternity Leave (AML). If you decide to take AML, you won't be paid for it unless it's your employer's policy to offer extra maternity pay, and you may lose other contractual rights as well. Check with your employer for full details.

What is Statutory Maternity Pay?

Statutory Maternity Pay (SMP) is a state benefit amounting to 90 per cent of your average weekly earnings during the qualifying period for the first six weeks of your Ordinary Maternity Leave (OML), then £117.18 a week or 90 per cent of your salary, whichever is less, for the remainder. To get SMP you must currently earn an average £90 a week; if you qualify, you can get SMP for up to 39 weeks, as long as you meet the conditions. Even if you decide not to return to work, you'll still be entitled to keep all of your SMP.

What is Maternity Allowance?

If you're not entitled to SMP – that is, if you are self-employed; are on a low income; have recently become unemployed; or have recently changed employer – you might be able to claim Maternity Allowance (MA) from Jobcentre Plus. To qualify for MA you have to fulfil one of the following criteria:

- you're employed, but ineligible for SMP
- you're registered self-employed and you pay Class 2 National Insurance Contributions or hold a Small Earnings Exception certificate
- you've recently become employed or self-employed.

You might also qualify if you've been employed and/or self-employed for at least 26 weeks of the 66 weeks up to and including the week before your EDD (part weeks count as full weeks); and you earned £30 per week taken as an average over any 13 weeks in the same period.

Maternity Allowance pays a standard weekly rate of £117.18 or 90 per cent of your average gross weekly earnings (before tax), whichever is less. MA is paid for a maximum of 39 weeks, but you might be able to get extra money for your husband, civil partner or other main childcarer if that person is on a very low income.

What is a Sure Start Maternity Grant?

The Sure Start Maternity Grant (SSMG) is a lump sum of £500 given to people on a low income and intended to help with buying things you'll need for your newborn: however, in effect you can spend the money on anything. It's payable if either you or your partner receive Income Support or income-based Jobseeker's Allowance. If you get Child Tax Credit or Working Tax Credit you might also be eligible, depending on your circumstances. Your personal savings aren't taken into account. An SSMG can be claimed any time from Week 29 of pregnancy until your baby is three months old.

You can find out lots more about your maternity entitlements by visiting www.direct.gov.uk

Visiting the delivery suite

If you've opted to have your baby in hospital or at a birthing centre, you should have a tour of the delivery suite around now. If you're not offered this tour as a matter of routine, contact the maternity unit and ask when it would be convenient for you to come. Some mums find the visit all a bit scary and daunting; others find it reassuring to be able to envisage exactly where they'll be on the big day. If you're a bit on the squeamish side, your visit will be particularly important for you as you'll be facing your fears head on. There's no getting around it: somehow your baby is going to make his appearance into the world and you're going to have to be there, so you may as well start trying to get your head around it now! This is also an opportunity to ask anything you might want to clarify in advance of the birth, so go armed with a list of questions. Try to take your planned birth partner with you so that they'll be familiar with what's what and where's where, too.

Here's a list of the sorts of questions you might want to ask. Take this book with you so you can tick off each question as it's answered.

- What pain relief options are there? □
- How soon would I need to say if I wanted an epidural? □
- What is your rate of emergency Caesarean deliveries? □
- What's your policy on episiotomies versus tears? □
- Under what circumstances might you induce labour? □
- Is there a birthing pool available? □
- May I bring my own birthing pool? □
- May I bring a complementary therapist with me? □
- May I bring my own music/beanbag/TV/pillows etc? □
- How many people may I bring to the birth? □
- How do we get into the delivery suite if it's the middle of the night? □
- Is it OK to eat and drink in the delivery suite? □
- Can my partner stay overnight if necessary? □
- How long can my partner stay with me after the birth? □
- What support can you offer me with breastfeeding? □
- Under what circumstances might my baby be transferred to a Special Care Baby Unit (SCBU)? □
- If my baby goes to a SCBU, for how long can I stay in hospital with him? □

It's a good idea for you or your birth partner to take a notepad and pen with you to jot down the answers as you might otherwise feel a bit overwhelmed and promptly forget the information.

What the netmums say

'Visiting the labour suite'

I found my visit to the labour ward really helpful: it was great to know where to go when things kicked off; seeing the rooms and equipment was good, too, though the sight of the forceps certainly made my eyes water! The best bit of the visit was hearing a woman in labour followed by her baby's first cry – ahhh!
Heather from Hull, mum to Daniel, 16 months

It was reassuring to go on to the ward and see everything in place and ready. When I had my son it was in the room I'd been shown round, which made it more comfortable somehow. I was also transferred to the same room to be examined after having my daughter at home: it was very surreal being there for a third time.
Julie from Leeds, mum to Morgan, 17 months and Paige, three months

The offer to visit my labour ward was made, but I was only given one time to visit, and as it was a midweek evening, my partner was working a shift, we live in the country and I don't drive, I wasn't able to go. When I asked if I'd get another opportunity, I was flatly told 'no'.
Amanda from Barnstaple, mum to Tristan, 23 months

It was fantastic as a first-time mum-to-be to be able to see the place where my baby would be born. I was six months pregnant and got to see where everything was and the layout of the rooms. I was able to view the equipment they use for the baby after delivery, and I got to check out the birthing pool, too, which I was told would be heavily booked as it was so popular. I think all pregnant women should have a tour of the labour ward, even if they have planned a home birth. After all, it's best to keep an open mind as you could end up being transferred to hospital.
Alicia from London, mum to Kyrus, two, Demiyah, one, and 14 weeks pregnant

Who'd have thought?

You're more susceptible to sunburn whilst you're expecting than when you're not pregnant, as your skin is more sensitive to sunlight.

Your mission this week: Think about a water birth

If you're considering a water birth, now's the time to investigate more fully and put the wheels in motion. Medics have long been in dispute about delivering a baby into water, with some maintaining that it's a potentially dangerous practice, whilst others insist that it's the most natural way to give birth as it eases a baby from the tranquillity of the amniotic sac into another warm-water environment, making the transition into the world less traumatic.

If you're planning to use a birthing pool, it's an issue you'll need to discuss in detail with your midwife. Much will depend on how experienced he or she is at delivering babies into water: a less experienced midwife may feel reluctant, whereas someone who has delivered many babies safely this way should be able to reassure and encourage you. Your baby won't breathe until he emerges from the water. Until then, he'll receive oxygen through the umbilical cord, as happened during your pregnancy. Most midwives are happy for a baby to stay under water for the length of time it takes for the new mum to reach down and pick him up. Any longer than about half a minute isn't recommended as it's difficult to predict when the placenta will begin to separate from the wall of the uterus and deprive the baby of oxygen.

Using a birthing pool doesn't mean having to deliver your baby into water, though: lots of mums use the warm water for pain relief and relaxation during labour, but emerge on to 'dry land' to give birth. Even if you plan to deliver into the water, it's important you keep an open mind as complications may mean you need to come out.

Thinking ahead

- If there's a birthing pool available at your hospital or birthing centre, make sure you book it ahead of time. Obviously, the timings will be subject to change, unless your baby is so obliging as to arrive on his EDD.

- Bear in mind that someone else might be occupying the birthing pool at the time when you need it.
- If there's no pool but you want to hire and bring in your own, book this early, too. Most companies will hire a pool for two weeks either side of your EDD. Prices vary from around £100–£300, depending on the length of hire and the calibre of pool.
- If you're planning a water birth at home, first make sure that your floor is strong enough to take the weight of a filled pool (around 500–1500kg, depending on size); that you can keep the room sufficiently warm for when you get out; and that your hot-water tank can hold enough water to fill the pool (around 500–1200 litres, depending on size).

Look no further

What happens to my maternity benefits if my baby comes early?
If your baby is born earlier than your EDD, your maternity leave and pay will be triggered the day after the delivery. Similarly, if you have a pregnancy-related illness that keeps you off work during any part of the last four weeks before your EDD, your employer can trigger your leave and pay on the day after your first day of absence.

I've heard that babies born into water are susceptible to infections. Is that right?
There's no evidence to support this belief. As long as the water in the birthing pool is perfectly clean at the outset, there's no more risk of infection in water than there is during a normal delivery. Hospital pools should be thoroughly cleaned and disinfected between births (and if you're in any doubt, get your partner to roll his sleeves up and give it a scrub first); if you're hiring a pool you'll need to buy a new liner to go in it, so the risk of infection is minimal.

What if the birthing pool isn't available on the day?
It's a chance you have to take really. If you're pinning all your hopes on a water birth, it might be better to make your own arrangements to hire a pool instead of relying on the hospital's facility (but check first that they're happy for you to do so). Otherwise, try to keep an open mind about the birth, and keep the pool in the back of your mind as an option should the opportunity arise.

Week 26 105 days to go!

Don't forget: Snatch as much daytime sleep as you can

With almost two-thirds of your pregnancy under your belt, is the finishing line is starting to hove into view? The increased pressure in your belly from your growing baby might be exacerbating problems like leg cramps, piles, backache, rib and side pain and headaches – or, on the other hand, you might be lucky and breeze your way through your entire pregnancy without so much as a minor niggle! (Keep it quiet when you're amongst other pregnant ladies, though – who wants to hear how much better they could be feeling at a time when they're going through the mill?) One of the key things to do is to rest as much as possible, day and night – not just to sleep, but to relax your muscles and take the pressure off your organs and joints. Prop yourself up with pillows and cushions to make yourself as comfy as possible. Maybe now would be a good time to start experimenting with different relaxation tapes: try the library first until you find one that you like enough to buy.

Hey baby!

Your baby weighs just over 900g (almost 2lb) this week and measures around 23cm (9.2 inches) crown to rump. Although your baby's veins are still visible through his skin, it's rapidly becoming more opaque. Don't forget that your baby is very aware of certain external sounds and will be accustoming himself to your voice as well as your favourite TV show theme tunes! He's also got used to all sorts of sounds that are unique to living in your uterus, like your heartbeat, your digestive system, and other bodily functions! He's likely to jump at sudden loud noises, too – see if you notice this.

All about you

You might feel a bit cumbersome about now – and you're perfectly entitled to challenge anyone who accuses you of being clumsy to try to maintain a graceful stance with the equivalent of an army training body pack strapped to their torsos!

The other thing you can expect around this time is an outbreak of spots, hives or some other skin complaint – yes, charming! Although there's often no obvious cause for these irritations, it's thought that increased hormone levels can make you more sensitive to contact with substances you'd normally tolerate without any problems. Some mums find they have a reaction to chlorine in pregnancy, for example. Although modern antihistamines are not safe to take in pregnancy, some of the older (sedating) types are usually considered safe. However, you should never take any medication in pregnancy without your doctor's advice and consent. Self-help for hives includes wearing natural fibres and applying calamine lotion to ease the itch.

Add to uncomfortable skin conditions the increasing difficulty you might have finding a comfy sleeping position – in between middle-of-the-night trips to the loo – and you're getting the picture: in other words, just when you thought that 'blooming' phase would last forever, you could find yourself slightly less enchanted by this whole state of pregnancy. You won't be alone, that's for sure. Be reassured, though, with two-thirds of pregnancy under your belt by the end of this week, the day when you finally meet your baby is not too far off now.

Leg cramps

Although it's still not really clear why mums-to-be get more leg cramps than other mere mortals, with theories abounding from extra pressure on your blood vessels to general muscle fatigue, in a way it's not that relevant – the fact is, if you get them you get them, and what you'll want to know most is how to ease them. For some reason they seem to be more frequent at night time.

What you can do about it
You might find that some of the following tips help to keep leg cramps to a minimum:

- try to massage and stretch your calf muscles regularly, especially during the hour or so before bedtime
- try having a warm bath before bed to relax your muscles, then massage them just before you get in
- avoid sitting with your legs crossed, or standing for long periods
- keep as mobile as possible, walking around rather than standing still
- whenever you think of it, keep your feet moving whilst sitting down: ankle circling, toe wiggling and leg shaking are all good
- lie down on your left side for rests and night-time sleep to improve circulation to and from your legs. Lying on your left takes pressure off the big vein that brings blood back up to your heart from your legs

- wear maternity support tights, especially if you have to stand for long periods
- drink plenty of fluids – around two litres per day. Water is best, but your intake could also include tea, squash and other non-alcoholic – and preferably decaffeinated – drinks.

There's currently no evidence to support the view that taking calcium supplements in pregnancy can help to ease leg cramps. However, it's important to ensure you have enough calcium in your diet, and it's found not just in dairy products, but also in tofu, pulses and tinned fish (with bones) or fish whose bones you can eat such as sardines, mackerel and whitebait.

How to relieve cramp

You should get some relief by immediately stretching out your calf muscle:

1 Straighten your leg and flex your heel so that your foot is at right angles to your shin.
2 Gently pull your toes backwards. It might take a minute for the spasm to subside, so keep holding.
3 Once the pain has subsided, walk around a bit and keep flexing your foot and rotating your ankle.
4 Massage the muscle again and lay a warm flannel or hot-water bottle over it.

NB If you notice that you get repeated cramps in the same leg, or if there is a hot, red or tender area, you might have a blood clot, so bring this to the attention of your doctor immediately. See p. 187 for more on blood clots in pregnancy.

Who'd have thought?

One baby in 2,000 is born with a tooth already visible!

What the netmums say

'Managing leg cramps'

I had bad cramps in my first two pregnancies, but while I was pregnant with Gemma I heard that having a boost of calcium and potassium can help prevent them, so I got into the habit of eating a banana mashed with some milk as a pre-bed snack. It seemed to help as I didn't have as many attacks this time round, but it didn't eliminate them altogether. My poor husband was probably just about ready to check into a hotel, as the only relief I could get was from him massaging my legs with cooling leg gel – which meant I had to wake him up in the middle of the night each time I got a cramp...!
Elise from Inverness, mum to Bobby, four-and-a-half, Lois, three and Gemma, 18 months

I used to stretch my calf muscles for five to 10 minutes before bedtime, then massage them really vigorously. This seemed to loosen the muscles up, at least for a time. I still got cramps, but once I'd started the stretching and massaging it would happen closer to the morning rather than almost as soon as I got into bed, so I could cope with that better. I also found it comforting to have a warm hot-water bottle in the bed to apply if I started feeling a twinge.
Lori from Caerphilly, mum to Louise, 16 months

Late breaks

If you haven't had a last holiday as a couple yet, it's not a bad idea to start planning for one around now. It might take a few weeks to get something organised – and to book some time off work if you're owed any – and most airlines won't want you flying after Week 35, so the latest you'll be able to take off is at the beginning of Week 33. You most probably won't feel quite as physically or emotionally enthusiastic about going away by then, though – and you'll have to keep in mind the possibility that your baby won't wait until you return home to put in an appearance! (How do you feel about a little Stavros rather than a little Stephen, for instance?)

If you're staying in the UK, try to plan to be close-ish to a hospital just in case of a medical emergency or a niggle you want sorting out. If you're planning a trip abroad, go for somewhere with a major city nearby so that you still have access to good medical services. It's always best to check with your airline how happy they are to take pregnant passengers, and how many weeks their cut-off point is, because this can vary. Whilst lots are happy to let you fly until Week 35 or even 36, others draw the line at 28 weeks in case of premature labour. Don't leave it to chance, because although you won't be asked if you're pregnant when you book your flight, you might be asked how far gone you are once you're actually at the boarding gate – and imagine the disappointment if you were to be refused permission to board at this point! Bear in mind, too, that some travel insurance companies won't insure pregnant women beyond Week 28, so shop around at the time of booking your holiday to ensure you're covered.

It's a good idea, too, to get a doctor's letter stating that you're fit to fly. This can help you to avoid delays. Make sure it's written only a day or so before your flight, though, or it might be considered invalid.

A few more points:

- don't fly on any small aircraft without pressurised cabins
- don't worry about your exposure to natural radiation while you're flying, as this is negligible unless you fly more than a few times a year
- get hold of some support stockings or socks to wear on the flight, to reduce your risk of deep vein thrombosis (DVT), to which you're more susceptible in pregnancy. For best results, put them on as you get up on the morning of the flight, and keep them on until you reach your accommodation
- keep well hydrated, as flying can dry you out.

What the netmums say

'Taking a late break'

When I found out I was pregnant we'd only been back from visiting my partner's family in Spain for just over a week. I flew again when I was about five months gone, but I made sure I packed my maternity notes just in case something happened. I'd fly whilst pregnant again, but I'm not too sure about in the later stages.
Sarah from Derby, mum to Lily-Mae, eight-and-a-half months

I flew at about five or six months in each pregnancy and had no problems either time. The first flight was with a budget airline that doesn't allocate seating so I just asked if I could have an aisle seat next to an emergency exit and they were great about it – they even let me board first, which is the only time I've ever felt like royalty! The second time around, I was so focused on keeping my 14-month-old entertained I forgot to ask about priority seating. My only advice is not to sit next to the window: you'll be up and down to the toilet every five minutes and will have to clamber across everyone else each time!
Debra from south Yorkshire, mum to Finn, four and Louis, two

My husband and I honeymooned in Jamaica when I was 32 weeks pregnant! I was a little nervous about flying, but then I am usually anyway. I wasn't overly worried as I'd had a trouble-free pregnancy. The only downsides were that I couldn't make use of the all-inclusive alcohol; I couldn't sunbathe on my stomach, and they wouldn't let me do any water sports. I did, however, still wear my bikini!
Sarah from south Essex, mum to Emilie, six months

Your mission this week: Think about complementary therapy during labour

If you think you might want to take a complementary therapist such as an aromatherapist, reflexologist or herbalist, to the birth with you to help ease labour and delivery – and your hospital or birth centre are happy for you to do so – but you haven't yet made the arrangements, now's the time to do it. A good therapist may be booked well in advance and you'll want to know you're taking someone you trust with you, so secure her services early. If you haven't tried all the therapies available and think it might still be an option you'd like to research, use the next week or so as a great excuse to treat yourself, expense permitting. If money is tight, perhaps your parents or in-laws might prefer to chip in for a session or two rather than buying your baby a costly present. Things to try include reflexology, acupuncture, aromatherapy, hypnosis and massage. It's worth asking first whether your midwife is qualified to practise any of these therapies – or if there is another midwife in your area who does.

Who'd have thought?

There's a school of thought that says if your nose gets bigger in pregnancy you're expecting a girl. In fact, there's not an ounce of truth in that assertion: more likely if your nose gets bigger it's because the blood flow to your mucus membranes has increased. If anything, you're more likely to get nosebleeds. Hmph! On the plus side, your nose will revert to its pre-pregnancy size when your hormones readjust after the birth.

Look no further

I'm suffering from constipation more than ever now. I've tried all the usual things like stepping up the fibre in my diet and drinking more fluids. What else can I do?

It's no coincidence that many mums find themselves a bit 'bunged up' again at around this stage of pregnancy. There are a few reasons why: you're starting to produce more relaxin again now, in preparation for the birth, and this will make your bowel still more sluggish; as your baby gets bigger, your digestive tract is becoming more compressed, meaning that the whole process is slower; and you are probably feeling less like exercising now that you're heavier. You're doing all the right things: now try to exercise a bit more, even if it's just taking a brisk walk once or twice a day. You'll be surprised how this can have a knock-on effect. Also, drinking something hot first thing in the morning can help get things moving. If you become very uncomfortable, however, speak to your midwife, doctor or pharmacist, who might recommend a laxative such as Fybogel. Don't just go ahead and take laxatives without talking to a healthcare professional first, though: some aren't compatible with pregnancy as they can stimulate the muscles of the uterus.

My baby often kicks in response to particular CD tracks I play. Does this mean he likes or hates them?

It's impossible to tell, really – except that it's unlikely hatred is yet a part of your baby's emotional vocabulary! Anything that triggers movement in your baby is stimulating him in some way, and this can only be a good thing for your peace of mind. Unless you're playing thrash metal (or any other frenetic sounds) at extremely high volumes that might be disturbing your baby – and who's to say he might not be enjoying it?! – why not continue to play the tracks that get your baby moving on a regular basis: you might find that they're soothing to him after the birth, as many babies can recognise music and voices they heard from within the uterus and find these reassuring.

I've always had inverted nipples, but my midwife has said they might 'pop out' as my breasts get fuller. So far, nothing's happened. Does it mean I won't be able to breastfeed?

To check whether your nipples are truly inverted, gently press down on the surrounding breast tissue. If your nipples don't protrude from beyond your breast tissue as you do this, then things are unlikely to change further along in pregnancy. There's no reason for alarm, though – milk doesn't come from your nipple, but from ducts in the areola (the skin surrounding it), and your baby will get the milk out by squeezing a good mouthful of breast tissue rather than by chomping on your nipples. You might need a little help from your midwife or a breastfeeding counsellor to get your baby latched on at first, but once you've got feeding established, you should get along just fine. You might even find that your baby's sucking eventually encourages the nipples to protrude a little.

Who'd have thought?

You're better off with a low-heeled shoe than a completely flat shoe or flipflops, particularly in your final trimester. This is because flats will encourage you to arch the small of your back to compensate for your bump, and this will play havoc with your back, especially if it's sore already. A low wedge is a good bet as it's a solid, stable design and will also support your feet more than a standard low heel.

Week 27 98 days to go!

Don't forget: Keep positive about the birth

Some experts consider Week 27 as the beginning of the third trimester; others, like us, split the trimesters into handy, three-month chunks. Either way, you're well and truly on the home strait and will inevitably start to focus more now on the birth itself.

Try to stay objective, despite the fact that you may be accosted by more people than ever who want to share their horror stories with you: some other mums can forget that wearing their birth experiences like a badge could be upsetting for someone like you! Shut your ears to all but the most positive birth stories: there's often no accounting for why some women have easier experiences than others, and unless you have a known problem that could result in intervention or a Caesarean, you have just as good a chance of an entirely straightforward birth as anyone else.

Hey baby!

Your baby has hit the 1kg (2.2lb) mark. This means your little sweetie weighs about the same as a standard bag of sugar! When you consider this, it's easy to see that there's a lot more growing to be done – by both of you – before he can emerge at a healthy weight. By now he measures 24cm (9½ inches) from crown to rump. About now your baby's eyes, which have been fused shut all this time so far, may open, and he'll get a glimpse of his watery environment for the first time. From now on he'll be practising blinking his eyelids as well as doing the swallowing thing! Should you happen to have a late scan for any reason, you might even catch him doing one or other – or both!

All about you

The top of your uterus is now around 7cm (almost 2 inches) above your belly button, although your bump may have pushed up to near your breasts by now! You might still be a bit of a banshee one minute, and a weeping, wailing baby the next. Don't worry, this is still to be expected, not just because of hormonal upheaval but because of the sheer stress of being pregnant, both physical and psychological. It's not unusual for some mums to burst into floods of tears over a news item or fly into a rage because the washing up hasn't been done. Do take time out to explain to the people whose feelings could be hurt or upset in the process, though – they deserve an explanation of sorts, if only so that they know what to expect!

Falls in late pregnancy

Although the effect of a minor fall in pregnancy is likely to be minor itself (see p. 200), at this stage of pregnancy a heavier fall could have some implications, either for your baby or for the placenta (see *Placental abruption*, p. 243), as well as for your own wellbeing. Falls are more likely, too, as your centre of gravity shifts with your growing bump, so it's good to be aware of this and to take steps to avoid falling over: for example, wearing flatter (although not completely flat) shoes with gripper soles; avoiding walking on slippery or icy surfaces; using a handrail when going up or down stairs; steadying yourself on furniture as you move from room to room; asking your partner to stand in front of you on escalators; taking a lift instead of stairs or escalators; carrying your shopping evenly distributed between your two hands.

Try to move around more slowly and take a little time to judge distances and spaces: a change in balance can also make you feel a little giddy or lightheaded, and what would normally be a small stumble could turn into a major tumble.

If you do fall, contact your doctor, who will probably want to examine you to make sure all is still well. You'll find it reassuring to be strapped on to a monitor and hear your baby's heartbeat and see evidence of his movements. You may even be offered an ultrasound scan to check on your baby more thoroughly.

Warning signs after a fall include:
- bleeding from the vagina
- a sudden gush of amniotic fluid from the vagina
- severe abdominal pain.

Who'd have thought?

According to the US Academy of Science, the healthiest babies are born to mums who gain at least 15.8kg (35lb) – but that's not a licence to pile on the stones...!

What the netmums say

'Falling in pregnancy'

It was my due date and we had workmen in the house working on the central heating. They offered to put the landing floorboards back when I went to the loo, but I said, 'No, don't worry, I'll be fine on the joists.' Talk about famous last words! As I fell my leg hooked over the joist, which saved me. The terrified workmen tried to pull me up but it was my hubby who managed to get me up. He'd been in the living room and rushed out as he heard me shout: all he could see was my legs dangling and my slipper on the downstairs hall floor! He phoned the doctor's, which was only a two-minute walk from the house, and got an appointment straightaway. The doctor felt my belly and thought everything was OK. I was told to watch out for bleeding, but there wasn't any. As it was, the shock didn't jog things along, and Rory was born 10 days later. The midwife did ask about the massive bruise on the back of my thigh! Looking back, I just dread to think what could have happened.

Joanna from Aberdeenshire, mum to Rory, almost three and Maisie, 16 months

I took a tumble at five months pregnant with my first baby: it was New Year's Eve and we'd decided to go out for a nice meal with friends. It was raining really heavily and freezing cold so I made a dash for the restaurant. I slipped on a patch of wet black ice and fell really heavily on my behind. I was so embarrassed and my poor hubby got a real fright. I didn't want a fuss, but I did spend the rest of the evening following the baby's movements, and the restaurant happened to be right next to our local A&E department, which was reassuring. As it was, our little one was fine and I was left with a black-and-blue backside as a souvenir. My next tumble came when I was nine months pregnant with Tom. My middle child had fallen, so I bent down to cuddle her. She cuddled me back just a little too enthusiastically and I fell backwards into a puddle – and couldn't get back up! My hubby was on the other side of the car and I didn't want to attract attention to myself, so I made my daughter shout,

'Daddy, I'm stuck' so he would rush to help her and find me floundering!
Nicola from south Glasgow, mum to Amy, four, Lucy, two and Tom, six months

I fell when I was six months pregnant with my son: I grazed my hands and pulled my back, all because of a stupid pothole in the pavement. My partner insisted on taking me to A&E to be checked out, and whilst there I realised that Morgan had stopped moving. As he was regular as clockwork normally, this was really worrying. Things got worse in A&E when they couldn't find a heartbeat as they didn't have the right equipment; they tried using some kind of scanning equipment that was unfamiliar to them, and they couldn't work it, so in the end they transferred us to the labour ward to be monitored. As soon as we were hooked up to the machine there was this loud 'whoosh' of Morgan's heartbeat, and we could hear him kicking away, too. At that point I started to feel relaxed again.
Julie from Leeds, mum to Morgan, 17 months and Paige, three months

Placental abruption

One of the complications of a serious fall in pregnancy is when the placenta starts to separate from the wall of the uterus. This is known as 'placental abruption' and will mean your baby could be at risk of not getting sufficient nutrients and oxygen. Depending on the degree of placental separation from the uterine wall and the amount of blood lost as a result, you will either be admitted to hospital for observation and foetal monitoring, or you will be given a blood transfusion and your baby will be delivered immediately. Failure to deliver the baby promptly in the case of a severe abruption could prove fatal.

Placental abruption occurs in only about 1 in 200 pregnancies, and can also be caused by drug use, smoking, injury other than from a fall, and complications arising from medical procedures (although rarely). You are also at risk if you have had placental abruption in a previous pregnancy.

Itching in pregnancy

As your abdomen grows bigger and the skin becomes more stretched, you may experience the further indignity of an itchy belly, which can give rise to some fairly unladylike scratching. A degree of itching is pretty normal – although, again, not everyone will get it. Sorry, but it can also be an indication that you're getting some stretch marks. Things that might help relieve the itching include spraying your belly with a cool, misting spray, rubbing some cocoa butter into it or soaking in a tepid bath, then moisturising afterwards. Wearing loose-fitting clothes in natural fibres without a restrictive waistband might also help, as may avoiding irritants such as perfumed toiletries and biological washing powders.

Other causes of itching

The most common itchy-skin condition of pregnancy – which still only affects one mum in a hundred, and usually only first-timers – has a very complicated name: Pruritic Urticarial Papules and Plaques (or PUPP)! This simply means itchy hives and flaky skin. It's unclear why PUPP occurs, but it seldom affects subsequent pregnancies, is usually in the family and can often be traced back through the father's side. It usually starts around the navel and can spread to the thighs, arms and extremities, although it never involves the face. It's harmless to your baby, but will be extremely distracting to you. In some cases, moisturising regularly can help, but in more severe cases your doctor might prescribe a special topical cream or even steroid tablets to help lessen the itching, although oral medication would be a last resort.

There's another condition, which is even rarer, called prurigo, which can occur early or late in pregnancy. Characterised by small raised spots over the body and especially on the upper trunk and upper parts of arms and legs in its early onset form (whilst late onset prurigo more commonly affects the abdomen), it's also no threat to your baby, but could drive you bonkers as it can be as itchy as a load of insect bites. You might get some relief from calamine lotion or bicarb baths.

Who'd have thought?

Just under two-thirds of first babies are born after their EDDs; just over a third arrive early – but only five babies in a hundred are actually delivered on their due dates.

Obstetric cholestasis

If you have all the itching of prurigo without the rash – in other words you have itching over your body, but most severely on your extremities – this could be a sign of a more serious condition of pregnancy called obstetric cholestasis (OC). It's a condition of the liver that affects about 2 per cent of mums-to-be, usually in the last trimester of pregnancy, and results from an excess of bile building up in the body because of a decrease in liver function. The itching from OC is much more severe than any other itchy pregnancy condition and can even cause scratching that results in broken skin that's open to infection. Diagnosis is made by two blood tests, and treatment is with drugs to improve liver function. If you have OC you'll be monitored closely for the rest of your pregnancy and, depending on the severity, your doctors might want to induce you early as the condition could have an adverse affect on your baby. Because the liver is affected, the blood is not effectively cleansed of potentially dangerous toxins, and if untreated can lead to stillbirth. It's thought that OC could account for around 5 per cent of unexplained stillbirths.

OC disappears within a short time of the delivery of your baby. If you have it once, you're quite likely to have it in subsequent pregnancies – but at least you'll be alert to the symptoms and can get early treatment.

What the netmums say

'That awful itching'

Around Week 27, I started itching like crazy across my bump but also down my arms and legs. It was so bad it was debilitating, and I was also suffering from a reduced appetite and had dark urine but pale poo. A blood test showed I had obstetric cholestasis. I'd never heard of it before, but when I read up on it I was really worried as it can cause stillbirth and major haemorrhaging after delivery. My doctors said they'd give me regular scans and monitor my baby more than they normally would to keep tabs on things. I was warned that I'd have to deliver at 38 weeks, so I was ready for being induced and it was managed well when it happened. I was given a vitamin K injection in advance of the birth to reduce the risk of bleeding. After the birth, things quickly got back to normal.

Barbara from York, mum to Abigail, 23 months

Who'd have thought?

Statistically, your chance of giving birth to a left-handed child increases with your own age at the time of conception, and mums over 40 are 128 per cent more likely to have a left-hander than younger mums!

Your mission this week: Prepare to start your antenatal classes

Start getting prepared for your antenatal classes, which should start in the next few weeks, by making a list of all the things you hope will be covered. You might have lots of things to ask that won't necessarily be covered, so it's as well to keep your list handy so you can tick things off as you get the answers. Ask your birth partner if there's anything they particularly want to raise, from practicalities to anxieties and worries – and reassure them that it's absolutely OK to feel squeamish, daunted or even frightened of being responsible for helping see you through the birth. Don't bombard your midwives with your list of questions as soon as you arrive, though: you'll probably be given a schedule outlining what will be covered at each session. The idea of your list is to prompt you to remember anything that doesn't come up.

Have a think about whether you might be able to instigate a few social meetings between yourselves and the other people at the group (if you find anyone you might particularly want to befriend!). That way you can communicate up to the birth about anything that's on your minds, and you'll already know each other better by the time your babies are born. Again, your midwife might pass round a list of names for you to add your phone numbers to, so don't jump the gun – but it's something you could do yourself if this doesn't happen. The feeling of support you can get from being in contact with others who are going through the same things you are at the same time is invaluable.

Who'd have thought?

The average woman loses around 6kg (13.5lb) within an hour of delivering her baby. This is made up of the weight of the baby, the amniotic fluid, the placenta and blood loss.

What the netmums say

'What we got from our antenatal classes'

There's a real lack of NHS antenatal classes in our area so we booked an NCT course of four evenings with six other couples. The classes were very focused on breastfeeding along with some other topics, and the blokes were often taken off in different groups to discuss things so we could then come back together to 'share'. The best bit was the friends we made: all of us, apart from one couple, became really close friends. We see each other at least once a week and have even been on holiday together. It's lovely watching our ever-expanding groups of children grow up together.
Shelley from Hornchurch, mum to Isabella, three

I went to the NHS classes. The best thing was meeting a network of people who have children the same age. Five years on, around eight of us are in regular contact: we meet a couple of times a week; we've been on holiday with one couple, and two are now godparents to my youngest.
Jen from Hertfordshire, mum to Jack, four and Theo, 17 months

Look no further

My mum said that I should be keeping a kick chart to record my baby's movements. Why would I need to do this?
A kick chart is a device for recording your baby's movements over a set period of time. There's no reason at all to keep a kick chart unless you've noticed a significant reduction in your baby's activity – and even then, it's a device that's used less and less now as it's thought to cause extra anxiety amongst mums who might forget to record every movement, sleep through some movements or fail to feel movements whilst they're concentrating on something else. If your baby is moving around to his usual pattern – or thereabouts, given that the space inside your uterus is starting to become a little more limited – then you have no need for concern on this score. If you do notice a drop-off in his activity and feel concerned, contact your midwife immediately. She'll be able to advise you and, if necessary, arrange for you to be monitored to set your mind at rest.

At the tour of the delivery suite, a midwife mentioned the resuscitation trolley they sometimes have to use on newborns, but I didn't really take in what she said. When might this have to be used?

This special unit – sometimes known as the Resuscitaire® – has oxygen and suction for your baby if his air passages are blocked with mucus at birth. If he's having trouble getting breathing after delivery, your midwife will take him to the resuscitation unit and clear his passages of mucus using a small suction tube, then give him a little oxygen to revive him. There's also a special warmer to stabilise your baby's body temperature if necessary. There's no need to panic if your baby goes to the resuscitation unit – it doesn't mean he's unconscious, just that he needs a little help to acclimatise to life outside of you.

I thought swimming was supposed to be good exercise in pregnancy. If this is the case, why does it hurt my back so much?

It's best to avoid swimming breaststroke in late pregnancy, especially if you have any pain in your pelvis or lower back. This is because, even though the stroke itself is gentle and rhythmic, the position you adopt for it can put a strain on your lower body as you curve the small of your back to stay level. Try backstroke instead – it should give you a fantastic feeling of weightlessness whilst being lovely and relaxing and keeping you supple and mobile. Some mums also enjoy special 'aquanatal' classes, which involve gentle aerobic exercise in warm water. If swimming doesn't suit you, you could check out this option at your local leisure centre or health club. Make sure the tutor is properly qualified to teach pregnant women, though.

Who'd have thought?

There's evidence to suggest that babies may dream in the uterus. How do we know this? Because, according to scientists at the Loughborough Sleep Research Centre, rapid eye movement (REM), which happens during dreaming, has been detected in unborn babies – and in the month before birth they may have as much as 10 hours' REM sleep in 24. Ahhh...

Week 28 *91 days to go!*

Don't forget: Start thinking about positions for labour

Obviously, the gods (or your medical team) will, to some extent, influence whether or not you end up as fully mobile as you'd like in labour, but if you've decided that you'll have as active a birth as is available to you, it's a good idea to start trying out positions for labour with your partner now. There are several reasons for this: firstly, it will be more comfy to check out positions and decide which you might want to practise nearer the time before you get much heavier; secondly, you'll get a good idea of positions you probably won't want to practise; thirdly, you'll be able to identify what sort of props might come in handy – like beanbags, body pillows and a couple of Chippendales, for example (and we're not talking armchairs here!). For details of positions to have a first go at, see *Positions for labour*, pp. 276–7.

Hey baby!

Your baby is now more than 10 times heavier than he was at Week 17, weighing in at just over 1kg (around 2.4lb). (Not that it'll feel like all you're carting around with you is little more than a standard bag of sugar: what with the added weight of the placenta, amniotic fluid and extra blood that's coursing round your system, you're more likely to feel like a pack donkey at this stage, and may have put on more like 10kg or 22lb.) Your baby's brain is forming grooves and channels, and his brain tissue is increasing in volume. He's growing plumper, too, and is no longer as wrinkly as he was earlier in pregnancy. Hair is continuing to grow as eyelashes, eyebrows and on his scalp. All in all, he's coming on in leaps and bounds!

All about you

This is a stage of pregnancy when you might be offered more tests to check for gestational diabetes or anaemia, both of which can occur around now if they haven't already – although it's by no means a given that you'll get either: plenty of mums sail through their whole pregnancy without incident. You'll only be offered a diagnostic test for gestational diabetes if glucose is found in your urine or blood, or if you are predisposed to developing it. Influencing factors include:

- having a family history of gestational diabetes
- having previously given birth to a large baby (weighing over 4.5kg/9lb 14oz)
- having previously had a stillbirth
- being overweight or obese
- having polycystic ovarian syndrome (PCOS).

You can read more about gestational diabetes on p. 212.

Anaemia

It's not uncommon for mums-to-be to become anaemic – which means lacking in sufficient red blood cells. Not only do you need more red cells yourself as your blood volume increases; your baby and placenta also need an independent supply of iron, which can only be got from you. So it's a case of supply and demand, and sometimes the demand outweighs the available supply, especially between Weeks 25 and 30 of pregnancy when the concentration of red cells to plasma is at its lowest.

Symptoms are relatively unusual in pregnancy unless the red cell count is very low, but can include unusual tiredness, pallor and – more rarely – dizziness, breathlessness, and palpitations. Anaemia is usually routinely screened for in the second half of pregnancy via a simple blood test, and might need treatment with iron supplements.

Avoiding anaemia

The most important factor in avoiding anaemia in pregnancy is to eat a varied diet that's rich in iron. Best dietary sources of iron include red meat (although avoid liver because of the high vitamin A content which could be harmful to your baby); green leafy veg like spinach and kale; fortified breakfast cereals, well-cooked eggs and baked beans. Iron is absorbed much more efficiently when eaten alongside vitamin C, so drink a small glass of orange juice or include some raw veg or citrus fruits with your meal.

Who'd have thought?

Just as when you're not pregnant, a little exercise can help to lift you out of the dumps when you're feeling a bit down, it will also make it easier to regain your shape post-pregnancy, so try to find something that suits you, and keep it going.

What the netmums say

'Discovering I was anaemic'

I had no idea I was anaemic until I had a routine blood test, which showed I was low on iron. I knew I was tired all the time, but just assumed this was normal. My midwife told me that the demands of the baby were draining me of iron. I was offered iron tablets, but as I was already suffering from constipation I decided to take the dietary route instead and stocked up on leafy greens and all the other iron-rich foods, washed down with orange or grapefruit juice. My iron levels went up gradually and I felt 100 per cent better!
Sheila from Inverness, mum to Angus, four and Linsay, 18 months

I was put on tablets during the second half of pregnancy and at first I ended up really constipated. I didn't know what was worse – knowing I was short of iron or the real pain of the constipation. I didn't realise there were different iron tablets you could take, but the third one I was prescribed seemed to agree with me more. I still think it was worth having the extra iron, especially as I find it hard to eat lots of vegetables.
Inez from Cheltenham, mum to Izzie, four months

What to expect in labour

OK, so maybe you've been avoiding thinking about the onset of labour itself up till now, but you're going to have to face it sooner or later – and, as with all areas of uncertainty in life, forewarned is forearmed so it's well worth mugging up on what to expect.

Early signs of labour

Not all mums experience all the signs of the onset of labour; some don't get any warning at all but just go straight into contractions. (This is relatively unusual, though, so don't get your knickers in a twist about the possibility!) Some of the stuff you might notice happening includes:

- having a 'show'. This means that the thick, often pinkish, blood-stained plug of mucus that's been sealing your cervix (and acting somewhat like a bathplug) comes away and is expelled via your vagina. Some mums notice this in their underwear or when they go to the toilet; for others, it happens while they're actually having a pee and is flushed away without incident! In some mums the plug comes away all in one piece; in others it's expelled in small fragments. A 'show' can happen weeks or hours before the onset of true labour

• your waters breaking. This is when the amniotic sac that's been cushioning your baby throughout pregnancy ruptures and the fluid escapes, again via your vagina. For some mums, this happens in a slow but steady trickle; for others it comes in a big, uncontrollable gush. Either way, it's not worth worrying too much about as there's no way of knowing which will happen to you. You should contact your midwife straightaway after your waters break as you and your baby become vulnerable to infection from this point on and you'll need to be admitted within 12–24 hours if you're having a hospital birth. Some mums' waters don't break until right at the end of their first stage, athough this is relatively unusual. Sometimes your midwife will break your waters with an instrument a bit like a crochet hook to kick-start a slow labour.

True labour

True labour is characterised by the onset of regularly spaced contractions. These start as period-like cramps, and are sometimes accompanied by backache or loose stools. The gap between contractions gets smaller and smaller, and the contractions themselves become more and more powerful as you approach the delivery of your baby. (For information about 'false labour', see p. 257.)

Three stages of labour

Labour happens in three stages: the first, which goes on until you're ready to push; the second, when you deliver your baby; and the third, which is the delivery of the placenta.

The first stage

The first stage of labour is usually the longest, starting from when your cervix begins to dilate – usually with the onset of true contractions – and coming to an end as you reach the pushing stage. Just to complicate things further, there are three phases to the first stage of labour. They are:

The latent phase. This describes the period of time when your contractions are fairly mild, manageable and widely spaced. Lots of mums are able to continue doing light chores during the latent phase: maybe you'll have a bath and wash your hair; change into the clothes you want to wear for the delivery; do a bit of washing up and make a final check that everything's ready for when you bring your baby home. Your waters may already have broken – in which case you'll need to have contacted your midwife to arrange to be admitted to hospital if that's where you're giving birth; some mums' waters don't break until the second stage, sometimes quite close to delivery.

The active phase. Doesn't sound quite so appealing, does it? Actually, though, this is the phase that most mums feel proudest of after the birth. OK, it's the phase that brings the true meaning of the word 'labour' to life, but it's also an engagement between you and your baby, when you are both working together to achieve a successful delivery. During this usually shorter and more intense phase of labour your contractions will be coming thick and fast, at intervals of only three or four minutes, and your waters should break. Once this phase is underway, it's time to call your midwife or doctor if you haven't done so already. If you're having a hospital birth, you'll need to start making your way there.

Transition phase. Once your cervix has dilated to around 8cm – which your midwife or obstetrician will confirm – you'll enter a phase of this first stage of labour known as 'transition'. Your contractions will be even more intense and closely spaced, with a new one coming every couple of minutes and lasting 60–90 seconds. Most mums find themselves in considerably more pain during this phase. As your cervix reaches its full 10cm dilation to allow your baby an escape route, you'll probably have a strong urge to push, which can feel a bit like really needing a poo. It's important that you listen to your midwife closely at this point – or that your birth partner communicates the midwife's instructions to you – as you should only push when she gives you the go-ahead. Some mums experience uncontrollable shaking and nausea during transition caused by a sudden big surge in hormones.

What the netmums say

'How my contractions felt'

I'd had an epidural, but before that the contractions were unlike anything I have ever experienced. I found myself very shocked, surprised and extremely unprepared for how strong they really were. I had my waters broken and within 30 minutes I was in full labour. The only way to describe it is as truly shocking! The anaesthetist did get the epidural going again, but it had worn off a bit by the time I got to the second stage. Whilst it meant most of the pain was gone, I could still feel the contractions, which was a good thing.
Erin from Leeds, mum to Connor, 11 months

To me, the contractions in the first stage felt like someone tightening a belt really hard around my middle and holding it there for ages. I found the pain literally breathtaking and also spooky, as my uterus was doing all these manoeuvres by itself and everything was out of my control. I did panic at first, which made things much worse, but then my boyfriend remembered the breathing exercises and did them with me, close to my face, so I was able to focus on those more. I had to have an epidural about halfway through, but looking back I'm kind of glad to have felt what contractions are really like.
Hayley from Manchester, mum to Harley, 13 months

The second stage

This stage describes the actual delivery of your baby and starts when you get the go-ahead from your midwife to push. First she'll make a final check that your cervix is fully open, then she'll encourage you to push and practise your breathing techniques in between pushes. You might feel burning or stretching sensations in your perineum during this stage, which can last up to an hour or more in first-time mums, but could also be over in as little as 10 minutes (so fingers crossed!). The second stage ends when the midwife or doctor cuts your baby's cord. This is the event you've been working towards all your pregnancy; you may feel overwhelming elation due to a rush of endorphins (or 'happy hormones') relief, exhaustion, fear of the future or a combination of the lot.

The third stage

You may find it hard to believe, but plenty of mums have no recollection of the third stage of labour, which is the delivery of the placenta (also known as the 'afterbirth'). You'll usually be given an injection of Syntometrine into your upper thigh to speed the process up, and this is known as a 'managed' third stage. It usually takes around 10 minutes.

It's your choice whether or not to have a managed third stage, but if you opt for 'unmanaged' – where the placenta is delivered naturally – you'll be more involved as you will have to push your placenta out; the process can take around half an hour or longer, and the average amount of blood loss is greater than in a managed third stage.

Don't feel pressurised into having a managed third stage if you'd prefer not to: as with all aspects of pregnancy, labour and delivery, you really do have a choice, so speak up and remain in control of your experience as far as you feel able. This is another situation where your birth partner could speak up for you if you don't feel able to.

What the netmums say

'What happened during the third stage'

With Caitlin I had the injection and didn't really feel anything, but to be honest I think the birth had left me numb down there anyway. With Lucy there were complications. I can't actually remember having the injection, but the cord was very short and wrapped around her leg, and it broke as the midwife pulled on it. I almost ended up in surgery to have the placenta removed, but they managed to fish it out in the end!
Donna from Manchester, mum to Caitlin, four-and-a-half and Lucy, three-and-a-half

I had an emergency Caesarean, so the placenta was removed at the same time as Natasha. I suppose it's one way of getting out of a normal third stage, but not necessarily one I'd recommend! I guess missing the third stage is something of a positive to come out of a negative, though.
Hilary from Carshalton, mum to Natasha, three

Your mission this week: Think about places to go when you've had your baby

Go out and make a recce of the high-street shops and cafés you might want to visit once you've had your baby. Note down whether or not they encourage breastfeeding; whether there are automatic doors to allow for the smooth passage of your buggy; whether the babycare departments are at ground-floor level; whether or not there's a lift to take you to upstairs; how friendly and helpful the staff are (you'll probably get a good gauge of this when you ask about breastfeeding policies!); whether there are many mums with babies making use of the facilities (this one is always a good indicator of how family-friendly an establishment is); whether there are baby changing facilities and so on. Once you're ready to go out and about with your baby, you'll be glad you've already sussed out where to meet your postnatal chums and where to avoid like the plague (and so will they)!

The Netmums can also give you loads of pointers as to where to go in your area: just log on to your local branch and look for recommendations and warnings. Don't forget to use this fantastic resource of new friends at your fingertips; we Netmums are an invaluable mine of information on just about anything you can think of! And if you can't find answers to your questions, make a posting yourself and watch the answers come flooding in!

Who'd have thought?

Endorphins, sometimes known as 'happy hormones' are released by your brain during labour, and can help to ease the pain and reduce stress. These are also responsible for the natural high lots of mums experience immediately after birth. However, the sudden drop-off of endorphins shortly after birth is thought to be in part responsible for the 'baby blues'.

Look no further

What do real contractions feel like?
It can be hard to distinguish true labour from false labour (see p. 206) – and what with Braxton Hicks contractions thrown into the mix as well, you could be forgiven for worrying about recognising the real deal! The main point of

difference is how long the contractions last and how much time there is in between them. At first, they'll come more or less sporadically, but instead of tailing off or petering out altogether, true labour contractions will gradually increase in length, intensity and frequency. In the beginning they'll feel just like Braxton Hicks – like your uterus tightening involuntarily, then relaxing again. As labour progresses, however, you'll begin to feel some real pain or discomfort as your cervix starts to dilate. Your contractions in the second stage of labour will build and build in intensity, reach a peak, then gradually die back down again. Obviously, the level of pain and discomfort will vary from woman to woman, but it's relatively rare for any mum to escape without noticing a thing! (See also *How my contractions felt*, p. 254.)

What is 'false labour'?
False labour is the onset of contractions that don't get stronger or more frequent, and that don't progress to established labour, eventually petering out. The contractions could either be genuine ones or 'Braxton Hicks' contractions. One reason this condition is called 'false labour' is that some mums do experience pain with the contractions and become convinced that true labour is underway. In reality, these contractions will probably have little effect on your cervix.

Some women have a very long latent phase of labour, where the contractions have some effect on the cervix but it takes days before they become regular and strong. It can be very hard to tell false labour from a long latent phase, and if you're in any doubt, you should seek medical advice from the hospital or midwife. In either case you should get as much rest in as possible before true labour begins.

What exactly is Syntometrine?
Syntometrine is a combination of two drugs: synthetically made oxytocin, which acts like naturally occurring oxytocin in that it encourages strong contractions of the uterus to expel the placenta; and ergometrine, a drug that ensures the contractions close the cervix. Syntometrine is given routinely to new mums to reduce the risk of excessive blood loss after delivery.

In mums who opt for a non-managed third stage of labour, putting their babies to the breast immediately after delivery stimulates the release of the hormone oxytocin which is necessary for the natural delivery of the placenta.

How long will I be in labour?

It's impossible to predict an individual's expected labouring time as there are a number of factors at play in each mum's individual case. Length of labour is influenced by whether or not this is your first delivery; how active you are during labour (and this may not be entirely down to you); how relaxed and in control you are (again this can be hard to influence); whether or not you are confined to a bed for continuous monitoring (ditto!); whether or not you've had an epidural; the way your baby is lying; how active or sleepy your baby is; the size of your pelvis – and any number of other outside factors. Currently, however, the average length of a first labour is around 12–14 hours. Because you have a long, hard job ahead of you, it's well worth trying to get as much rest and nutrition as possible in the last days of pregnancy.

How are you feeling?

Tick the box that most closely represents how you feel about the given statements, then look back to the charts in previous chapters to see how you've changed over the months.

Physically	Emotionally
I've noticed a definite shift from floating to bloating! Strongly agree ☐ Agree ☐ Neither agree nor disagree ☐ Disagree ☐ Strongly disagree ☐	I feel as if I've been pregnant for ever! Strongly agree ☐ Agree ☐ Neither agree nor disagree ☐ Disagree ☐ Strongly disagree ☐
It's getting harder to sleep at night Strongly agree ☐ Agree ☐ Neither agree nor disagree ☐ Disagree ☐ Strongly disagree ☐	I'm closer to my mum than ever before Strongly agree ☐ Agree ☐ Neither agree nor disagree ☐ Disagree ☐ Strongly disagree ☐
I feel sleepy during the day again Strongly agree ☐ Agree ☐ Neither agree nor disagree ☐ Disagree ☐ Strongly disagree ☐	I still don't feel ready to be a parent Strongly agree ☐ Agree ☐ Neither agree nor disagree ☐ Disagree ☐ Strongly disagree ☐
I'm happier eating small meals more frequently Strongly agree ☐ Agree ☐ Neither agree nor disagree ☐ Disagree ☐ Strongly disagree ☐	My partner feels a bit distant Strongly agree ☐ Agree ☐ Neither agree nor disagree ☐ Disagree ☐ Strongly disagree ☐

My boobs are taking over the world!	My mood is more 'up' than 'down' now
Strongly agree ☐ Agree ☐ Neither agree nor disagree ☐ Disagree ☐ Strongly disagree ☐	Strongly agree ☐ Agree ☐ Neither agree nor disagree ☐ Disagree ☐ Strongly disagree ☐
I've got stretch marks Strongly agree ☐ Agree ☐ Neither agree nor disagree ☐ Disagree ☐ Strongly disagree ☐	I'm feeling overwhelmed with decisions to make about the birth itself Strongly agree ☐ Agree ☐ Neither agree nor disagree ☐ Disagree ☐ Strongly disagree ☐

Quick quiz

How well do you know your hormones?

1 What's relaxin?

a. Sittin' down listenin' to my fave sounds

b. A hormone that makes your ligaments and joints go slack

c. The hormone that makes your pregnancy test positive

2 What is Syntometrine used for?

a. To ease a midwife's backache

b. To help deliver the placenta after the birth

c. To kick-start labour

3 What do endorphins do?

a. Help sperm swim up through your cervix

b. Provide you with a natural high in labour

c. Make you pee more

4 What is oxytocin?

a. A cream for reducing stretch marks

b. A naturally occurring hormone that encourages the uterus to contract

c. A pain-relieving drug for labour

5 What's ergometrine?

a. When someone comes to check your workstation is safe for pregnancy

b. A hormone that encourages your cervix to close after birth

c. An injection to help you sleep

Answers: The answers to this quiz are all 'b'.

Mostly a: Oh-dear-oh-dear-oh-dear. Are you serious? These answers aren't even about hormones! They might not be the easiest terms to learn and remember, we agree, but all the same your hormones are responsible for nearly everything that happens to you in pregnancy, so it might just be worth mugging up on them again (see the Glossary, starting on p. 381).

Mostly b: Hooray! Someone's done her homework. You actually deserve to award yourself a gold star as some of the hormones sound very similar to each other and act in similar ways, so well done for paying full attention.

Mostly c: It's kind of endearing that you've tried hard to pick the right answer – but we suspect that you're adopting more of a 'hit and hope' strategy than actually demonstrating your knowledge. Visit the Glossary for a chance to recap!

Part Three

The Third Trimester:
Months 7–9

Chapter 7
Weeks 29–32

Remember when you were waiting to get your first 12 weeks of pregnancy under your belt so you could relax a bit, knowing that the greatest dangers to your baby had passed? It probably seemed like an eternity because you wanted it so much. Now, depending on whether you're desperate to meet your baby at last or whether you're dreading the day when you have to give birth, the same period of time will either drag interminably or race past at the speed of knots! (It goes without saying that those of you who want to get to the end of pregnancy quickly will feel like you're waiting the longest and vice versa!)

During this final trimester, you'll probably begin antenatal classes (if you haven't already); you'll begin practising your breathing techniques and positions for birth (if you haven't already); you'll make your baby's room ready (if you... OK, you can take it as read in each instance!); you'll pack your bags if you're having a hospital birth and receive a midwives' sterile pack if you're planning to deliver your baby at home – and, if you're a working girl, you'll start your maternity leave (yippee!). In short, it's all happening over this next three months – and from a busy-busy point of view, this trimester will make the last one look like a walk in the park!

Week 29 84 days to go!

Don't forget: Be kind to your feet

Plenty of mums find they need shoes another half-size bigger during this last trimester of pregnancy, so get your foot size re-checked. Having uncomfortable feet can make for a miserable life at the best of times, but when you're pregnant it's even worse, so treat your feet kindly and make yourself as comfy as possible. A pair of low heels or low wedges, rather than completely flat shoes, will probably be most comfortable as flat shoes put extra strain on your shins and calf muscles. Remember, it's not just that your feet are retaining water that's making them larger: they may actually be wider and longer because your increased weight means they are slightly flattened and have spread a little.

Try to go for leather shoes or boots, even if it seems a bit of a costly exercise for a relatively short period of time. Actually, your feet may never go back to their pre-pregnancy size, but if they do you can always keep your shoes for subsequent pregnancies; in winter, invest in boots that you can wear afterwards with thicker socks or insoles.

Buy a soothing foot cream and ask your partner to massage your feet for you. It's best done after a lovely soak in a warm bath when the skin is at its softest. Show him how to massage firmly enough that he's not tickling you: maybe you could do his feet first. (OK, maybe not!)

Hey baby!

Your little bundle now weighs around 1.25kg (almost 3lb) and measures around 26cm (just over 10in) from crown to rump. Overall, he measures around 37cm (just under 15in). He's breathing much more rhythmically now and looking more and more like a fully developed baby. He's most likely still tossing and turning about inside you, utilising the available space to the full and reminding you of his presence (as if you could forget!). He'll also be fiddling with his umbilical cord and noticing bright lights with his ever-improving eyesight. In fact, if you shine a powerful torch directly at your bump, you may even get a response from your baby: it's a great party trick when it works!

Who'd have thought?

Microwaves are believed to be safe to use in pregnancy as the amount of radiation emitted is thought to be insignificant.

All about you

Your uterus continues onwards and upwards and the top of it is now about 10cm (4in) above your belly button – and rising! What with the amount of relaxin that's coursing through your veins, you might find you have more twinges in your joints, especially your pelvis, than in recent times. Conversely, though, you might find you can adopt some positions you'd have found difficult or uncomfortable before. Make the most of this while you're still reasonably agile…

Breathing techniques

OK, you probably don't feel in the least ready to start practising breathing exercises for birth, but as we discussed in the last chapter, it's always best to be prepared – and to practise so often that your breathing technique becomes second nature if possible. (There will be plenty of stuff going on once you're in labour without you suddenly finding yourself unable to remember what it was you were supposed to be doing on the breathing front!) Give your birth partner a sharp prod in the ribs when breathing is covered in your antenatal classes, as coaching you to breathe properly is one of the single most important jobs he or she can perform on the big day.

Very much depends on your own individual pain threshold – and for some women, the pain of contractions is too overwhelming to cope with without some serious pain relief – but as you won't know until you're actually in labour, you'll be better equipped if you learn the techniques than if you don't. If it turns out you're one of the lucky mums for whom breathing exercises are a powerful antidote to the pain of contractions, then the right techniques could help see you through the first stage as well as the second, lessening the pain, giving you a focal point and helping to relax you. They're a source of comfort to lots of labouring mums, at least early on, because this is one area of labour they feel they can maintain some control over; breathing exercises can also help to prevent or minimise the risk of a tear during the delivery by controlling the speed at which your baby emerges into the world.

There are different techniques for different stages of labour. Start by practising those that help to ease the pain of the first stage of labour and give you something to focus on:

Breathing for the first stage

- Sit or lie somewhere as comfortably as possible, then shut your eyes and make yourself aware of your own breathing: notice its rhythm and the pattern of your in- and out-breaths. Now start breathing so that your out-breaths are a little longer than your in-breaths, keeping them rhythmical. Try to breathe fairly slowly and steadily. It might help if you repeat the word 're-la-ax' to yourself as you breathe. The 'la-ax' part should last around twice the length of time as the 're' part. Although you might breathe less deeply once a contraction is underway, it's important that the rhythm remains controlled so that you don't start hyperventilating (overbreathing triggered by panic).
- Continue breathing in this way, focusing more on your out-breaths than on breathing in. (Breathing in will happen automatically!) Each time you exhale, visualise your muscles all relaxing, and picture yourself somewhere tranquil and beautiful.
- Try SOS ('sighing out slowly') breathing. Breathe in through your nose, then sigh through your open mouth: don't force your breath out, just allow it to escape gently through your relaxed lips. This technique is helpful in both the first and second stages of labour.

Breathing for the second stage

The second stage of labour is the point at which you'll be ready to push your baby out, and lots of mums have to fight the inclination to hold their breath. It's a very common response to pain, discomfort or anxiety – but as it involves tensing up your muscles, it will only make things worse for you. This is why it's so crucial to practise, practise and practise some more so that you'll be able to breathe more or less automatically when the time comes. If you do end up holding your breath, though, it won't do you or your baby any harm as long as you don't do it for more than a few seconds at a time as prolonged breath-holding can reduce bloodflow to the placenta.

- Imagine your contraction is beginning, and take a deep breath in through your nose. Then breathe out slowly as you push, making sure the effort of pushing is concentrated on your pelvis and not in your throat!
- It can help to visualise your baby progressing down the birth canal so that you push in the correct area.
- Don't try to push for a long period of time whilst holding your breath: this will not only deprive you and your baby of oxygen – it will result in you becoming exhausted very quickly.

Resisting the urge to push

Lots of mums feel they want to push before the cervix has dilated fully, but it's important that you're fully dilated to 10cm before you do push, because until this point there's simply not a wide enough space for your baby to pass through. Your midwife will tell you to resist the urge to push before you reach 10cm; this can be really hard, but you might find that panting helps you to hold off. Practise drawing a sharp breath in, then panting four or five times before breathing in again and repeating the process. Get your birth partner to coach you by saying 'Pant, pant, pant, pant, breathe; pant, pant, pant, pant, breathe' or by doing the breathing technique with you. Some mums find that trying to defy gravity can also help them resist the urge to push, so practise this technique whilst kneeling on all fours with your cheek to the floor and your backside in the air!

Next week, you can start practising positions for labour and delivery (see p. 276): then you'll be able to bring your breathing exercises in, too.

Who'd have thought?

You're likely to remember your dreams better now than at any other time of pregnancy as you're waking from REM sleep more frequently – either to go to the loo or because you're not comfortable. Mums often report vivid or disturbing dreams in the third trimester, but these are nothing to worry about – just your subconscious finding outlets for any fears and anxieties you may have.

What the netmums say

'How breathing helped in labour'

I was a Hospital Play Specialist prior to getting pregnant – a job which had involved being trained in relaxation and breathing techniques. I used breathing techniques from early labour through until I was 8cm dilated. With each contraction I managed to concentrate on slowing down my breathing rather than focusing on the pain, and it certainly helped me to remain calm. The midwives were shocked by how far gone I was when I arrived at the hospital as I was that relaxed! Unfortunately, I then had complications and had to have gas and air, pethidine and an assisted delivery, but had my baby not got stuck I think I would have managed the whole labour with just relaxation and breathing techniques.
Niki from Liverpool, mum to Zak, 23 months

I didn't learn any specific breathing techniques before going into labour, but with my second baby I tried to concentrate on breathing through the contractions, which did help a lot. I still decided to have some pain relief but I didn't feel I needed it as early on. I used the same technique with my third baby, but ended up having a Caesarean, so I'm not sure how long I would have lasted. I found it really useful to concentrate on exhaling and imagining I was blowing the pain away; it still hurt, but concentrating on that took my mind off it a bit.
Fiona from Doncaster, mum to Emma, five, Samuel, three and Holly, seven months

I used breathing and relaxation techniques, and these saw me through to the actual birth after a 10-hour first stage. It was only then that complications made things a bit difficult. Having said that, my daughter didn't make an appearance until I relaxed again. I would have had some pethidine if there'd been time, but by the time I wanted it, it wouldn't have kicked in until after the birth.
Danie from Ipswich, mum to Amelie, seven weeks

Restless Legs Syndrome (RLS)

If you've ever experienced an irresistible urge to move your legs about, which can occur at any time when you're resting (and not just in pregnant mums!) but is especially common at night, you'll know just how infuriating the condition known as Restless Legs Syndrome (RLS) can be. If you've never experienced it, it can be hard to understand what RLS feels like, but some mums have described it as being like a reflex: imagine having your knee reflex tested repeatedly against your will and you'll have some idea of the feeling of helpless discomfort involved: it's a bit like having an itch you can't locate or can't reach. Some mums who've suffered with it before find that RLS comes on more frequently in pregnancy; although the reasons for this remain inconclusive, it's thought that the condition might be linked to anaemia and low iron levels. It's an area where more research is needed, especially as it's thought to affect around 25 per cent of mums-to-be.

Symptoms of RLS

- An uncomfortable or unpleasant urge to move the legs which occurs when you're resting.
- Temporary relief after moving the legs, but a rapid return to symptoms when you stop and rest again.
- A need to move the legs every 10 seconds to a minute.
- Sudden jerks in the legs, especially when dropping off to sleep or whilst asleep.

Around a quarter of pregnant mums get RLS, and it can be worse if you are anaemic. Iron tablets can help in this instance; otherwise, you'll be relieved to learn that symptoms usually disappear after the birth.

Who'd have thought?

The metal-detecting archways you have to walk through at airports are not thought to be harmful to pregnant mums: it's the machines used for scanning hand luggage that utilise X-rays. The passenger scanners utilise low-frequency electromagnetic fields.

Self-help for RLS

You can help to ease or reduce attacks of RLS by:

- keeping to a regular bedtime and not allowing yourself to become overtired before sleeping
- trying not to drop off to sleep before you go to bed
- avoiding caffeinated drinks in the last hour or so before bed
- practising a relaxation technique
- having a warm bath and massaging your legs with baby oil before bed.

What the netmums say

'How I coped with Restless Legs Syndrome'

I had restless legs with all of my pregnancies and it drove me to distraction! Every night was the same – and it's not pretty seeing a nine-months-pregnant lady having a tantrum! I tried all the remedies I'd read about, including drinking tonic water, wearing socks to bed, massaging my legs and walking around before bedtime – all to no avail. With my last pregnancy I discovered that if I drank a large class of cold water, sprayed my legs with cooling foot spray and tried not to get overtired it really helped.

Nicola from Glasgow, mum to Amy, four, Lucy, two and Tom, six months

I've suffered with this since I was pregnant with my first daughter, and it's never gone away totally, but it's 100 times worse when I'm pregnant, particularly towards the end. It put a real damper on being pregnant, and some nights I would lie awake with it for hours getting so cross I actually felt like chopping my legs off! I find I get some relief by putting my legs in the air and doing exercises, like pretending to ride a bike. This gets the circulation going, and it made my legs feel less heavy and irritable – at least for a while anyway!

Emma from Nottingham, mum to Lauren, seven, Katie, five and Chloe, one

Your mission this week: Think about childcare

If you know you'll be needing childcare but still haven't sorted out a place for your child, have another think now. It's well worth paying a few visits to childminders and nurseries so you can get a feel for which option you think would best suit you and your baby. Of course it might be that things change after the birth, but if you wait until then to organise a childcare place, you'll most likely be disappointed, especially as all the best providers have long waiting lists for places. Ask friends for recommendations of childcarers; go to www.childcarelink.gov.uk to find providers in your area; draw up a shortlist once you've made some visits; work out how much each option would cost you and how flexible you'll need your childcarer to be; consider whether you'll have contingency childcare in place (such as a friend or family member) should your arrangements not work out in time.

Look no further

My legs feel really heavy and tired. Is there anything I can do to relieve them?
Lots of mums liken the feelings in their legs in later pregnancy to like walking in leaden boots! The cause is usually sluggish circulation, and is often made worse after sitting or standing for prolonged periods. It's a debilitating feeling, and one which can make you feel very unenergetic and reluctant to walk. You can get cooling gels and lotions to rub into your legs, which can bring some temporary relief to heavy, aching legs. You might also find that using cool compresses on your calf muscles during the evening, and massaging your calves gently – or better still getting your partner to do it for you – will also help. Some mums feel better when wearing support tights; others swear by misting their legs with a cool-water spray. You might also get some relief by resting with your legs elevated to just above hip height, to make circulation easier and reduce swelling due to water retention. Try everything until you find something that works for you.

Who'd have thought?

The pressure in your legs in pregnancy increases to three times what it was before because of the extra volume of blood you're carrying. This can help account for heavy, tired-feeling legs.

What can I do in advance to prepare for a home birth?
Your midwife will be able to advise you on what equipment she'll need you to provide, but often all that's required is a bright, angle-adjustable lamp and a large piece of sheeting to protect your furniture and carpet. Once you've got these at the ready, other ways in which you can prepare are by:

- having a compilation of suitably soothing music ready if you think it will help
- having any special aromatherapy oils for burning or massage at the ready (but make sure you've taken advice from a qualified aromatherapist)
- having food and drinks ready prepared or needing minimal preparation: even if your partner is a champion cook, you'll want him or her with you, not in the kitchen preparing a Michelin-standard meal! There should be enough food for a couple of meals for you and your partner plus snacks and drinks. Don't forget your midwife, either: she could be with you across a couple of mealtimes, so cater for her, too
- having your birthing ball (see *What is a birthing ball?*, p. 280) or other support device at the ready
- having your TENS machine set up, and a supply of fresh batteries at the ready
- having a hospital bag packed just in case you end up transferring for any reason (see p. 307 for what to pack).

Is it safe for me to use an electric foot spa?
Lots of mums do find great relief from foot soreness from using a foot spa. An ordinary foot spa is OK as long as you check that any aromatherapy oils supplied with it are safe to use in pregnancy; otherwise you can use it without oils or add some of your own (having checked for safety with a qualified aromatherapist). Ionic foot spas, however, which claim to counteract the effects of toxins in the body, are not suitable for use in pregnancy, so do read the small print before you purchase a foot spa.

Who'd have thought?

Not drinking enough in late pregnancy can cause more frequent bouts of Braxton Hicks contractions. This condition is referred to by some experts as 'irritable uterus'.

Week 30 77 days to go!

Don't forget: You're three-quarters of the way there at the end of this week!

Reaching and completing Week 30 of pregnancy is another cause for celebration, as the great news is that your baby would have a 90 per cent chance of survival if he were to be born now. The definition of a premature baby is one who is born before the end of Week 37, and there are, of course, degrees of prematurity, but from now on his chances improve all the time. OK, he'd need to spend some time in a special care baby unit (SCBU) if he turned up any time soon, but babies born at this level of maturity are usually sufficiently well developed to come out the other side of the SCBU without further complications.

Hey baby!

Your baby now weighs somewhere in the region of 1.35kg (3lb) and measures around 27cm (just over 10.5in) from crown to rump. His total length from head to foot is now around 38cm (just over 15in), so you can imagine that he's now looking even more like a full-term baby. From now he'll go on growing at a rate of almost 1cm (just under half an inch) a week, and he'll be laying down more and more fat under his skin so that he'll be all plumped out by the time he's ready to emerge into the world. He'll continue opening and closing his eyes and breathing rhythmically in readiness for birth. You might notice more attacks of hiccups in your baby, which may result in more noticeable small jerks or 'jumps' felt in your bump.

All about you

You may well imagine that you can't have much more growing to do yourself, but you'd be surprised! From now you'll put on around 500g (1lb) in weight per week, and this week the top of your uterus is around 10cm (4in) above your belly button. You might experience more heartburn or indigestion now that your uterus has invaded the space usually occupied exclusively by your stomach! Eating small, nutritious snacks regularly, rather than struggling with three main meals each day can help. As in earlier pregnancy, you might also find it helps to avoid eating late in the evening, and to prop yourself up with pillows so you're not lying flat at night. If you were discovered to have a low-lying placenta at an early scan (see p. 282), you might have another around now to check whether or not it has risen up out of your pelvis and away from your cervix.

Pre-eclampsia

This is the commonest of the serious conditions of pregnancy, affecting around 10 per cent of first-time mums-to-be, but as long as you attend all your antenatal screening appointments, it will usually be caught sufficiently early to prevent harm to you or your baby. Signs can begin to emerge at any time, usually after Week 20, often in the third trimester, although you may not have any actual symptoms yourself and the cause is unknown. The signs your midwife and medical team will be looking out for include: oedema (swelling, particularly of the ankles, hands and face, due to abnormal water retention); a rise in blood pressure and protein in the urine – hence the need for regular blood pressure and urine checks, and the reason why you should keep all your antenatal appointments. If you have any of these symptoms in isolation, however, it doesn't necessarily mean you have pre-eclampsia.

Symptoms of more serious problems may develop if pre-eclampsia continues unchecked. These include:

- headaches
- blurred or distorted vision
- nausea and/or vomiting
- shortness of breath
- pain in the shoulder or abdomen
- general confusion.

If you become aware of any of the above symptoms, you should report them to your midwife or doctor as soon as possible. If left untreated, pre-eclampsia can lead to eclampsia – or convulsions – which although rare can prove deadly, with one in 50 mums and one in 14 babies dying as a result. Around 44 per cent of mums who develop eclampsia have their first convulsion soon after delivery rather than in pregnancy itself; 38 per cent are first affected in pregnancy and 18 per cent experience fits during labour.

If you do develop pre-eclampsia, you may be admitted to hospital for complete rest whilst the symptoms are attended to, and may need medication – although this is by no means inevitable. Once you've been diagnosed, you can expect to have more frequent antenatal appointments and extra monitoring of your health and your baby's wellbeing to keep tabs on the progress of the condition. This will mean more blood-pressure checks and blood tests, as well as possible scans of your placenta and extra checks on your baby's heartbeat. The high blood pressure associated with pre-eclampsia often forces doctors to deliver babies early, as sustained high blood pressure can cause oxygen deficiency in the newborn. Most mums with pre-eclampsia still deliver perfectly healthy babies.

Who'd have thought?

Although paracetamol is considered safe to take in pregnancy (on medical advice), you should avoid ibuprofen as it can cause heart and kidney problems in your baby during this final trimester.

What the netmums say

'Coping with pre-eclampsia'

My blood pressure was normal right through my pregnancy until Week 36. My doctor then found it was very high, so they decided to keep me in hospital overnight. It didn't improve, though, and I was at the hospital every second day to have blood and urine tests. Each time the results were different, so nothing was done, but I was told I was borderline pre-eclampsia. At 37 weeks, the baby's growth slowed down, and was found to be below the normal rate, but still nothing was done. I decided at 38 weeks to stop going into hospital every second day, as they obviously weren't going to do anything about it. Consequently, at my 40-week check-up appointment, my blood pressure was sky high and I was experiencing blurry, spotty vision, dizziness and headaches. The doctor decided to break my waters, and within eight hours Connor was born.

Erin from Leeds, mum to Connor, 11 months

At 26 weeks I began to suffer from migraines and morning sickness. I went to a routine antenatal appointment and the midwife found protein in my urine sample, and very high blood pressure. I was sent straight to hospital, where I was admitted and given steroids to mature my baby's lungs in case I had to deliver. I also had a scan and everything seemed OK. My blood pressure yo-yoed from normal to extreme for four weeks, and I spent most of this time in hospital. I was scanned again at 30 weeks while in hospital, and they found that the blood flow through the umbilical cord was reduced. The doctors were concerned the baby wasn't getting enough oxygen; also she hadn't grown at all in four weeks. I went back up to the ward and was told by a consultant to expect to have to deliver within 48 hours. That afternoon, while being monitored, my blood pressure went up to 180 over 125 and I began to see black shadowy shapes in front of my eyes. My hubby was phoned and I was taken down to theatre for an emergency Caesarean. Charlotte was born, weighing 2lb 6 oz, and was rushed straight into the neonatal unit, hooked up to a ventilator and put in an incubator. I was told in recovery that the cord had broken down significantly and, had I remained pregnant for much longer, I would have haemorrhaged. I remained in hospital for two weeks until my blood pressure came down, and Charlotte was in for a whole month. Although small, she did fantastically well and came home weighing just 3½lb.

Berni from Stoke-on-Trent, mum to Charlotte, five, Alex, four, Rosie, two and Jack, seven months

Positions for labour

Now you've got into practising breathing techniques for labour (see p. 265) it's time to turn your attention to positions you can adopt during labour that may make you more comfortable and help accelerate the whole process. It's a really good idea to start trying out positions now whilst you're still relatively agile and not yet too heavy for your partner to practise supporting. As long as you practise often, when the time comes you'll be able to move around between positions without having to refer to a manual, and your partner will have got used to your increasing weight, so that it won't come as so much of a strain when labour is underway. Try to practise a couple of times a week from now until the birth.

Positions to try

There's nothing complicated about positions for labour: the important thing is that you give yourself options. Once strong contractions are underway, you'll probably want to move around to try to alleviate the pain, and some positions will feel more comfortable at different stages than others. Try:

- sitting back-to-front on a chair, with a cushion or pillow to rest your forearms and head on
- standing leaning against your partner, facing towards them, with your arms around his or her neck and your head on his or her shoulder
- leaning forwards on to a work surface (in the delivery suite this could be the bed) with your head down on your forearms
- kneeling – on all fours on a large floor cushion or pillow, leaning on to a birthing ball, your partner's lap or a chair
- going down on one knee
- sitting on a birthing ball, rocking backwards and forwards
- lying on your left side (to allow optimum blood flow from your legs back to your heart), with your right leg and arm slung over pillows or a full body bolster
- squatting supported under the arms by your partner, or with your back against a bed or sofa and your elbows and forearms on the surface. This is particularly helpful in the later stages of labour, to help encourage the pelvis to open up more fully
- rocking your pelvis backwards and forwards in any position: this will help to distract you from the pain as well as encourage your baby down the birth canal.

If you have severe backache, your baby might be lying with his spine against yours. This position, known as a 'posterior lie' can be extremely uncomfortable, but you can help to ease the pain by getting into one of the all-fours positions described previously.

Resisting the urge to push

Trying to resist the urge to push, even with breathing techniques (see p. 267), can be incredibly difficult – a bit like trying not to poo once you're already on the toilet. One way you can help yourself is to adopt an 'anti gravity' position on all fours, but with your head down on your forearms and your bottom in the air.

Positions for pushing

It makes sense to try to remain as upright as possible when it comes to pushing your baby out, as you'll be going with gravity. Kneeling or squatting with your arms around your birth partner's neck are proven to be effective for lots of mums, and going on to all fours is a good position for the actual delivery as it reduces the speed of your baby's emergence into the world and will reduce the risk of your perineum tearing.

Epidurals and pushing

If you're totally numb from the waist down, your midwife can still encourage you to push at the right times by prompting you whenever a contraction comes: she'll know this is happening by keeping her hand on your bump so she can feel your uterus tightening. This doesn't mean, though, that there's only one position for you in labour: you could lie on your left side and ask your partner to lift your right leg during contractions as you push; if you want to turn on to your back in between times, you'll need some pillows under your lower back to make it easy for you to roll over on to your side again. If you have a mobile epidural (see p. 96), you should be able to move around more than with a normal epidural. As long as you do find yourself reasonably mobile, all the positions detailed above are open to you if you have enough sensation to be able to maintain them.

Who'd have thought?

Whilst the average length of pregnancy is 280 days, the duration of your own pregnancy will be down to chance and is not influenced by factors like your race, age, weight or number of previous pregnancies you've had.

What the netmums say

'Taking our positions!'

I hadn't really thought about positions – I always thought I'd just go with the flow when the time came and do whatever felt comfortable. The midwife suggested I turn on to my side to help with the pain, and I ended up staying that way, with one leg in the air and my arm wrapped around it holding on to hubby's hand for extra anchorage! In the other hand, of course, was the gas & air breathing pipe!'
Emma from Bedford, mum to Geordan, two

All I knew was that I did not want to give birth on my back. In the end, I had a water birth and switched between pushing on all fours then kneeling while hanging on to the side of the pool. I'd definitely do it that way again!
Amy from Enfield, north London, mum to Lola, eight months

Your mission this week: Keep exercising

Although you may feel that exertion is becoming more difficult and it would certainly be easier to just sit down and put your feet up whenever you have free time, keeping as toned as possible can only give you an advantage for labour and delivery. Even if you run into difficulties on the day of the birth, you'll have more stamina and flexibility if you manage to keep exercising to some extent.

You may have to re-think the form of exercise you take, especially if you've been continuing with pre-pregnancy activities, because now that more relaxin is flooding your system your joints will be more vulnerable. However, swimming, brisk walking (perhaps on a treadmill in a gym), using light weights (with the supervision of a gym instructor who is experienced in overseeing pregnant mums) and aquarobics (without over-stretching yourself) are all still good bets.

Look no further

Are some mums more likely to develop pre-eclampsia than others?
Yes, the condition is most common in first pregnancies and in mums with a
family history of pre-eclampsia. You're also more at risk if you're a teen
mum; if you're over the age of 40; if you're carrying more than one baby; if
you had high blood pressure before you became pregnant; if you have a body
mass index (BMI) over 30; if you're diabetic; or if you've suffered from kidney
disease. Around 5 per cent of mums who get pre-eclampsia in their first
pregnancy will develop it again in a subsequent pregnancy.

What is a birthing ball?
It's basically the same as an exercise ball you can find in a gym and that's
used in some exercise classes – a large PVC ball you inflate yourself to your
required size and rigidity using the pump provided. It allows you to sit
and rock your pelvis to and fro during labour, and also acts as a great
support when kneeling. If you like the sound of a birthing ball, you can
buy one for £20–£30 (including power pump) from pregnancy and
nursery outlets; some outlets do have them for hire for about £10 for five
weeks, and some hospitals also provide them free of charge. Make sure you
get one well in advance of your EDD as it's not only a good idea to practise
sitting and rocking on it – it's also a good aid to exercise before and after
the birth.

What is a birthing stool?
A birthing stool looks a bit like a frontless loo: it's a crescent-shaped chair
with a hole in the seat that allows a mum to stay in an upright position when
pushing her baby out. They are considered very old-fashioned and are rarely
used these days, although some hospitals do still have them available, so it's
worth making enquiries first if the idea appeals to you.

Who'd have thought?

Travel to countries where you need to be vaccinated against
disease is generally not recommended in pregnancy because of a
possible risk of transmission of the live vaccine to the baby.

Week 31 70 days to go!

Don't forget: Keep up those pelvic floor exercises

Have you been practising your pelvic floor exercises for the past 13 weeks since we last discussed them? (They're the special toning exercises that strengthen the girdle of muscles supporting the pelvis, and help to prevent stress incontinence and intercourse problems later on.) If you have, you'll have done yourself some huge favours, especially for after the birth. If you haven't, it's not too late to start. Turn to p. 158 to read up on the technique again, then start to exercise in earnest. It'll be harder to get your pelvic floor back into shape after the birth if you haven't primed the muscles in advance – and you'll have plenty of other things on your mind, too! However, starting well ahead of labour means they'll become second nature and won't seem such a chore after the event.

Hey baby!

Now your baby weighs around 1.6kg (3.5lb) and measures around 28cm (just over 11in) from crown to rump. His total length from head to toe is around 40cm (just under 16in). Given that the average birth weight in the UK in full-term babies is around 3.3kg – with boys weighing approximately 300g more than girls – you can see that your baby will roughly double his weight between now and the birth! In contrast he's already reached around 80 per cent of his birth length, so it's clear that the extra weight will be largely accounted for by your baby 'fleshing out'. Although your uterus might feel quite full by now, it's actually the pressure on your other organs you're feeling because it's still growing upwards: there's still enough room for your baby to continue moving fairly vigorously, even though you might have noticed that he's slowed down a bit compared with earlier activity. By now you'll probably be very familiar with his different sleepy and wakeful times.

All about you

The top of your uterus is now around 31cm (just over a foot!) from your pubic bone, and around 11cm (four-and-a-half inches) from your belly button. Your uterus is now filling most of your abdomen, meaning that your other organs will continue to feel the pressure until it drops slightly into your pelvis in the next few weeks; it also means your baby will gradually feel more restricted, and you may find you feel him moving around less vigorously from around now. As long as you still feel him moving every day, though, this isn't a cause for concern. By now you should have put on something between one-and-a-half to two stones).

Placenta praevia

In some mums the placenta attaches too low in the uterus and either partially or entirely covers the cervix. It's often discovered at the anomaly scan mums have at around 20 weeks, when it might have been described as a 'low-lying placenta'. This isn't necessarily a cause for concern, as the majority of low-lying placentas lift up and away from the cervix as pregnancy progresses. However, in 1 in 10 mums the placenta continues to obscure the cervix partially – blocking the baby's exit route. This is known as placenta praevia. If the cervix is covered entirely, it's known as major placenta praevia.

Diagnosis

The best way to confirm placenta praevia, one symptom of which can be vaginal bleeding in pregnancy, is with a transvaginal ultrasound scan. This is when a probe with a microscopic camera is inserted into your vagina whilst you lie on your side, and it allows a much clearer view of your placenta and uterus than your doctor would get from an ultrasound scan. It's not painful – at worst a little uncomfortable – and poses no risk to your baby. For more on transvaginal scans, see p. 69.

What happens next

If placenta praevia is diagnosed, you'll probably be offered a further scan at 32 to 36 weeks; if your placenta is less than two centimetres from the cervix at this time, you will almost certainly need a Caesarean section and might need a general anaesthetic. You are also more likely to need a blood transfusion after a Caesarean.

If you have major placenta praevia, your doctor might want to admit you to hospital after 34 weeks of pregnancy. Even if you haven't experienced any bleeding to date, there's a small risk that you could bleed suddenly and severely, which might mean an emergency Caesarean needs to be performed.

What the netmums say

'Coping with placenta praevia'

Placenta praevia was detected during an early scan, and although it didn't affect most of the pregnancy, the last six weeks were pretty boring as I wasn't allowed to do anything much or go anywhere. I had to stay close to the hospital and have someone on standby to rush me in if I started bleeding or went into labour. It felt a bit like being under house arrest! I was booked to have a Caesarean a week before my EDD. When I arrived at the hospital, I was not told it would have to be done under general anaesthetic because of the position of the placenta and the risk of rupture and heavy bleeding. This was very upsetting for me and my husband, but everything went OK and I had a wonderful baby boy, Owain, weighing 7lb 7oz. Having been sterilised nine years ago and having had a reversal five years ago but then taking all that time to become pregnant, Owain was the baby we thought we'd never have.

Lynette from Aberdare, south Wales, mum to Owain, two

'Small/large for dates' babies

Sometimes a baby's size might not seem to tie in with his gestational age (the date from which pregnancy was dated): some babies are significantly smaller or larger than expected. You might, in this case, be told that your baby is either 'small for dates' or 'large for dates'. Any discrepancy in a baby's size for dates is usually picked up at a routine antenatal check, when your midwife measures the height of your fundus in relation to your pelvic bone and feels your baby's size by palpating (manually investigating) your bump.

Small baby

When a baby grows at slower than the expected rate, this is sometimes referred to as Intra-Uterine Growth Retardation (IUGR), and if this is the case with your baby you'll probably be offered some investigations and more regular scans to check things out and plot his progress. Distinguishing between a small but healthy baby and one which is suffering from poor growth is an inexact science, so don't panic if you're sent for investigation. Most likely you'll be referred for a series of regularly spaced, detailed scans which will look at your baby's proportions, the amount of amniotic fluid you're carrying and how well the blood is flowing through the umbilical cord. If all is well, your dates may need to be re-calculated; if not, you might be advised to have your baby delivered early, in which case you'll probably be sent to a specialised premature baby unit where the team will oversee your delivery and care for your baby afterwards.

Large baby

Some babies are just big – and there can be a family trend here. Usually it's not a cause for concern, as your baby can't become overweight in the uterus through taking too many nutrients from you. If you're diabetic, however, your baby's growth will be monitored carefully throughout the remainder of your pregnancy, as sometimes too much glucose can cross the placenta making your baby overweight before he's even delivered. This can not only mean your birth may be more difficult; it can also put your baby at risk of a plummet in blood-sugar levels at birth, as his rich source of glucose is cut off from him. He might also have some respiratory problems at birth. Either way, if you're diabetic, you should expect your baby to spend a little time in a Special Care Baby Unit (SCBU), although it's not necessary in all cases. You can help your baby and yourself by following the strict low-fat, low-sugar diet you'll be prescribed for the rest of your pregnancy to reduce the adverse effect of your diabetes.

The growth rate of twins and multiples

Twins and multiple foetuses usually grow slower than single babies and don't always grow at the same rate as each other. In twins who share a placenta (monochorionic twins), this can be as a result of one twin being attached via more efficient blood vessels, and therefore enjoying better nutrition. If your twins are found to be growing at different rates, their progress will be monitored carefully to check on the growth rate of the smaller baby. In very rare cases, a major complication can occur in monochorionic twins: it's a condition called Twin to Twin Transfusion (TTT), and it happens when there's an imbalance of circulating blood and amniotic fluid. The condition is life-threatening for both twins and it needs prompt and expert treatment in utero.

What the netmums say

'Finding out my baby was the "wrong" size'

I measured small throughout my pregnancy and my midwife was convinced I was a closet smoker! There was no need for extra scans as I was only a couple of weeks behind my dates in terms of size. As it turned out I gave birth to an 8lb 3oz baby – not bad for someone with a very small frame!

Amy from Enfield, north London, mum to Lola, eight months

My baby was on the big side, so I was tested for gestational diabetes but the test came back negative. Then my community midwife said she reckoned the baby would be around 7lb – but three days before my due date I gave birth to Kiera and she weighed 9lb! I'm so glad I didn't go overdue as I'm only little!

Abbie from Norfolk, mum to Kiera, 10-and-a-half months

I was sent for a scan at 32 weeks as my midwife thought my baby was going to be on the large side. At the scan they told me my baby would probably be over 10lb at full term; they even told me I'd have to consider a Caesarean as I might not be able to deliver her vaginally. I was really scared and confused as to why my baby was growing so big: I thought maybe I'd eaten too much during the pregnancy or done something else wrong! I eventually had my baby at 42 weeks, delivering her vaginally without any pain relief – and she weighed 8lb 6oz.

Marie from Chorley, mum to Emily, 13 months

With my first pregnancy they found my son was big for 27 weeks and the hospital brought my due date forward by two weeks. Then at 33 weeks his growth slowed down and was averaging out, so they gave me my original due date back. In the end I went two weeks over my due date and had to be induced. The pregnancy was perfectly healthy, but I still reckon it was the craving for large quantities of full-fat milk a day from six months of pregnancy that made him grow so fast. After all, he was 9lb 3oz and 22 inches long!

Alicia from London, mum to Kyrus, two, Demiyah, one, and 14 weeks pregnant

I got halfway through my last pregnancy when they started questioning my dates: I didn't measure up for my weeks. At every appointment after that I'd be asked, 'Are you sure your dates are right? Do you smoke? Do you drink?' No, I didn't smoke or drink. I can't remember how many extra scans I had because of this. All I did was worry for the rest of my pregnancy, and then I was told I couldn't go to a birthing centre to have my baby as I was now high risk! Eventually I got to see a lovely doctor who told me that I wasn't to let anything worry me, and that I was a skinny girl who wasn't built to have a big baby. In the end, 16 days early, I gave birth to a very healthy 5lb 9½oz baby boy. This time around I won't let anyone worry me unless there is a really good reason.

Emma from Slough, mum to Charlie, 10, Aiden, one, and 25 weeks pregnant

Your mission this week: Think about taking off your jewellery

Remove any jewellery that's getting tight, and take steps to reduce swelling. You might find it hard to get your rings off, for instance – in which case it's sensible to take them off while you still can, and before they need to be cut off! If you're married or usually wear a ring and feel self-conscious or 'undressed' without your wedding ring or other jewellery, why not treat yourself to a couple of pieces of inexpensive dress jewellery just for now? Or how about asking your partner if you could wear his ring until your own fingers shrink back to normal size?

If you find that your shoes are tight after an hour or so's wear, or that you can't get them back on your feet once you've taken them off, and as long as you have no other symptoms (see p. 274), this is due to poor circulation and water retention: the good news is that you can help prevent this by drinking plenty of fluids and avoiding crossing your legs or ankles, and by wearing non-restrictive socks, stockings, tights and other clothing.

Who'd have thought?

Babies lay down two types of fat in late pregnancy: brown fat, which generates heat and is necessary from birth, and white fat, which provides energy.

Look no further

I've heard you can have too much or too little amniotic fluid. Why does this happen and is it dangerous?

Having too much amniotic fluid (or 'waters') is a condition known as polyhydramnios, and is usually picked up when your midwife finds your uterus is too large for your dates. She's more likely to suspect polyhydramnios if your uterus is big and yet she's finding it hard to feel your baby properly. There are several reasons why you might have too much fluid:

- it's more common in diabetic mums
- it can indicate a problem with your placenta
- it might mean your baby is having difficulty with his swallowing mechanism
- it's more common in mums who are carrying more than one baby.

Polyhydramnios can lead to your waters breaking early and your baby being delivered prematurely, so you might need to have some of the fluid drained off at regular intervals until the birth. If you're diabetic, improving your control of the condition can resolve the problem. If your baby's having problems swallowing, he might need surgery at birth.

Having too little amniotic fluid is called oligohydramnios. A lack of water can mean your placenta isn't functioning properly; your baby's kidneys or bladder aren't working properly; your baby is overdue (if you're in late pregnancy); your waters are leaking. Whatever the reason, you'll be offered a scan to check on your baby's growth and development. If all is well, you'll probably just be monitored more closely with more frequent scans and appointments. If you're nearing the end of pregnancy and there are potential problems with your baby, induction might be suggested to you. Some experts believe that increasing the amount of water you drink can help to increase your levels of amniotic fluid.

Who'd have thought?

Autumn- and winter-born babies are more likely to be at their best in the mornings, whilst those born in the spring and summer are more likely to be evening types.

Week 32 63 days to go!

Don't forget: Check out contingency maternity units

Sometimes the unthinkable happens and there's 'no room at the inn' on the day you go into labour. Although it's relatively unusual, some mums have been referred to maternity units many miles away – so, although it's probably the very last thing you want to contemplate, you should make a point of asking your medical team where else you might have to make your way to if they can't attend you. If there are other maternity units local to you, it's worth paying them a visit, introducing yourself and asking if it's possible to have a quick tour just so you are not completely unfamiliar with the set-up should you have to transfer there at the last minute.

Hey baby!

Your baby has now reached a weight of around 1.8kg (nearly 4lb) this week, having put on 200–250g (around half a pound) in a week! He's plumping out nicely and now measures about 29cm (only 1cm short of a foot) from crown to rump and is 42cm (just over 16.5in) long from head to toe. Your baby might adopt a head-down position in the uterus around now, although he could still shift back out of it again. With any luck, though, if he does perform a headstand he'll stay that way until the birth.

All about you

The top of your uterus has continued to rise upwards in your abdomen – but if you've been thinking it can't possibly get very much higher, the good news is that this time you're right! The top of the uterus is about 32cm (nearly 13 inches) above your pubic bone and it's about 12cm (5 inches) above your belly button. Around now, especially if your baby has turned head down, it'll be heading towards reaching its highest point. Enjoy it while you may: once the baby's head engages (drops into the pelvis in readiness for birth) at around Week 36, you'll feel the relief of having more space to breathe and more capacity for eating – but the pay-off for that might well be a heavy, uncomfortable feeling between your legs and a rather ungainly waddling gait!

Caesareans

We now have an average Caesarean rate in the UK of 15.3 per cent – that's one in every 6.5 births – with around 50 per cent of these performed as unplanned (or 'emergency') sections. Much as you probably hope and imagine that you won't be one of the mums who end up having a Caesarean delivery – especially if your particular NHS Trust has a generally low Caesarean rate – it's always best to be prepared. If you haven't read up on what could happen and what the procedure might be, it could be alarming – even frightening – to have to go through it unprepared on the day. With a bit of luck and a following wind you won't need the information, but as we've discussed before forewarned is forearmed, so do take in as much as you can, just in case.

What is a Caesarean?

A Caesarean, also known as a Caesarean section or C-section, is a major operation where a surgical incision is made through the abdomen and uterus – usually along the bikini line – in order to deliver a baby who cannot be born vaginally. The procedure can be carried out under local (epidural or spinal) anaesthetic if time allows, or under general anaesthetic in extreme emergencies or in other cases where a local anaesthetic is not appropriate.

'Emergency' Caesarean

Although around half of all Caesareans performed are classed as 'emergency' – a term that implies full-scale, red-light action – in many cases the term actually means 'unscheduled' or 'non-elective'. True, there are some situations which can be classed as emergencies, but in other cases there is time to consider the implications and other possibilities. Situations where an emergency Caesarean may be performed include:

- where mother and baby are becoming exhausted or distressed and labour is not progressing well
- where the baby is found to have moved into a transverse (sidelong) or difficult breech position (see p. 304)
- where there is previously undiagnosed pelvic disproportion (see p. 297), which means the baby's head is too large to pass through the birth canal
- where the placenta starts to come away from the wall of the uterus and there's a risk of heavy bleeding (haemorrhage).

If you have an epidural in place already, you will have this topped up for surgery; if not, you'll need to have a general anaesthetic, which will mean your partner won't be able to be present at the birth.

Elective Caesarean

In an 'elective' (pre-planned) Caesarean, the decision to deliver your baby surgically is made during pregnancy so that there is time to plan events. Situations where you might be counselled to have an elective Caesarean include:

- if you have serious pre-eclampsia which is threatening the wellbeing of you or your baby
- if you are having twins or more babies (although some hospitals are happy for you to try for a vaginal delivery with twins if the babies are in a compatible position)
- if you have a pre-existing condition that means labour could prove too stressful for you
- if your baby is in a transverse (sidelong) position and can't be manipulated
- if you have placenta praevia (see p. 282) or another placental complication
- if you have known pelvic disproportion (see p. 297), where your baby's head is too large to pass through the birth canal
- if your baby is in a difficult breech position which your medical team considers incompatible with vaginal delivery – although you may want to get a second opinion on this as many breech babies can be delivered perfectly safely vaginally. Go to www.rcmnormalbirth.org.uk to read about the Royal College of Midwives' Campaign for Normal Birth.

There are advantages to having an elective Caesarean: you'll not only know the date on which your baby will be born (unless he makes an unscheduled early appearance!), you'll also be able to arrive at the hospital in as calm and prepared a state as possible. You won't have to endure the pain of labour either – although some mums see this as a mixed blessing, as they can end up feeling that they haven't experienced childbirth 'properly' (see *How I recovered from a Caesarean*, p. 293–4).

First, an epidural or spinal will be set up (see p. 96) so that you can be awake and alert for the birth. (It's usually not an option to have general anaesthetic unless this is already known to be necessary. This is because of the inherent risks of general anaesthetic during any procedure.) Having a Caesarean under an epidural means your partner will be able to be present, too, which wouldn't be possible in the case of a general anaesthetic.

Physical recovery

A Caesarean is a major abdominal operation from which you'll need to allow yourself time to recover, both physically and emotionally. It usually takes a good six weeks for the wound to heal, and you'll probably be advised not to drive in that time (usually for insurance purposes, so it's worth having a word with your own insurer to see what their policy is on this). You should be visited by a midwife once you're back home, who'll check on your wound and change dressings if necessary – but as resources in some areas are woefully inadequate you might have to make trips up to the hospital or to your GP practice. Do make sure you get prompt medical attention if you're in any way unhappy with your wound or any other aspect of your Caesarean. You can always go back up to the maternity unit unannounced if necessary. Some mums have said that it took six months to a year before they felt fully back to their normal physical selves.

Ways in which you can help your own recovery include:

- delegating all jobs that require lifting, shifting, bending and stretching to someone else (hurrah!). If this isn't possible because your partner has had to return to work and you're alone with your baby during the daytime, make sure you have as much of the equipment as possible that you'll need for the day at hand, and let everything that doesn't need doing urgently wait!
- keeping tabs on your Caesarean wound: whilst you don't want to be getting it out and exposing it to infection all the time, if you experience undue pain or notice any redness, bleeding or oozing from or around the site, pain in your calves or fever, get medical advice straightaway as you may have contracted an infection. If it's late at night and you can't get to a doctor's or up to the maternity unit call NHS Direct on 0845 46 47
- supporting your wound when you stand, sit or lift your baby
- drinking peppermint tea to help ease the wind many mums experience after abdominal surgery
- eating a varied, nutrient-rich diet and drinking lots of water to keep your strength up and flush out your bladder regularly.

Emotional recovery

Some mums feel cheated of a normal birth after having a Caesarean; others feel that they are in some way inadequate because they've not managed a vaginal birth; if you've had an elective Caesarean, you might feel regretful that you haven't experienced labour at all; if your operation was performed under general anaesthetic, you might feel that you missed out on the birth altogether, and bonding with your baby could take longer. All of these feelings are perfectly normal, and you can help ease yourself over them by discussing them with your midwives, doctors and partner. You'll probably be encouraged to focus on the fact that you have successfully delivered a healthy baby – but don't allow yourself to be fobbed off with platitudes. If you feel depressed about your experience, say so: you are more vulnerable to postnatal depression, which can develop into a serious illness if left untreated.

You can help your own emotional recovery if you:

- talk over the circumstances of your Caesarean with your midwife or obstetrician: you might feel you need to do this more than once, especially if the decision to operate was taken quickly and suddenly
- ask to be referred to the Birth Afterthoughts Service if your hospital has one and you have had a particularly traumatic delivery: this can be tremendously useful in helping you come to terms with the experience. If the Service is unavailable to you, contact the Birth Trauma Association (www.birthtraumaassociation.org.uk) – a free service run by volunteer mums – or consult the Netmums for their experiences and advice: they're an invaluable resource, and there's nothing like communicating with other mums who've been through the same as you have.

Who'd have thought?

If you do end up travelling in your third trimester – whether to the UK or abroad – first check out the medical facilities in and around your destination. You should always carry your medical notes with you so that other doctors will have all of your medical information to hand.

What the netmums say

'How I recovered from a Caesarean'

I'd planned a water birth in a midwife-led unit, but as soon as my contractions started I just knew something wasn't right. I was 8cm dilated after four hours, and if everything had been the way it should have then Lara would have popped out into the water like a dream. It turned out she was breech and she'd opened her bowels and was inhaling meconium [a baby's first bowel movement]. This meant she was in danger and would have to be delivered immediately. The midwife told me we didn't even have time to wait for a wheelchair to take me down to the hospital's labour ward, so she and my husband carried me to the lift and down two flights of stairs. I wasn't frightened about having an emergency Caesarean as I knew I was in the best place, and I had complete trust in the nursing staff. Lara was taken away to Special Care to help her with her breathing. The next day I had to wait until the catheter was removed before I could get to see her. I bonded with her the first time I held her properly, although it was almost 12 hours after she was born. Luckily my husband was off work for six weeks, which was a huge help, but in any case I was walking and back on my feet the morning after the section. It was sore, not too painful, and I felt every time I stood up that my bottom half would come away from my top half – but surprisingly that didn't happen! I'm proud of my scar, and tell Lara, 'That's where the doctor had to cut Mummy to get you out because we couldn't wait to see you.' I don't feel a failure at all: there was absolutely nothing I could do about it and I've never once worried about it.
Ruth from Greenock, mum to Lara, two-and-a-half

When I was pregnant with my daughter, I was at high risk for pre-eclampsia, so the decision was taken to induce me at 38 weeks. Three days later there was still no sign of labour starting, so the doctors had no choice but to give me a section. The recovery was hard: I was in agony for a week and my scar wouldn't heal properly for months afterwards. I couldn't manage breastfeeding and felt like a failure. In the end I developed postnatal depression and my bond with Emma was definitely affected. We didn't really bond until she was around 18 months old. My son was born by elective Caesarean, which was a very different experience. I felt fine afterwards: I recovered very quickly and it wasn't half as bad as my first section. I bonded with my son straightaway and managed to breastfeed him. I've also managed to stay free of postnatal depression this time. *Susan from Dudley, mum to Emma, two and Nathan, eight months*

I was advised to have a planned Caesarean in my second pregnancy as I'd had an induced forceps delivery with Jacob, which was awful. I nearly died through loss of blood due to Jacob tearing my cervix badly: no one had realised I was bleeding as he was stuck and acting as a plug and the blood was flowing back into my uterus. I had very bad postnatal depression afterwards, although it didn't affect my bond with Jacob. As I'm a nurse and have spent years working in an obstetric theatre, I wasn't at all worried about the Caesarean: I'd rather a planned one than an emergency. The operation was planned for Week 39, but my waters broke late in Week 37, so I went into hospital and spent the morning waiting to go to theatre. The section was done under spinal and it was great. I was out of hospital 72 hours later, and the day after we came home I walked to the local park and around six football pitches! I bonded with both children equally, although my post-section recovery was a lot quicker than my recovery from Jacob's birth, and this time I didn't feel violated. In fact, I feel I lost out more with my vaginal delivery as none of it was in my control: my body wouldn't do what it was supposed to. Despite not being in control with the section, we were very involved – my husband cut the cord and the doctors chatted to us through the whole procedure.
Caroline from Northamptonshire, mum to Jacob, 10 and Sam, two

Honing your birth plan

It's often true for many mums that a birth plan turns out not to be entirely representative of their actual birth experience, but for some it's an important part of preparation for labour and delivery. If you know the way you'd prefer things to go, having your birth plan drawn up and distributed to your midwife and birth partner will give you a better chance of having your voice and preferences heard. Just putting things down on paper can help you to get your head round what lies ahead, too. So, even if nothing turns out the way you're planning – and it's important to keep an open mind and take advice from your medical team when there are difficult choices to be made – it's still worth having another look at it now. It may even be that you'll have changed your mind about certain aspects by this stage of your pregnancy.

Questions to ask yourself:
- Have I learned more about pain relief? If so, do I feel more or less flexible about it now?
- Have I decided whether or not to take a complementary therapist to the birth with me?
- Would I prefer a home birth? And has my medical team indicated that I could be a good candidate?
- Am I now considering a water birth?
- Do I want music during labour, and is this permissible by the hospital?
- Am I planning to use a birthing ball or stool, and have I checked with the hospital that this is OK?
- What position do I want to adopt for the delivery?
- Would I prefer to be cared for by women only? (This may be an option in some units, but you may not have a choice in others.)
- Do I want to avoid an episiotomy?
- How do I feel about other possible interventions?
- Does my birth partner want to cut the cord?
- Do I want my baby placed straight on to my chest after birth rather than being cleaned and wrapped up first?
- Do I want a managed or unmanaged third stage of labour (delivery of the placenta)?
- Am I happy to have a student midwife or doctor present at the birth?
- Do I want my baby to have vitamin K? (This is given routinely at birth – either by single injection or as three separate oral doses – because newborns have low levels and vitamin K is needed to help the blood clot. You don't have to agree to it, and there has been some controversy about it: two papers published in the early nineties

suggested a link between vitamin K and childhood leukaemia, but many subsequent studies have failed to establish this link. We do know that giving vitamin K prevents a potentially life-threatening disease called vitamin K deficiency bleeding, which occurs in around one in 10,000 babies.)

Other points to include on your birth plan are:

- your hospital number and the name(s) and telephone number(s) of your labour ward and/or midwifery team
- the phone number of whoever has volunteered to look after any older children when the time comes
- your birth partner's name and telephone number (if different from your partner).

It's best to print off several copies of your finalised birth plan and give one to your midwifery team; one to your obstetrician; one to your birth partner; one to your complementary therapist (if applicable); and leave one near your home phone. Make sure that if this is an updated plan everyone concerned destroys their previous drafts. For this reason, it's sensible to date each version.

Your mission this week: Do your homework on your choices for labour

Read up again on your choices for labour, even if you're planning an active birth without pain relief. The best-laid plans can go awry no matter how well prepared you feel you are and how relaxed you may be about the birth. Did you know, for instance, that half of all Caesareans are performed once labour is underway – in other words, as 'emergencies'? For this reason, it's best to read about Caesareans (see p. 289) as well as the pros and cons of various types of pain relief (see p. 93). That way, if you do need some help you'll know which types you'll feel most happy with. Don't forget to include your birth partner in your research and reading: on the big day you may not be best disposed to be making important decisions, and one of the roles of your birth partner is to be your spokesperson whenever necessary.

Look no further

If I have a Caesarean this time, does it mean I'll never be able to have a normal delivery in the future?
Not at all. Some mums have found themselves under pressure from medical staff to have subsequent Caesarean deliveries – especially in the case of pelvic disproportion (or CPD – cephalo-pelvic disproportion), where the baby's head is too large to pass through the pelvis – but in many cases there's no reason at all not to try for a normal birth next time round. CPD is difficult to diagnose accurately in any case, and the real reason why many babies get 'stuck' in the birth canal is that they've entered it awkwardly rather than that their heads are too large. Many mums who have a Caesarean for CPD in one pregnancy go on to deliver a baby with a larger head in a subsequent pregnancy.

There are support groups to help you achieve a vaginal birth subsequently (visit the site of Vaginal Birth After Caesarean, for instance, at www.vbac.org.uk). Your chances of a successful vaginal birth vary according to various factors, such as the reasons for your past Caesarean and the number of past Caesareans you've had. If, however, you do choose an elective Caesarean next time, hopefully you'll find that your experience is much more positive than if you previously underwent an emergency section.

Are twins always delivered by Caesarean?
No – although much will depend on how straightforward your pregnancy has been; how your twins are lying; whether both are thriving equally well; and whether or not there are any other complications. Sometimes when twins are monoamniotic (sharing an amniotic sac), the medical team prefers to perform an elective Caesarean because of the risk of the umbilical cords becoming entangled during a vaginal delivery. Keep communicating with your medical team about your birth options: if both babies are in a head-down position towards your EDD, you may be able to attempt a vaginal delivery. Keep an open mind though, as you might need an emergency Caesarean for one or both babies when the time comes: for this reason, it's worth considering having an epidural set up during labour so that it can be topped up for the delivery. In some cases, a general anaesthetic will be given for a twin Caesarean delivery.

I've heard that raspberry leaf tea is good to drink in late pregnancy. Why?
It's thought that raspberry leaf helps to stimulate and tone the uterus in preparation for labour, and mums who take it often report an easier or shorter second stage of labour than those who don't. Although more research needs to be done before this can be confirmed conclusively, this belief is backed up by an Australian study where some mums were given raspberry leaf tablets and others were given a placebo. You can take it in tablet or tea form, but shouldn't start before Week 32 because of its stimulating effect on the uterus. Start with one tablet or cup of tea a day and increase this gradually to a maximum of four doses of either. You can continue taking raspberry leaf throughout labour, too, and there's no evidence that it has any adverse effect on unborn babies.

I'm fed up being pregnant. How can I get through the next couple of months?
It's very common for mums in their third trimester to start flagging like this: you've probably begun to feel cumbersome; perhaps the simplest task now seems like too much effort; you might be struggling at work; maybe you're just losing patience for meeting your new baby. This is where your support network starts to kick in: keep in close touch with other mums from your antenatal group if you've found any likeminded people; if not, talk to friends who've had babies; ask your mum about her experiences of late pregnancy; arrange some home-based treats for yourself, like a takeaway with your mates or a girls-only pampering session; distract yourself by rearranging your baby's nursery and putting finishing touches to your home; go online and chat with the Netmums, who will offer you lots of support and encouragement. Don't despair: as the next couple of weeks pass you'll probably find yourself seemingly hurtling towards the birth!

Who'd have thought?

Research conducted in the Netherlands which charted the responses to repeated sounds of babies at 37–40 weeks' gestation over three different time intervals concluded that unborn babies have short-term memories of at least 10 minutes and long-term memories of at least 24 hours.*

*Source: Department of Obstetrics and Gynaecology, University Hospital, Maastricht

How are you feeling?

Tick the box that most closely represents how you feel about the given statements, then look back to the charts in previous chapters to see how you've changed over the months.

Physically	Emotionally
I'm finding it harder to breathe freely Strongly agree ☐ Agree ☐ Neither agree nor disagree ☐ Disagree ☐ Strongly disagree ☐	I'd love to go into labour right now! Strongly agree ☐ Agree ☐ Neither agree nor disagree ☐ Disagree ☐ Strongly disagree ☐
I'm beginning to feel like a heffalump Strongly agree ☐ Agree ☐ Neither agree nor disagree ☐ Disagree ☐ Strongly disagree ☐	I'm worried about losing control in labour Strongly agree ☐ Agree ☐ Neither agree nor disagree ☐ Disagree ☐ Strongly disagree ☐
I need to rest frequently and small exertions tire me out Strongly agree ☐ Agree ☐ Neither agree nor disagree ☐ Disagree ☐ Strongly disagree ☐	My mum is my new best friend Strongly agree ☐ Agree ☐ Neither agree nor disagree ☐ Disagree ☐ Strongly disagree ☐
I know I've got to get a nursery ready, but can't bring myself to do it yet Strongly agree ☐ Agree ☐ Neither agree nor disagree ☐ Disagree ☐ Strongly disagree ☐	My non-pregnant friends don't understand me Strongly agree ☐ Agree ☐ Neither agree nor disagree ☐ Disagree ☐ Strongly disagree ☐
I'm enjoying sex again now Strongly agree ☐ Agree ☐ Neither agree nor disagree ☐ Disagree ☐ Strongly disagree ☐	My partner seems as fed up with this pregnancy as I am! Strongly agree ☐ Agree ☐ Neither agree nor disagree ☐ Disagree ☐ Strongly disagree ☐
My beautifully clear skin's gone all pimply! Strongly agree ☐ Agree ☐ Neither agree nor disagree ☐ Disagree ☐ Strongly disagree ☐	I'm a bit worried about getting alienated by my colleagues once I've left work Strongly agree ☐ Agree ☐ Neither agree nor disagree ☐ Disagree ☐ Strongly disagree ☐

Quick quiz

What have you learnt so far?

1 How do breathing techniques help in labour?

a. They help you to control the intensity of contractions and your rate of pushing

b. They help you get a bit of a natural high

c. They help you to use gas & air properly

2　What are the main symptoms of pre-eclampsia?

a. High blood pressure; swelling; protein in the urine

b. Nausea; abdominal pain; itching

c. Hunger; thirst; cravings

3　Why do you need to exercise your pelvic floor?

a. To help prevent stress incontinence later

b. To help lose weight after the birth

c. To increase your repertoire of party tricks

4　What is placenta praevia?

a. A low-lying placenta that partially or wholly obstructs the cervix

b. A placenta that's stopped working

c. A placenta recipe for after the birth

5　What can put you at risk of having a larger-than-normal baby?

a. Diabetes

b. Not exercising enough in pregnancy

c. Having sex in pregnancy

Answers: The answers to this quiz are all 'a'.

Mostly a: Well done you: you've been taking it all in, haven't you? The best way of preparing for labour and childbirth, as well as adapting to new parenthood is to keep yourself as well informed as possible – and you're certainly doing that!

Mostly b: Well, you've certainly taken in some of the information in this book, but it seems you've got it all in the wrong order in your brain! It can be more dangerous to have the wrong information than none at all, so go over the sections in this chapter again so you'll have all the facts on board.

Mostly c: Have you thought of using this book as a doorstop? It seems you haven't had too much use for it so far! Maybe you're just focusing on the bits that apply to you at the particular time of reading, but this is a bit short-sighted: the more often you read and re-read the sections where your knowledge is lacking, the more ready you'll be for the big day and all that may happen to you and your baby.

Chapter 8
Weeks 33–36

Does it feel like you're getting a bit close to the end of pregnancy for comfort or are you champing at the bit to arrive at your Big Day? Some mums at this stage find themselves unable to bend down without squatting, uncomfortable in most positions, still rather breathless and with only a distant memory of how their feet used to look! Others remain serene, neatly bumped and glowing like Mother Nature herself. (How is that FAIR??) If you fall into the former category, you can probably look forward also to leaking breasts – prettily adorned with a haphazard blue pattern surprisingly similar to a map of Spaghetti Junction – leaden legs and bouts of flatulence. If you fall into the latter – well, whoop-di-do for you! Seriously, though, if you're positively breezing through pregnancy, you're fortunate indeed – and an example to the rest of us that it doesn't have to be a rolling series of physical assaults! If you're having a bit of a rough ride, on the other hand, try to think of each week to come as only $1/32$ of what you've been through already!

Who'd have thought?

From the moment of conception, there are 46 chromosomes and 30,000 genes at play which determine all your baby's physical characteristics.

Week 33 56 days to go!

Don't forget: Keep tabs on your blood pressure

Now you are at greater risk than before of developing high blood pressure – and, if you have a combination of oedema (swelling), protein in your urine and high blood pressure, you might be diagnosed with pre-eclampsia. It's by no means an inevitability as it affects only one in 10 mums, but as it's the commonest serious condition of pregnancy it's well worth ensuring that you attend all your antenatal checks from now on (and hopefully you've kept all your appointments to date in any case!). If for any reason you can't get to your midwives for an appointment, try to arrange a check at your GP's surgery instead. Don't rely on machines found in pharmacies and fitness clubs: your blood pressure should always be checked by a doctor or midwife, who can then check for other potential problems at the same time.

Hey baby!

Not an awful lot has happened since last week, except that your baby has put on still more weight and now weighs about 2kg (4.4lb). At this stage you might find you're putting on weight rather quicker than previously, and this is down to the fact that your baby's increasing his own weight by as much as 224g (½lb) a week! He measures around 30cm (a whole foot!) from crown to rump now and is about 43cm (17in) from top to toe. The hair on his head continues to grow, although the amount of hair a baby's born with varies a lot from case to case: some are more or less bald, and even babies with a thick shock of hair will often lose most of it shortly after birth. It's down to genetics, and nothing to do with how well your baby's been growing or how healthy you are. Your baby's hair colour at birth won't necessarily have any bearing on his true colouring either: some babies born with black locks grow into blondes, and some blondes-at-birth are actually redheads.

Who'd have thought?

The umbilical cord is like a kind of swap shop: you pass your baby nutrients and oxygen, and in exchange he passes you his carbon dioxide waste!

What the netmums say

'My newborn's hair colour'

Lauren was born with lots of jet-black hair which stuck up on end; it didn't fall out but went lighter to brown. Robert had dark-brown hair although there wasn't as much of it as Lauren had. This did fall out and grew back white-blond: I'm not sure where that came from as both my hubby and I are both dark haired. Robert's still got blond hair now.
Sharon from St Helens, mum to Lauren, 16, Robert, three, and 25 weeks pregnant

Amelia was born with a mop of black curly hair. It never fell out and now comes halfway down her back when wet. It's still curly, but now a lighter brown.
Kaleigh from Newmarket, mum to Amelia, nine months

My kids are mixed race, so it wasn't a surprise that they both had very black hair. James's was totally straight when he was born, but turned into a curly Mohican at around nine months! Kayla also had lots of straight black hair, and now has a curly Mohican too, although hers is much softer than James's.
Catherine from Erskine, mum to James, three and Kayla, nine months

Harriet was born with a small amount of very blonde hair all over her head – we kind of expected it really as both of us were born blonde. Now Harriet's six months old it's grown quite a lot on top, and is starting to grow more all over and around the sides now, as it was a little bald on the back from where she slept. She's still blonde, although it's not as white-blonde as when she was a newborn.
Carla from Poole, mum to Harriet, six months

All about you

OK, so last week you read that your uterus couldn't get much higher – and that remains true – but there's still a little rising up to be done nevertheless, and this week it'll have gained another centimetre in height, bringing your fundus up to around 33cm (just over 13 inches) from your pubic bone, and 13cm (just over 5 inches) above your belly button. Hold tight: it won't be too long now before it starts to drop!

Breech babies

You might have learned at your last antenatal check that your baby is lying in breech position. This can mean one of three things:

- he's lying upright with his head towards your ribcage and his legs extended upwards in front of his face. This happens in 85 per cent of breech presentations and is known as a 'frank' breech
- he's lying upright with his feet towards your cervix, but with his knees and arms tucked into his body. This is known as a 'complete' breech
- he's lying upright with one leg tucked into his body and the other dangling down. This is known as a 'footling' or 'incomplete' breech.

Because babies can move in and out of position throughout pregnancy, the percentage lying in breech position decreases as pregnancy goes on, so that although 15 per cent of babies are breech at 30 weeks, only 6 per cent present this way at 35 weeks and only 3–4 per cent remain breech at full term. There's no need to worry yet, as the majority of babies reported as lying in breech position this week will turn to a head-down presentation by 36 weeks – and even then, as long as your pregnancy is otherwise uncomplicated, the Royal College of Midwives recommends having an experienced obstetrician try to turn the baby by manipulating your bump externally. This is known as External Cephalic Version (ECV), and it's successful in an average 46 per cent of cases in the UK, with higher or lower success rates depending on the number of experienced doctors in your area. It's not considered a risky procedure, so it's worth allowing your obstetrician to have a try if you still find your baby is breech any time from 37 weeks onwards. The procedure should only be carried out by an experienced obstetrician using ultrasound screening as guidance, with monitoring of the foetal heart rate beforehand and afterwards.

What the netmums say

'Finding my baby was breech'

I got all the way to 10cm dilated and ready to push when the midwife made a last check to see if the baby's head was crowning and found that there was a different part presenting: it seems she'd managed to turn sideways during labour, even though she was a larger-than-average baby due to my gestational diabetes. Within minutes I was rushed into theatre for an emergency Caesarean. It felt like a real disappointment at the time as it was not only my worst fear, but I'd already been through 27 hours of induced labour! Luckily Natasha was born a healthy 8lb 12½oz without further complications, except that I lost a lot of blood and was kept in recovery for almost 16 hours. Even though we bonded straightaway, I did suffer from delayed postnatal depression, though, which I'm sure stemmed from her traumatic delivery.

Hilary from Carshalton, mum to Natasha, three

I was 35 weeks pregnant when my baby was found to be breech. I was really worried as I'd already had one Caesarean for breech and was really keen to try for a vaginal delivery this time. The midwife said not to worry as I had another two weeks for him to turn back again, but would I like an obstetrician to try to turn him in the meantime? I thought I might as well let someone have a go, and although it was quite uncomfortable with all the pushing and shoving, it proved worth it. Liam didn't turn back to breech position again but stayed head down until the birth at 39 weeks. I delivered him vaginally and felt overjoyed afterwards – which was quite a contrast to how I felt after having Lydia.

Helen from north London, mum to Lydia, two and Liam, three months

Elective Caesarean for breech

The most usual method of delivery for a breech baby is by elective (planned) Caesarean. This is considered safest, especially in the case of a footling breech, where the cord is in danger of preceding the baby down the birth canal. In most cases, a baby who is identified as lying in breech position at 37 weeks, and who doesn't respond to ECV, will be delivered at 38 weeks.

Who'd have thought?

In the second and third trimesters of pregnancy, your baby's urine is the main component of your amniotic fluid.

Vaginal delivery for breech

Sometimes, however, a baby will arrive in a hurry, leaving no time for a Caesarean. In this case, you'll probably be asked to adopt an 'all fours' position so that your baby isn't delivered too quickly, as a very rapid delivery could damage or traumatise his head.

You might decide that you want to try for a vaginal delivery even if you know in advance that your baby is in breech position at full term. You'll want to ensure that your medical team is experienced in delivering breech babies, and is happy to attempt to do so; you'll also need to keep an open mind about the possibility of having to have an emergency Caesarean. You may find you have to meet the following criteria before your medical team will attempt a vaginal breech delivery:

- your baby mustn't be either very large or very small
- you're not suspected of having pelvic disproportion (where the pelvis is too small for the baby's head to pass through)
- your baby shouldn't be in 'footling' breech position, with one or other foot dangling down. This is because of the risk of the cord falling out of the vagina prior to the baby's descent, known as a 'prolapsed cord'
- your baby shouldn't be 'stargazing' with his neck extended and his head facing skywards
- labour should start spontaneously: an induced labour is risky because of the often rapid delivery of the baby.

Assisted delivery for breech: forceps or ventouse

Having a breech baby – or a baby who becomes 'stuck' in the birth canal – means you might have to have an 'assisted' delivery. This means the midwife or obstetrician will use forceps or ventouse extraction to deliver your baby. Either procedure might mean you'll have to have an episiotomy, as the instruments themselves are fairly large and awkwardly shaped. If this is the case and your perineum can't stretch enough on its own, you'll be given a local anaesthetic or an injection called a 'pudendal block', which numbs a wider area. If you've got an epidural or have had a spinal, you won't need any more pain relief. You might also be asked to put your feet up in 'stirrups' to give the midwife or obstetrician more space in which to work, and you'll probably have a long, thin tube called a catheter inserted into your urethra (the hole you pee through) to drain your bladder of urine prior to the procedure.

Forceps look like two large, hollow salad servers that are inserted separately into the vagina, then clipped together to cradle your baby's head and pull him down through the birth canal. This can take some force, and your midwife will need you to push to her cue to get the maximum effect. Ventouse extraction involves placing an electrically powered suction cup on to your baby's scalp and trying to 'vacuum' him out of the birth canal with each contraction. Ventouse-delivered babies are usually born with very pointy heads, but don't worry: the effect isn't permanent and your baby's head will settle into a normal shape within a few weeks of the birth.

Pack your bag

Any time from now is a good time to have your bag packed and ready to go to hospital, especially because of the increased risk of pre-eclampsia, but also because you could potentially go into premature labour. Another possibility is that you could be called in for bed rest or observation at a moment's notice; or you might, in some circumstances, even be advised not to leave the hospital after your antenatal appointment (and do you really want your other half to be in charge of packing for you? If you can trust him to do that all by himself, perhaps you'd like to share him around a bit...). You can't be sure in advance how long you'll stay in hospital, but it could be as little as 24 hours for a straightforward delivery or three days for an uncomplicated Caesarean, so keep this in mind when packing. Having a bag ready applies, too, if you're planning a home birth, as you may have to transfer to hospital in an emergency. You won't regret it even if you don't end up going anywhere: having a bag close to hand full of what is essentially a babycare starter kit can't be a bad thing!

You'll need a sizeable bag or small suitcase – but try to stick to one plus a small hand-luggage-size holdall as there won't be storage space in hospital and you could end up with paraphernalia taking up all the floor space, which will be considered dangerous. (Your hospital might have a policy on the number and size of bag/s you can bring, so it's worth asking about this.) Choose a bag with plenty of compartments and pockets so you can lay hands on all your different bits and pieces with relative ease: otherwise everything will get all churned up as you root around for a specific item and you'll never find anything quickly.

What to pack
For you
Hospital notes and birth plan Top of the list as they're of prime importance!

Disposable pants All mums have quite significant postnatal bleeding as the lining of the uterus is expelled, and for some it's heavier than others (see *Look no further*, p. 313). You'll need around seven to ten pairs of disposable pants, depending on how many come in a pack. You can't do laundry in hospital and you won't want a bag of bloodied knickers lying around, even if you have enough 'period pants' to see you through your hospital stay, so don't overlook these!

Maternity sanitary pads Take two packs of 10 or 12. If your hospital stay is prolonged for any reason you can always get your partner, a family member or friend to bring in some more – and you'll probably find them in the hospital shop in any case.

Two long T-shirts or old nightdresses The chances are whatever you wear will end up with some blood or milk stains on it, so don't take your favourite negligee or best pyjamas into hospital: something loose-fitting, long enough to cover you to mid-thigh at least and preferably with a front opening for breastfeeding is your best bet.

Socks One of the commonest discomforts mums in labour complain of is cold feet! You might think it's a small consideration, but why make yourself more uncomfortable than you're already likely to be when a cosy pair of socks could make all the difference!

Slippers You're bound to find yourself wandering the corridors at some stage, whether to keep active in labour or to make a trip to the loo or payphone. Hospital corridors can be highly polished, so take warm, comfy slippers with a good grip.

Dressing gown Essential for when you're cosying up out of bed or making trips to and from the shower.

Lip balm Lots of mums find they get very dry lips in labour and that lip balm (or a small tin of petroleum jelly) helps.

Cool-water spray This can be soothing during labour and after the birth if you get hot.

Facecloth Some mums like a cool facecloth applied to their foreheads or necks during labour. (This is another duty for your birth partner.)

A hairband To tie your hair back in labour.

Cartons of juice or bottles of water

Glucose tablets Some mums swear by these for giving them an extra energy boost in labour when they start flagging.

Snacks Pack enough for you and your partner – and try to make them nutritious rather than anything too sugary or fatty which will satisfy you instantly but leave you hungry again quickly afterwards.

Toiletries Travel-size shower gel, shampoo and deodorant are a good idea; you might also want to pack body lotion and/or face and hand cream.

Spare toothbrush and paste It's worth buying a spare set of these so you're not reliant on remembering to pack your usual set when the time comes.

Tissues You never know when you'll need one!

Hairbrush and towel

Make-up and remover If make-up makes you feel better, then go for it!

Maternity bra and breastpads Once your milk comes in properly, a few days after the birth you'll know all about it, so be prepared.

A phonecard Some hospitals prefer mobile phone use to be restricted to outside the building; others are happy for them to be used in the corridors. In any case it's worth keeping a phonecard in case you can't get a signal or your battery dies.

Some loose change About £10 in coins is all you should need to buy drinks, papers, maybe a snack and perhaps some extra sanitary towels. You can always ask someone to bring more money in for you; if you keep more on you and it goes missing, the hospital won't be liable.

Your address book You'll want everyone's phone number close to hand after the birth!

Laundry bag For your dirty clothes.

Going home outfit You might want to wear day clothes if you're kept in for longer than 24 hours in any case. Remember, you'll still be wearing maternity clothes for a little while yet, so don't pack those skinny jeans!

A camera and spare batteries (and film if it's not digital)

A camcorder (if allowed) and film/ batteries

Your mobile phone

A portable battery-operated stereo/radio player and tapes or CDs (if you want them for the birth) plus spare batteries

An MP3 player and spare batteries

A few books/magazines/games for both of you

Pen and paper

A pillow, blanket and change of clothes for your partner (in case he or she's in for an overnight stay) Some hospitals will provide these; others are short on supplies.

A gift for your older child You can give this from your baby, to help prevent jealousy.

For your baby

A pack of newborn nappies

A pack of cotton wool balls

A towel You could buy a hooded type which helps prevent heat loss through your baby's head.

Six stretchsuits

Six vests

A cardigan

Socks

Hat

Blanket (plus coat in winter)

A few muslin cloths (you can buy these in packs from nursery outlets)

A pack of disposable bibs or six cloth bibs

A soft toy Check it's safe for newborns.

What the netmums say

'What I wish I'd packed...'

I wish I'd had a big bottle of drinking water. I had a water spray and fan, but we only took a small bottle of mineral water. Between my husband and myself I could have done with one of those two-litre bottles, as it was thirsty work!

Kari from Exeter, mum to Jennifer, three months

I wish I had taken more pairs of pyjamas as my waters broke all over my only pair, so after the birth I spent the night in a delightful pink old-lady-style hospital nightie!
Nicola from Norwich, mum to Jacob, three

Baby wipes: cotton wool and water just doesn't cut it on the sticky newborn poo!
Rosie from Southampton, mum to Bethany, 21 months

I was booked to have a home birth but had to transfer to hospital after two-and-a-half hours of pushing! Although I had packed a 'just in case' bag I'd forgotten to put in contact lenses or glasses, so I spent the night in hospital completely unable to see, until my husband brought me my glasses in the morning! I also wish I'd taken some food, as the ham sandwich I was given after the birth didn't touch the sides – and some lighter pyjamas, because it felt like it was over 100 degrees on the ward!
Frances from Bristol, mum to Nathaniel, 17 weeks

Straws! I took plenty of water but couldn't really lift my head up to drink, so I didn't – at all! I was so thirsty. I also wish I'd packed some food for my husband to eat during labour and something for me to have after the birth: my hubby nipped out to get some food during the first stage and it was the longest 20 minutes of my life. Finally, a pair of scratch mitts. Lucy was a scratcher right from the word go.
Sam from Hants, mum to Nathan, 13 and Lucy, 21 months

I wish I'd taken lollipops to suck on in labour as I'm sure I wouldn't have got so dehydrated and sick if I'd just had some to hand. Oh, and I forgot to bring a bar of soap, so I had to wash with just plain water, which isn't nice when you've just delivered and are covered in blood, vomit and sweat!
Alicia from London, mum to Kyrus, two, Demiyah, one, and 14 weeks pregnant

Who'd have thought?

Your baby absorbs a gallon of amniotic fluid every 24 hours and it's replaced completely every three hours!

Your mission this week: Get your baby's car seat

Buy a baby car seat if you haven't done so already. You'll need to check first that it's compatible with your make and model of car: some outlets that sell the seats now offer a free fitting service, so do take advantage of this as a recent survey* of 1,000 car seats found that a shocking 75 per cent were fitted incorrectly, with 20 per cent of these needing major adjustment to make them safe and 16 per cent incompatible with the vehicle for which they were bought. Having a seat but fitting it incorrectly will put your baby's life at serious risk if you're involved in an accident.

What you want is a Stage 1 rearward-facing baby seat that can be used forward facing once your baby weighs at least 9kg or his head reaches the top of the seat. Some will see your child through to around nine months; others will be usable up to around 15 months. Some come as part of a pram/pushchair/car seat three-way combination – but again you must check that the car seat element is compatible with your motor (or motors if you are a two-car family) before you purchase the product.

Don't use a secondhand seat unless you are 100 per cent sure of its origin and are certain that it hasn't been involved in any accidents or damaged in any way, and it comes with the original instructions. Finally, check that the seat meets the United Nations Standard Regulation 44.03 or 44.04: look for the 'E' mark.

- For more advice on choosing and using car seats, visit RoSPA's dedicated website at www.childcarseats.org.uk/choosing

Look no further

If my baby's found to be breech and has to be turned, will it hurt?
As you can imagine, having anyone heave your bump around is probably

*Survey published by GMTV, February 2008.

not the way you'd choose to spend your spare time, but if your baby is easy to turn it shouldn't be too uncomfortable and should be over fairly quickly. Sometimes babies are a bit more stubborn and difficult to turn, and then the procedure can be a bit uncomfortable – but it's worth a try, given that it could facilitate an easier birth. You'll have an ultrasound scan before and after your obstetrician attempts ECV so he or she can see exactly how your baby is lying and where your placenta is positioned; you might also be given a muscle relaxant to help your uterus to yield to the pressure of turning. If the procedure is successful, your baby is unlikely to turn back into a breech position again... although a small number still do!

What percentage of mums who book a home birth end up transferring to hospital?
According to one extensive study*, 60 per cent of first-time mums who had planned to deliver at home did so and 40 per cent transferred to hospital. The figures for subsequent home births were more encouraging, with 90 per cent of mums who'd had previous births managing to deliver at home. Some mums transferred before labour actually started, whilst others transferred during labour. The biggest reason for transfer was slow or no progress, which happened in 37 per cent of cases. Just under a quarter transferred because of their waters breaking prematurely – mostly before the onset of labour – and distress in the baby accounted for around 15 per cent.

What is lochia?
The discharge that follows childbirth, known as lochia, can keep on coming for anything between two and six weeks, and is heavier for some mums than others, but eventually turns from bright red to browny pink before tailing off altogether. You'll need to let your midwife or obstetrician know if you pass any clots larger in size than a 50p piece. This indicates that small pieces of placenta may still be inside your uterus. This can cause heavy bleeding and infection later on. If fragments of placenta have been retained, they'll need to be removed under general, spinal or epidural anaesthetic and you'll probably be given a course of antibiotics.

*Home Births: The Report of the 1994 Confidential Enquiry by the National Birthday Trust Fund

Week 34 *49 days to go!*

Don't forget: Take the weight off your bump

You might feel as if you're hauling a heavy shopping bag out in front of you and that your belly is under pressure from the weight of your baby – and this is especially true for those mums whose babies have 'engaged' (dropped into the pelvis in readiness for birth, see p. 332). Although this doesn't happen to most first-time mums quite yet, being more usual at around 36 weeks, you might be one of those mums who find themselves waddling along like Jemima Puddleduck any time from this week. You can buy special bump supports to make you feel more comfy and less like your baby is going to 'fall out'! These are deep, elasticated fabric bands that act like a kind of sling under your belly. They're generally higher at the front than at the back so that there's room for even more expansion, and they can also make your clothes more comfortable. Go to www.bumpband.co.uk to find out more. You can also find devices that allow you to expand the waistbands of your maternity clothes even more, so if you're busting out of your best preggie jeans, check out www.bumpto3.com.

Hey baby!

Still laying down fat to keep him warm after birth, your baby is a good weight now at around 2.3kg (5lb). He's almost the length of a newborn at about 32cm (nearly 13 inches) from crown to rump and around 44cm (almost 17.5 inches) from top to toe. The other main development taking place is the maturation of your baby's lungs between now and the birth. A substance called surfactant, which is a liquid that lubricates the lungs so they don't stick together when we breathe out, needs to line the lungs before your baby is born, as one of the commonest problems amongst premature babies is a lack of surfactant. If a routine scan highlights the fact that your baby's lungs are underdeveloped, you might be offered a one-off steroid injection, thought to be harmless, which encourages the lungs to mature.

Who'd have thought?

Your baby is developing a sweet tooth while inside you. No wonder so many of us would rather eat a chocolate bar than a bowl of steamed veg...

All about you

Your uterus has grown to around 34cm (just over 13.5in) up from your pubic bone and about 14cm (just over 5.5in) above your belly button. You probably feel like it's bursting up through your ribcage and forcing your boobs upwards and outwards like a couple of barrage balloons! If you had thought in previous months that pregnancy was the most natural thing in the world, you might now be reviewing this attitude... Lots of mums report being plagued by strangers saying things like, 'You must be due any day now!' and 'Don't have that baby here, will you?' daily from now until the end of pregnancy, which can be aggravating, especially if nothing would please you more than to get on with the birth!

You might be feeling secretly resentful about the sacrifices and indignities you've had to endure in pregnancy (don't worry: plenty of mums do!) with no real reward – yet! Try to focus on meeting your baby for the first time; and chat to new mums about whether or not they feel the end result was worth the wait (we think you'll be pleasantly surprised).

Premature labour

About 50,000 babies are born prematurely each year in the UK – that's around 7 per cent of all births. Much as you might be getting tired of pregnancy, going into labour early isn't by any means an easy option, especially for your baby. Premature labour is classed as the onset of labour before 37 weeks of pregnancy. Although your baby's chances of survival are excellent at 34 weeks, he will probably still need to go to Special Care if born this early. The main reason is that his lungs might not be mature enough for him to breathe independently (see p. 322).

Although many cases of premature labour happen for no known reason, there is some evidence to suggest that particular bacteria found in the urine of mums-to-be are associated with the early onset of labour. For this reason, tests are carried out for the bacteria in early pregnancy as treating the infection does seem to reduce the risk of premature labour in these mums. Complications of pregnancy such as diabetes, pre-eclampsia, placental problems, cervical incompetence – a condition where the cervix starts to stretch and thin prematurely – and multiple pregnancy, where more than one baby is due, can also mean babies either arrive early spontaneously or need to be induced or delivered early by Caesarean.

Although there are inherent problems when babies are born early, sometimes the risks outweigh those associated with letting pregnancy progress further. Babies born before 34 weeks are at risk of complications including hypothermia; low blood-sugar levels; jaundice; infection; damage to the retina causing problems with vision, and even death – but these risks diminish with every passing day your baby remains in the uterus.

For some mums the first sign that labour is going to start early is their waters breaking spontaneously. This is called Pre-labour Premature Rupture of Membranes (PPROM) and is usually followed quickly by contractions as the cervix begins to dilate: once this point has been reached, there's usually no going back. Drugs to stop contractions only help about 25 per cent of mums and usually stop being effective after 48 hours, so they're not considered a viable option in most cases.

What to do if labour starts early

If your waters break before Week 37 of labour, contact your midwife or doctor straightaway as this could mean that labour is imminent, and you're at risk of infection once the protective amniotic sac surrounding your baby has ruptured. You'll need to get to hospital urgently – even if it means phoning for an ambulance – or call your midwife to your home if you are planning a home birth (although many health authorities will not agree to attend a home birth before 37 weeks of pregnancy because of the risks to the baby, so you may have no alternative but to go into hospital if labour starts before then). Similarly, if you start having contractions that get closer and closer in interval and that are increasing in intensity, contact your midwifery team or get yourself to the hospital.

What happens next

First it will need to be established whether or not you are in true labour. Tests for this include a urine test to check for the bacteria mentioned above which are sometimes associated with premature labour; a vaginal ultrasound scan to assess your cervix; a vaginal swab, blood test or even amniocentesis to check for infections associated with the early onset of labour. If your doctors aren't sure whether or not it's true labour, you'll probably be admitted to the antenatal ward for observation.

If you're 34 or more weeks pregnant and in true labour, your medical team probably won't intervene, but will let things progress as they would have done at full term. Your baby will probably need a little help with his breathing as his lungs aren't really mature enough to cope alone until Week 36, but other than this he's unlikely to suffer any serious complications.

How you might feel

It's bound to be a big shock if your baby suddenly makes an appearance before you're mentally or physically prepared for his arrival. Some mums of prem babies have reported feeling that their bodies have let them down; that their babies are spending time in SCBUs when they should be inside them still; that they're not emotionally ready to bond with their babies. Others have described the unexpected joy of meeting their babies early; the anxiety about their newborns' welfare; the overwhelming sense of love and protectiveness they felt towards their vulnerable infants. All of these emotions are completely normal. If you feel you're struggling to come to terms with a premature labour and delivery, however, do ask to talk things through with your medical team until you feel more able to accept what has happened. The Netmums have plenty of experiences to share with you, too, so don't forget to make use of this fantastic free resource.

How a prem baby might look

Your baby would still be considered premature if born any time now, and he'd look quite different from a full-term newborn, depending on how prematurely he arrived. Prem babies can look thin, scrawny and wrinkly with transparent skin and underdeveloped eyelashes, fingernails and hair. They are often red in appearance with very swollen-looking genitalia. They may be quite downy and very 'curled up'. The closer a baby gets to full term, the less extreme his appearance will be.

Who'd have thought?

Brain activity, measured by electroencephalography (EEG), has been recorded in unborn babies as early as 40 days of gestation.

What the netmums say

'The early arrival of my baby!'

I was caught on the hop with my youngest, as I went into labour at 36 weeks and five days. I was out for a walk and my waters went, so I phoned the hospital and they asked me to come in to be checked over. It turned out that I was in labour and 3cm dilated. I had a straightforward labour and delivery and Theo was 7lb 4oz, so they treated him as full term as he was only a couple of days premature. The worse thing was, I just wasn't ready! I didn't have a bag packed, and didn't even have anywhere for him to sleep, as I had a big consignment of baby goods due to be delivered the next day. I had to beg and borrow from friends for the first 24 hours until my stuff arrived.
Jen from Hertfordshire, mum to Jack, four and Theo, 17 months

In my first pregnancy I went into labour spontaneously at 31 weeks and two days, but didn't actually realise I was in labour as the pains were all in my back and not really that sore. When I spoke to my mum the following morning she whisked me straight to hospital where I was found to be 5cm dilated. The doctors were unable to stop labour at that point, and Emma was born six hours later, weighing 3lb 8½oz. She was in Special Care for a month. My second child was four days late, but in my third pregnancy I went into labour in Week 29. I had a 'show' in the afternoon, so I was able to be on top of this one and went straight to the hospital where I was found to be 2cm dilated. I was given steroids to mature the baby's lungs, and a drip to try to stop labour. It worked for eight days, during which time the SCBU filled up and I had to be transferred to a hospital 50 miles further from home. I went into labour again but it was stopped again, and Ryan was finally born at 31 weeks and two days, just like his sister. He weighed 4lb 3oz and was in Special Care for two weeks. He has a small hole in the heart and had two groin hernias which were repaired when he was six months old. I'm expecting my fourth baby in January so I hope this time I'll go to term, but I'll be fully prepared for another early baby.
Joanne from Tayside, mum to Emma, 12, Jack, four, Ryan, two, and three months pregnant

Perineal massage

Who'd have thought that massaging that tiny area between your vagina and your anus with some oil could help to prevent you from tearing or needing an episiotomy during the delivery of your baby? Sounds unlikely, maybe, but it's true – at least for some mums. It's not just a case of rubbing the skin, though: there's a special technique you need to repeat often. If you find it difficult to reach that area of yourself in late pregnancy, you could ask your partner to do it for you (although if he's the sort of chap who thinks your G-spot resides somewhere close to your left earhole, or who dons latex gloves to stuff a chicken, you might want to think again…).

You can start massaging any time from now as the technique is made more effective by a surge in progesterone and relaxin which help to soften your tissues. One word of caution: if you suffer from genital herpes or any other vaginal infection, check first with your midwife, as you might make matters worse.

How to massage

- First have a warm bath to soften and relax the tissue of your perineum. Then go to the loo: the action of massaging this area can give you the urge to empty your bowel, and you don't want to have to stop for a pee halfway through, either!
- Make sure your hands are perfectly clean and your nails are short and filed smooth.
- Find the position in which you can most easily access your perineum, bearing in mind you'll need to be able to insert your fingers part way into your vagina and sustain the position for a few minutes at a time. For some mums, it's sitting on the loo; for others, it's lying on their sides (remember to stay on your left to allow for optimum circulation).
- Choose a vegetable oil, baby oil or specially formulated perineal massage oil (although this will cost more for no real extra benefit) and – using a well-placed mirror so you can see what you're doing – massage the skin of the perineum with your fingers, going into your vagina by a couple of centimetres and concentrating on the vaginal walls without pushing your fingers right up inside yourself.

NB Avoid nut oils if there's any history of nut allergy in your family.

- Insert your thumbs into your vagina up to the first joint, and pull gently downwards towards your anus, then upwards in a U shape to ease and stretch the perineal muscles. Avoid the area near your urethra and clitoris: you're only trying to stretch the area between your vagina and anus, not give yourself an orgasm!
- Keeping your thumbs just inside your vagina, massage the perineum with your index and middle fingers.
- Repeat the massage for around five minutes per day: after a week or so you should notice how much more flexible your perineum has become.

What the netmums say

'Massaging my perineum'

At first I found it really hard to be able to reach my perineum comfortably so I got my boyfriend to do it for me. But he was a bit uncomfortable with this (so was I!) so I got round things by doing it with one leg up on the side of the bath. Although this wasn't exactly easy either, it did mean I could reach and do it in privacy. I didn't have a tear or a cut, and I like to think it's down to the massage – which I did every day. It might just have been that I'm young, though, as I'm only 18. If we have another baby I'll definitely do it again anyway. After all, there's nothing to lose, is there?
Hayley from Manchester, mum to Harley, 13 months

I started off with really good intentions, rubbing oil into the area morning and night. I carried on until about Week 28, but then I gave up because things didn't feel any different. I reckon I had the technique wrong as I only realised you were supposed to stretch the skin from the inside after I'd had a bad tear with William! When I was pregnant with Anna it wasn't even suggested to me. I might give it a go again if I have another baby.
Julia from Swanage, mum to Anna, six and William, one

Who'd have thought?

There's some evidence to suggest that mums who experience mild sickness in early pregnancy are less likely to go into premature labour. It seems that moderate nausea and vomiting are related to the production of hCG (the hormone indicating the presence of human life) and that the resulting restriction of nutrients during critical periods of an unborn baby's development may ensure the production of hCG at optimal levels*.

*Study carried out by the Department of Biomedical Sciences, Queens Medical Centre, University of Nottingham.

Your mission this week: Hang out with mums and babies

Immerse yourself in the world you're about to enter. Check out your local mother-and-baby clubs and ask if you can sit and observe for a little while; revisit your childcare provider; find out about postnatal mum-and-baby exercise classes and swim sessions: it's a fairly safe bet that you'll find some of the attendees in the nearest coffee shop afterwards, where you might be able to infiltrate a group and get chatting about new motherhood! If you're uncomfortable about approaching strangers, see if you can get some of your antenatal group together for a social so you can all chat about how you're feeling. There's no need to make elaborate arrangements: a picnic in the local park in fine weather or a get-together in the local pub are good plans as you can stay as long (or as short) a time as you like. Get partners involved if you can: your partner might well appreciate the company of other new dads after your baby's born. He'll probably have the urge to talk fatherhood but might feel uncomfortable about bringing it up with his usual crowd, especially if some or all of them are not dads. Log on to your local Netmums website as a fantastic starting point for all of the above!

Look no further

It can't be good for me to put my fingers inside my vagina, even for perineal massage, can it?

As long as you are scrupulous about cleanliness and follow the instructions given on p. 320, there's no need to worry – neither you nor your baby are in danger of coming to any harm. The key points are to wash your hands thoroughly before each massage and keep your fingernails short and clean (or wear latex exam gloves); avoid inserting your fingers so far inside yourself that you can feel your cervix; stop if you feel uncomfortable at any time; choose a plain, non-nut oil; make sure your partner follows the same rules if you are handing the massaging over to him.

What would make me more at risk of premature labour than other mums?
Most cases of premature labour happen for no identifiable reason. However, there is evidence to support the idea that some groups of mums are more at risk than others. According to research, you're most at risk of going into premature labour if you're:

- a young or single, unsupported mum
- underweight
- a smoker.

Some mums have admitted smoking and dieting throughout pregnancy in order to try to have a smaller baby or to give birth earlier whilst their babies are still small: this is highly dangerous and will only put a baby's life and welfare at great risk.

How long will my premature baby stay in Special Care?
For many babies, it will be for a short period of observation only – and the closer your baby is delivered to your EDD, the shorter the time he's likely to have to spend in Special Care. Depending on how premature they are, or what problems they are born with, some babies just need a little extra oxygen to revive them after birth, whereas others will need to be attached to a ventilator to breathe for them until their lungs have matured. This can take hours, days or sometimes weeks. So it's impossible to predict how long an individual baby will spend in Special Care, if any time at all, but you can be sure your newborn won't be kept away from you for any longer than is necessary – and that you'll be encouraged to have as full a part in his care as is possible whilst he's in the SCBU (Special Care Baby Unit).

Week 35 *42 days to go!*

Don't forget: Catnap whenever you can

Now that you're about as cumbersome as it's possible to be, you're probably having renewed trouble sleeping, and a lack of decent sleep coupled with the mood swings lots of mums seem to experience around now again might make you quite challenging company to be around... The best antidote is to catnap as frequently as you can. Now, as in earlier pregnancy, take your eyes off the housework and put your feet up instead. If you have a mobile phone with an alarm you can set, you'd be surprised how refreshed even the odd 10 minutes on a bus or train can leave you feeling. If you're still working, try to find somewhere you can put your head down during your lunch break or at other break times. At weekends, sleep as much as you feel like and don't struggle to get out of bed early in the mornings: the time for seriously disturbed nights and early mornings is not far off!

Hey baby!

Your baby now weighs over 2.5kg (around 5.5lb). From crown to rump he measures around 33cm (just over 13in) and his total length from top to toe is about 45cm (around 18in). You might be able to feel your baby's position yourself at this point: ask your midwife to place your hands around his head at your next antenatal appointment. You may have been aware of his feet, knees and elbows for some time already as they've jabbed your belly during his intra-uterine acrobatics! By now, though, there is very little space for your baby to move around in. If he's head down, he's likely to stay that way; if not, he still has time to turn.

All about you

Your fundus now measures a substantial 35cm (14in) from your pubic bone and about 15cm (6in) from your belly button. Most mums at this stage of pregnancy have put on around 10–13kg (23–29lb). If it feels like all your insides have been rearranged by your burgeoning bump, to an extent you're right! Your other organs – your bladder, stomach, intestines and lungs have all been forced to one side or compressed, which is why you are likely to be feeling even more breathless and generally uncomfortable than ever. You'll probably be peeing more again, eating tiny meals throughout the day, huffing, puffing and generally heaving yourself about the place. If you have just the one baby in there, spare a thought for mums of multiples: there's always someone worse off somewhere!

Relaxation techniques

The idea of relaxation in labour might sound like something of a contradiction in terms, and it's certainly not a state that most mums slip into automatically! But being able to relax has been proven to help ease labour and delivery because it helps the muscles of the uterus – and elsewhere – to work more effectively without tensing up and over-straining. It will also help you to conserve energy and prevent stress hormones from crossing the placenta and distressing your baby. That's why it's really helpful to practise a few techniques regularly in late pregnancy so that they come more naturally once labour's underway. Try out the following techniques to find which ones you feel most comfortable with.

Visualisation

Sometimes known as 'guided imagery', the idea of visualisation is that you transport yourself away from a situation mentally by visualising a more pleasurable environment, or a good outcome in a given situation:

- find a quiet, relaxing place where you can get 5–10 minutes by yourself, uninterrupted
- breathe deeply, concentrating on your out-breaths
- imagine yourself in a beautiful setting: a tropical beach; breathtaking gardens; exhilarating mountain scenery; or flying through the clouds
- focus on really being there, homing in on every little detail to immerse yourself in the situation: bring to mind the sounds, smells and feelings associated with your special place
- try to stay in this scene, without becoming distracted, for at least five minutes. (Set an alarm if you don't think you can time five minutes without checking your watch – which would be a distraction in itself)
- some mums find it helpful to visualise the cervix as a flower bud opening up more and more with each contraction – but go with whatever works for you
- instead of visualising a beautiful setting, you can focus on visualising your labour and birth going calmly, smoothly, painlessly and without intervention.

Meditation

Whilst you can attend some really excellent courses for meditation, it's possible to emulate the state of meditation by practising similar techniques:

- sit comfortably in a peaceful room where you can be alone, uninterrupted, for 20 minutes
- relax your hands in your lap and close your eyes
- focus on breathing deeply and regularly, concentrating on your out-breaths
- think of a two-syllable sound you feel comfortable repeating: it doesn't have to be meaningful – in fact, it's helpful if it isn't (perhaps something like 'ah-um'). Begin repeating this chant to yourself as you breathe, stressing the second syllable with each out-breath
- let other thoughts float away from your mind and bring your focus back gently to your chant whenever your mind strays
- continue for about 20 minutes once or twice a day – but be warned: you might very well fall asleep, so you might want to set an alarm!

For details on getting full instruction in Transcendental Meditation – a specialist meditation technique – visit. www.t-m.org.uk.

Self-hypnosis

You could put yourself on a course of self-hypnosis which can help you to take full control of your labour. Mums have reported having an empowering experience with an uplifting and even pain-free labour as a result of learning the HypnoBirthing® technique (also known as the Mongan method), for example. Practitioners usually advise attending as a couple, and courses cost around £200–£450 for the two of you, depending on whether you are coached in a group or privately. There are other courses available, too, including Natal Hypnotherapy™. For full details, visit these websites:

- www.hypnobirthing.co.uk
- www.birthwithoutfear.co.uk.
- www.natalhypnotherapy.co.uk

Breathing techniques

Breathing techniques are the single most widely used relaxation technique for labour, and are taught at National Childbirth Trust (NCT) and NHS antenatal classes. Focusing on your breathing helps you to maintain some control over your contractions, and also allows you to utilise your energy more efficiently. In the third stage of labour, panting can prevent pushing until your midwife instructs you to do so, meaning your baby isn't delivered too quickly. This can help reduce the trauma to your baby's head as well as reducing the risk of your perineum tearing or of the need for an episiotomy. For full details on breathing techniques, see p. 265.

What the netmums say

'My own relaxation technique!'

I found biting the nozzle on the gas & air breathing pipe helped, as well as screaming and sucking ice cubes whilst inhaling the gas & air. This was definitely a much more painful experience than when I'd had an epidural with my first child, but I managed fine with gas & air second time around. I think you just need to listen to what your body wants you to do, whether it's deep breathing or howling like a werewolf: go with the flow and you'll cope fine, even if your birth partner ends up with one arm after it all!
Alicia from London, mum to Kyrus, two, Demiyah, one, and 14 weeks pregnant

We already knew we were having a little girl and that we wanted to call her Louisa, so I used her name to help me with my breathing towards the end of the second stage. I'd repeat, 'Come on, Louisa' each time, stretching 'Lou-i-sa' to fill each out-breath. It really helped to connect with her as it kept me focused on the fact that we were going through this difficult experience together. At the moment she was delivered the two midwives in the room said, 'Hello, Louisa!', which was just lovely. I already loved her before I even held her.
Maya from east Sussex, mum to Louisa, eight weeks

Make your own baby book

Here's another nice-to-do exercise, and one that'll give you a lasting, personalised memory of your pregnancy, labour and birth, as well as the early days with your new baby!

1 First, find a beautiful blank A4 notebook or album: you'll find bejewelled, ornate ones in some specialist stationers and department stores – or you could find something plainer and fix a laminated photograph of your baby to the front later on.
2 Decide on sections for your book. They could include: 'Finding out!'; 'My scans and test results'; 'Thoughts and feelings'; 'My pregnancy'; 'Baby's first footprint' – or whatever you like.
3 Stick envelopes on to some of the pages for keepsakes such as your positive pregnancy test (or you could just include a photograph); your scan photos; your baby's hospital identity bracelets; photos of the birth and so on.
4 Fill in the written sections as far as you can: you can use the *How are you feeling?* charts in this book to transfer and record your thoughts and feelings at various stages of pregnancy.
5 Encourage your partner to contribute to the book, too. Perhaps you could have a 'Dad's thoughts' section here and there throughout the book?
6 Let your imagination run riot: perhaps you want to record your favourite foods in pregnancy; your best and worst moments; a list of the music you listened to in labour (or a compilation CD); how your relationships with your parents, friends and partner have changed; a few photographs of your work leaving do, or whatever else occurs to you.
7 Find a box to keep your special baby book in and decorate it however you like.

Your mission this week: Indulge yourself!

Have a little of what you fancy whenever you fancy it: enjoy a curry; have a night out with your partner; get together with girlfriends; treat yourself to a massage or a haircut; take your mum or a friend on a spa day at your local health club; buy a new lipstick; have a manicure – just don't buy a new 'signature' perfume as you might well go straight off it once your hormones start to normalise after the birth! Make a point of really enjoying whatever treats you choose, and not in a last-minute, now-or-never kind of desperation. Remember, although you'll be pretty busy for a few months after the birth, you'll probably be so immersed in babycare you won't really miss your usual treats for a while; and, in any case, although admittedly your life is about to change forever, your baby's arrival certainly doesn't have to coincide with a permanent end to all fun! Don't worry, you'll naturally find a new rhythm to life and new ways to enjoy yourself – as well as time to go out as a couple or with friends in your own good time.

What the netmums say

'Those little last-minute treats'

I had a feeling Connor would come when he was due, so I made sure me and my husband went out to my favourite restaurants, went to the movies loads of times and did all the things I was worried about not getting to do again for a long time. I'm glad I did!
Erin from Leeds, mum to Connor, 11 months

I'd always really wanted to go to the theatre, so although it was really expensive my other half surprised me with tickets when I was about 32 weeks pregnant. It was perfect, actually: any later and I think I'd have been too uncomfortable to stay in the seat, but any sooner and it wouldn't have felt like a 'last-minute' treat, which was quite important to me. Otherwise I'd have been looking for some other big treat nearer the time. Call me spoilt, but that's me!
Claire from Bristol, mum to Sadie, six months

I booked me and my boyfriend into our favourite guesthouse by the sea for a 'dirty weekend' in my 37th week! I can safely say that nothing dirtier happened than eating our dinner in bed and spilling chocolate ice cream on the duvet – but it was great fun in any case.

We spent the first day on the pier (with me sitting and walking alternately every 15 minutes!); went to the Sea Life centre on the second day (which made me decide to take our little one when he's old enough!) and enjoyed a fish-and-chip lunch on the seafront. Marvellous!

Francesca from Dorking, mum to Louis, seven months

Look no further

I feel absolutely exhausted after a daytime sleep, so how is catnapping a good thing?

You're probably falling into the trap of sleeping for too long so that your body enters the deep sleep phase usually only achieved during night-time sleep. Dragging yourself back from deep sleep will leave you feeling groggy, headachy and as if you've just woken from 100 years' kip like Sleeping Beauty (with the probable omission of a handsome prince waking you gently with a kiss!). The key is to sleep for short bursts – say 10–20 minutes, but no longer: set an alarm if you need to. These shorter naps allow you to sleep lightly, but just enough to recharge your batteries. When you wake up from a nap, splash your face with water, have a cool drink and, if it's practical, go for a short walk to revive yourself fully.

If I hypnotise myself in labour, won't I be out of control and miss the birth?

No: hypnosis is not at all as it's portrayed in old movies, where a person enters a zombie-like state (any more than sleepwalkers tend to roam the house with arms outstretched, shuffling around like Frankenstein's monster!). When you enter a hypnotic state, you remain fully aware of all that's going on around you, but you can distance yourself from the intensity of the experience so that you're a kind of 'observer' rather than a participant. You might be unaware of how much time is passing, but in labour that's a good thing! It's easy to bring yourself out of your hypnotic state simply by opening your eyes: remember, you're totally in control just as if you were daydreaming. If you feel a bit 'spacey' coming back from hypnosis so abruptly, however, you can count yourself back by chanting 'five, four, three, two, one' vigorously in your mind and opening your eyes on the count of 'one'.

Can we bring a professional photographer to the birth?

The regulations on how many people can attend a birth and whether or not photographic equipment can be set up vary between different hospital trusts, so you'll need to ask your midwife in advance of the birth. If they agree, you'll probably have to get written permission. If you're having a home birth, it'll be up to you who's there and how much paraphernalia is brought in; however, it's courteous to inform your midwife in advance and for her to have a say in where and how things are set up so that she has optimum space and working conditions. Either way, you'll have to get permission from any hospital staff, including your midwife, if they are to appear in photography.

Who'd have thought?

Although identical twins share the same genes, they don't have identical fingerprints*. This is because fingerprints aren't only dictated by DNA, but by the physical environment in the uterus, too: so a twin's position in the uterus, for example, can cause differences in the way the whorls and arches on the fingers develop.

*Research published in New Scientist, October 2005

Week 36 35 days to go!

Don't forget: Look for a nursing bra

If you're planning to breastfeed your baby, round about now is a good time to get fitted for a couple of nursing bras. There are lots of different types: the best have 'drop down' cups with simple clips, or zippable cups, both of which are easy to open and close one-handed. The most important things to consider are fit, comfort and flexibility as you'll need even more room for growth once your milk comes in a few days after the birth, and space for breastpads too. Go for 100 per cent cotton if possible for comfort and 'breathability'; ensure the bra has wide straps to support your breasts and prevent shoulder and neck pain; look for a deep band at the back to help keep the bra from slipping and sliding; ask to be fitted – and remember that different styles will fit you differently so you may end up with bras in various sizes. It's worth having at least two bras so you'll always have a spare when one is in the wash. Trying to manage with an ordinary bra probably won't be something you'll want to try twice!

What the netmums say

'How much my boobs grew!'

Pre-pregnancy I was a 38E; within the first few weeks I went up to an F cup, and I was a G by the time I gave birth. There seemed to be a growth spurt at the beginning and end of my pregnancy and not much happening in the middle. I'm now a 38FF so never really went all the way back down.

Emma from Bedford, mum to Geordan, two

I was really looking forward to great big boobs for once (or rather twice!) in my life, but my rather neat 32Bs only actually went up to a 32C in each pregnancy, which was a bit disappointing! I did have a little bit of a cleavage, but nothing really dramatic. I suppose I saved on buying new bras and new tops! After breastfeeding two babies, my boobs seem to be even flatter than before, but I don't mind. I'm lucky still to be able to go bra-less if I really want to – not bad for a 35-year-old.

Roberta from Hendon, mum to Lucy, two and William, four months

Hey baby!

At 2.75kg (around 6lb), your baby is a very good size now. He measures around 34cm (around 13.5in) from crown to rump, and 46cm (almost 18.5in) from head to toe. His latest growth spurt is coming to an end now, although he'll still put on weight at a slower rate over the next few weeks. There's no room for any more amniotic fluid in your uterus and very little room for any contortions either, so your baby might seem to fidget and 'rumble' around rather than make big movements. This restriction of movement will be compounded by the fact that your body will now begin to reabsorb some of the amniotic fluid that's given your baby space for manoeuvre. If your baby's head down or breech you might feel him 'drop' into your pelvis this week if this hasn't happened already. This process is known as 'engagement'. This is the last week that your baby would be considered premature if he were born now.

All about you

Now we've discussed previously just how much higher your uterus can possibly grow under your ribcage, and you'll be relieved to know that this week is more or less the pinnacle for many mums because of the likelihood of the baby's head engaging (see below). So your uterus measures around 36cm (about 14.5in) upwards from your pubic bone and just over 14cm (around 5.5in) from your belly button. You're likely to feel like a balloon about to burst, and are probably more likely to be dreaming of a lovely refreshing sorbet than a full-on curry. Even if you do fancy a substantial meal, chances are you won't be able to finish it!

Engagement

Also known as 'dropping' and 'lightening', the term 'engaging' refers to your baby's head dropping down and fitting into your pelvis ready for the onset of labour. From now on you'll start to feel the weight of your baby's head shift away from your ribs and down into your pelvis, and you might well begin to adopt the waddling walk associated with late pregnancy (so why isn't it called 'weightening'?). You might have a gnawing worry that your baby will suddenly drop out of you without warning once the process of engagement has started (you should be so lucky!). OK, so it all sounds like just so much more discomfort – but the compensation of being able to breathe more freely (ah, hence 'lightening'!), get a little respite from indigestion and enjoy the odd pig-out at one sitting should even things out a little. Oh, and early engagement doesn't have anything to do with early labour, although it's definitely another sign that labour isn't too far off.

Not all babies will engage yet: sometimes it happens at Week 37 or 38; sometimes it doesn't happen until the onset of labour – although this is unusual in a first pregnancy. There are several factors that can mean engagement is delayed:

- mums in sedentary jobs or who spend lots of time sitting down are more likely to find that their babies have adopted a 'posterior lie' – where the baby's spine is lying against their own. This can make for a really uncomfortable labour with severe back pain, so it's worth doing all you can to encourage your baby to turn and face your spine: you can try sitting in an upright, firm chair leaning forwards with your knees apart (very attractive!); kneeling with your palms against a wall and 'walking' your knees backwards so that you are propped leaning forward with your thighs further back than your hips; or using a kneeling chair (often used by people with lower back problems), where you appear to kneel 'suspended'

- mums with strong, toned abs may find that their babies are slow to engage. If this applies to you, there's not a lot you can do, but take heart: you're only likely to experience this phenomenon in your first pregnancy!
- if you're carrying a large baby – or if your pelvis is a tight fit for your baby's head – he may simply need the force of contractions to push him down into your pelvis.

If your baby's head doesn't engage over the next couple of weeks, your midwife will probably want to investigate with an extra scan just in case a fibroid or your placenta is causing an obstruction, but it may be all that she needs to do is give him a bit of a shove!

What the netmums say

'Feeling my baby's head engage'

I remember a distinct feeling of the head being engaged: it was very uncomfortable. I had SPD [see p. 117], which was made worse by it, but also it felt as though my son was going to fall out of me if I walked around for too long. I had sharp pains in my cervix, as if he was poking at me, and there was a really full feeling down there like he was going to pop his head out any second to say hello. I now understand why women waddle in late pregnancy!
Erin from Leeds, mum to Connor, 11 months

Leaving work

Lots of mums choose the end of this week as their date to leave work – and, in any case, if you're off work with any pregnancy-related condition, from now on your employer can theoretically enforce your maternity leave.

To make the most of your leave, try to plan it out a little. If you still have chores to do in preparation for the birth – decorating to finish; things to buy;

bags to pack; furniture to set up – then schedule them in order of priority, taking on one thing every couple of days and resting or doing something else pleasurable on the alternate days. Your main priority has to be to rest and enjoy your time alone. If you have family or friends elsewhere in the UK, why not pay them a visit for a night or two? (Don't forget to take your maternity notes with you, though, and check there's a maternity unit close by just in case!) Have a last girls' night out if you feel like it – or organise a 'baby party' where you ask your friends round to your home (but if you're setting it up yourself, make it clear you're not asking for presents!).

Enjoy lie-ins if you're comfy staying in bed; take some long, relaxing baths; listen to music – maybe make that compilation CD for the labour room. Record your thoughts and feelings in the chart at the end of this chapter and in your baby book if you've made one. Get your partner to take some more photos of you in your heavily pregnant state; sort out your pre-pregnancy wardrobe so you have some clothes laundered and ready for when you no longer need your maternity clothes (although don't expect this necessarily to be any time soon!); cook for the freezer, if you enjoy doing it, so that there are meals at the ready for your partner when you're in hospital, or for both of you when you're home. If you're not the cook of the household, then delegate to your partner – but whoever does it, you'll save time and money as well as enjoying nutritious meals if you cook ahead.

If you don't fancy an all-out evening 'leaving do' with colleagues – and, let's face it, who wants to try to drag home late at night? – then warn them in advance that if they're planning anything at all, a lunch or afternoon tea party would be nice. It's an idea to organise for your partner to come and pick you up in the car afterwards if possible: you might have too many gifts to carry comfortably (well, let's hope so!) and, if not, you've got the great excuse that you don't feel like travelling any more in any case.

Most of all, enjoy yourself: there's a whole world of new experiences ahead of you, but it's lovely to indulge in some of your favourite, most familiar comforts while you can.

Who'd have thought?

As from May 2008, fertility clinics no longer have to consider a child's need for a father when treating single and lesbian women.

What the netmums say

'My feelings about leaving work'

With my first pregnancy I was relieved to have finished work but also upset, as I knew I wouldn't be going back to the job I loved (and I would have got promotion if I had stayed). I couldn't afford to go back as all my wages would have gone on childcare, and I worked right up to 37 weeks. With my second pregnancy I was working in a pub/club and went on maternity leave as soon as I could because I was working two shifts from 5 p.m. till 3 a.m. and I was knackered from being on my feet for so long. That time I finished at 31 weeks. I was glad to leave, but knew I would be going back. I left without a backward glance and went back six months later to nearly all new faces.
Gail from Glasgow, mum to Brodie, six and Zoe, four

I wasn't working in my first pregnancy, but with my second I couldn't wait to finish. I was fed up for ages before I even got pregnant and was getting tired of the job altogether. I do miss some of the people and friends, but not the nature of my job, which was as a property manager in a letting agent's. I won't be going back for two reasons: I can't afford the childcare and I don't really want to!
Michelle from Brighton, mum to Emily, nine and Finlay, six weeks

I had to keep up the pretence that I was going back to work when I left, even though I was 99 per cent certain I wouldn't be. I wanted to keep my options open in case they came up with a really good part-time offer. Because of that I had to keep my feelings a bit low-key, which was tricky. I really loved my team mates in the customer services department of a big department store, and would have loved to buy them each a little something and say a proper goodbye. As it turned out I was able to have a few of them round for dinner once I'd finally confirmed my resignation, which was lovely. They hadn't forgotten all about me, even though my replacement sounded enviously popular...
Grace from Cardiff, mum to twins Sam and Jack, two

Your mission this week: Enjoy some special times

Plan a couple of family occasions as well as some pleasurable time alone: perhaps an evening out with your partner (whilst you still don't need a babysitter); or a lunch with both sets of parents (maybe all together, or maybe not...!); find a lovely peaceful setting for a walk if the weather's good (National Trust gardens are a good choice and tend to have lovely tearooms and gift shops as a reward at the end!); if you can afford to splash out a bit, why not do an overnighter in a country pub or have a spa day with your partner or a girlfriend.

Look no further

Will my baby drop down into my pelvis in one go?
No, there's no need to expect a sudden shock that'll have you clenching your knees shut and freezing to the spot! Engagement usually happens by degrees over a number of weeks. Your midwife will record how far down your baby has descended in terms of 'fifths to brim', meaning how many fifths of your baby's skull she can feel above the brim (or edge) of your pelvis when she palpates your abdomen – so 5/5 means your baby's head hasn't descended at all, whilst 0/5 means she can no longer feel any of the head and your baby is fully engaged.

Is it safe to keep wearing jewellery in my body piercings?
By now – if not earlier in pregnancy – you may find that the skin around your piercings, especially if you have a pierced navel or nipples, is becoming overstretched and tight feeling. The danger here is that if the skin splits you are at risk of an infection setting in. Luckily there's a solution that means you don't have to remove your body jewellery and risk having to have the piercings done again after the birth: you can buy special maternity body jewellery with extra long bars that's made from flexible plastic, with plastic end caps. This means you should be able to keep them on for scans too! Some websites to visit include www.bellybar.co.uk, www.bodyjewelleryshop.com and www.ouchbodyjewellery.co.uk.

My belly button is so sore. What can I do?
It's a common problem once your belly button becomes an 'outie' and is a similar affliction to the rather comically named 'jogger's nipple'! The soreness is caused by the friction of your clothes rubbing against your belly

button, so the simple answer is to keep it covered with a breathable dressing – but keep a supply with you as these can rub off too. If it looks sticky as well as feeling sore, clean your belly button with warm salty water and cotton wool, then dry with your hairdryer on a cool setting. Apply a little antiseptic cream and cover with a gauze dressing. If it's inflamed, red, hot or painful, contact your midwife or GP for advice. You may be prescribed an antibiotic cream that's safe to use in pregnancy.

How are you feeling?

Tick the box that most closely represents how you feel about the given statements, then look back to the charts in previous chapters to see how you've changed over the months.

Physically	Emotionally
Phew! I can breathe more easily! Strongly agree ☐ Agree ☐ Neither agree nor disagree ☐ Disagree ☐ Strongly disagree ☐	I'm going to miss my colleagues Strongly agree ☐ Agree ☐ Neither agree nor disagree ☐ Disagree ☐ Strongly disagree ☐
I'm enjoying food again – lots of it! Strongly agree ☐ Agree ☐ Neither agree nor disagree ☐ Disagree ☐ Strongly disagree ☐	I'm terrified of having a Caesarean Strongly agree ☐ Agree ☐ Neither agree nor disagree ☐ Disagree ☐ Strongly disagree ☐
I'm finding it hard to bend from the 'waist' Strongly agree ☐ Agree ☐ Neither agree nor disagree ☐ Disagree ☐ Strongly disagree ☐	I don't want my relationship with my midwife to end Strongly agree ☐ Agree ☐ Neither agree nor disagree ☐ Disagree ☐ Strongly disagree ☐
My feet feel fat and clumpy Strongly agree ☐ Agree ☐ Neither agree nor disagree ☐ Disagree ☐ Strongly disagree ☐	I feel I know my baby's sex Strongly agree ☐ Agree ☐ Neither agree nor disagree ☐ Disagree ☐ Strongly disagree ☐
I'm getting more flushed than ever Strongly agree ☐ Agree ☐ Neither agree nor disagree ☐ Disagree ☐ Strongly disagree ☐	I feel too young/old to be a mum Strongly agree ☐ Agree ☐ Neither agree nor disagree ☐ Disagree ☐ Strongly disagree ☐
I feel like I've got a football between my legs! Strongly agree ☐ Agree ☐ Neither agree nor disagree ☐ Disagree ☐ Strongly disagree ☐	I'm torn between going for a natural birth or an epidural Strongly agree ☐ Agree ☐ Neither agree nor disagree ☐ Disagree ☐ Strongly disagree ☐

Who'd have thought?

US researchers believe that the sound of an ultrasound scan is as loud to an unborn baby as an underground train coming into a station is to us – although it's not thought to harm the baby.

Quick quiz

What do you know about labour?

1 Which of the following conditions most often leads to a Caesarean?
a. Gestational diabetes
b. Placenta praevia
c. Fear of labour

2 What is a 'show'?
a. The gush of water when the amniotic sac breaks
b. A plug of mucus that breaks away from your cervix
c. The start of a good night out

3 What is your perineum?
a. The top of your uterus
b. The area of tissue between the vagina and the anus
c. That's a very good question...

4 How late can a baby's head engage?
a. 38 weeks
b. In labour
c. It might not engage at all

5 What is delivered during the third stage of labour?
a. Your baby
b. Your placenta
c. A huge bouquet hopefully!

Answers: The answers to this quiz are all 'b'.

Mostly a: You've put two and two together, but unfortunately made five. It seems as if you've got your wires crossed a little bit and, although you've definitely taken a lot of information on board, you've got it all slightly confused along the way. Have another read over the sections you weren't so sure about and you'll be fine.

Mostly b: It seems you're all equipped and ready for labour, having taken in everything you've read. This is the best preparation you can make, so keep reading all the way to your big day for lots more useful information.

Mostly c: Still burying your head in the sand? Your lighthearted approach is refreshing, but you might find yourself feeling a little bit vulnerable on the day labour finally starts, unless you read over some of the previous chapters again. Go on, it can't hurt to be prepared – and it's going to happen whatever you do, so you may as well be as knowledgeable as possible.

Who'd have thought?

You should avoid having any new piercings in pregnancy because of the risk of infection and the fact that most oral antibiotics are not recommended. Also, nipple piercings may not heal properly because the breasts continue to grow, opening the wound up further.

Who'd have thought?

It's unwise to get a tattoo in pregnancy for several reasons: you may feel differently about it emotionally once your hormones have normalised after the birth; your skin may be stretched right now so the appearance of the tattoo might change considerably when it shrinks back; and tattooists are reluctant in any case because the effect of tattooists' ink if absorbed into the bloodstream is unknown.

Chapter 9
Weeks 37–40

You are so nearly there now! In fact, let's face it, even though around two-thirds of first-time mums go overdue, you could go into labour any day (yikes!) – and if you're expecting twins, you're actually considered to have reached full term by the end of this week (cripes!).

What a long way you've come since Chapter 1 when you first discovered you were pregnant. Back then you were probably full of trepidation about staying pregnant; now you're probably full of anxiety about the implications of going overdue…

This next four weeks (or so) will either seem to drag by in slow motion or whizz past in a flurry, and much depends on your attitude to the birth: it's almost a law of nature that if you want to get it over with it'll feel as if this last lap is as long as your entire pregnancy to date, whereas if you'd rather stay pregnant for the foreseeable future you'll seemingly find yourself in that labour suite by this time tomorrow!

From now until your delivery date you'll be making all your final preparations, physically, mentally and practically; you'll be looking forward to the arrival of your newborn and anticipating your new life together; you may be grieving for your fancy-free past already or celebrating the start of a brand-new phase. Above all, you'll be getting ready to be someone's mum – a lifelong role and your most important job ever.

Week 37 *28 days to go!*

Don't forget: Make a phone list

Once your baby's born you'll want to tell the world! (Well, maybe not the world – but everyone who's important enough to be on your 'friends and family' phone list.) It's a good idea to make an actual paper list of names and numbers for your partner to ring: you won't necessarily have the presence of mind to think of them all straight after the birth and your partner won't necessarily remember who he's rung and who he hasn't unless he has a list of names to put ticks, crosses or 'left a message' next to. Give one copy to him; give another to someone like your mum who can be trusted to keep it safe in case your partner loses his or leaves it at home; and put a third in your hospital bag. You might want to discuss the order he rings people in as well, as some relatives and friends can get incredibly sniffy if they think they're not high enough up the pecking order! (Remember any head-scratching over who to tell first when announcing your pregnancy all those months ago?)

Hey baby!

Your baby's not up to a whole lot except bulking up now, and he's only going to grow by about another 2cm (¾in) in length between now and your EDD. He weighs almost 2.95kg (6.5lb) now and he measures about 35cm (14in) from crown to rump. His total length is around 47cm (almost 19in). Although your baby has very little room for manoeuvre in your uterus now and you'll feel less movement generally, he's quite capable of delivering a sharp dig or poke that might take your breath away! Part of the reason for all the fat he's storing up is that he'll need it to keep him going as he adapts to accepting milk from you in place of the nutrients he's been receiving via the placenta. He'll use the surplus to keep his energy levels up: this is why most babies lose weight after birth.

Who'd have thought?

Your baby's arrival date is closely tied in with the length of your normal menstrual cycle: if you have a short cycle, you're likely to deliver your baby earlier than if you had a longer cycle. If you have a cycle close to the average 28 days, you'll probably have your baby close to your due date.

All about you

You might get a bit of a surprise if you happen to have an antenatal appointment this week when you find that your uterus has stayed in position from last week! It varies from mum to mum, but lots do find that they don't grow 'upwards' any more. If you have grown, you may find that the top of your uterus is around 37cm (almost 15in) from your pubic bone and around 16.5cm (6.5in) from your belly button. Your weight should have peaked around now, too, and although weight gain also varies enormously (no pun intended!) from mum to mum, the average gain by now is around 11–13.5kg (25–35lb). Your breasts will feel full and tender, and the areolas may continue to darken. If your baby's head has engaged, your pelvis may feel quite 'full' and uncomfortable.

What the netmums say

'My total pregnancy weight gain'

I'd been ill before I became pregnant and lost weight, so I was under my normal weight at about eight-and-a-half stone. After finding out I was pregnant I just ate whatever I wanted when I wanted, although for most of the pregnancy I was so sick I could only face certain things. At eight months pregnant I weighed myself and found I was 15-and-a-half stone! I didn't get on the scales after that, but I was like a big balloon and I'm sure most of it was water retention as it all seemed to come off (or out!) after the birth when I deflated quite quickly. My family and friends think it's hilarious that my weight nearly doubled. I was lucky I dropped quickly to my pre-pregnancy size, but if I was to do it again I would definitely watch what I ate. I might not be so lucky second time around.
Carrie from north Lincolnshire, mum to Ruby, three

I put on about three stone in my first pregnancy and lost it quite quickly afterwards. With my second I put on five-and-a -half stone, then lost about three after I had him. I found losing the three stone very hard, though, and have now ballooned back up to 16 stone. Argghh!
Rachel from Northumberland, mum to Hollie, seven and Lewis, two

I was eight stone before I fell pregnant, but by about my eighth month I weighed 13-and-a-half stone! I didn't eat much for the first five months or so as I had very bad sickness and couldn't even keep water down – but I suppose towards the end I did eat quite a lot of junk food as I just didn't have the energy to cook. I now weigh 13 and a half stone and my son is three years old. I'm finding it very hard to diet, as before I was pregnant I ate whatever I liked and never put on any weight.

Nadine from Berkshire, mum to Riley, three

Group B strep test

You might be offered a Group B strep test during pregnancy Week 37, although usually only if you are displaying any symptoms such as fever or vaginal discharge. Otherwise you can pay to have it done privately at a cost of around £30 if you're worried. The test detects a type of bacteria (Group B streptococcus) that can live in or around the vagina and is present in about 35 per cent of healthy adults. You're more at risk for Group B infection if you've had a urinary tract infection caused by Group B; if your waters break before 37 weeks or if you've already had a baby infected with Group B. Researchers are working on developing a vaccine to treat Group B strep. Group B is usually harmless, but if your vagina is swabbed and found to contain the bacteria in late pregnancy, it means your baby might become infected during labour and delivery. If you're found to have Group B strep in late pregnancy, or if you're considered at risk of carrying the bacteria, you'll be given antibiotics in labour to help prevent this. If it does happen, however, your baby will be given antibiotics at birth and will need to be observed because Group B can cause serious infections in newborns such as blood infections, meningitis or pneumonia.

True labour

From around now it can be quite tricky to tell if real labour has begun or not, especially as Braxton-Hicks contractions can confuse the issue. Many's the mum who's turned up at hospital only to be sent home again because she's experiencing 'false labour' (see p. 206). There are some signs that you're in true labour, although they can happen at different stages from mum to mum. Here are some pointers to look out for:

- you've had a 'show' (see pp. 251–2). Not all mums notice they've had a show, however, as the mucus plug can come away in bits and pieces or it might be passed down the loo without you noticing it. So just because you haven't had a show that you know about, it doesn't mean you can't be in labour
- your waters have broken (see p. 252). The waters should be clear or honey-coloured. If they're stained greenish-black, contact your midwife straightaway as this usually indicates that the baby is in distress and may need delivering sooner rather than later. In many cases, the waters don't break until labour is already underway and a midwife might rupture them artificially with an 'amnihook' in order to speed things up. This is known as Artificial Rupture of Membranes (ARM) and involves the sac being pierced with the amnihook (an implement that looks like a crochet hook). Because it has to pass through the cervix, the procedure can be quite uncomfortable, but it shouldn't take long
- you're having regular contractions. Once labour has really started you'll experience contractions that come in regular waves, last more than 40 seconds each and happen every 10 minutes or so to begin with. Contractions during the first stage are commonly described as feeling like severe, involuntary tightenings of the belly and can be quite breathtaking for some mums. Once labour is underway, your contractions will continue relentlessly, gradually getting longer and closer together – so if you've been in any doubt as to whether or not you've felt a contraction of true labour to date, you'll know now what you're looking for.

When to go to hospital

It's fine to stay at home in the early stages of labour, so you don't have to panic and rush off to the hospital. Plan to go when your contractions are coming about every five minutes and lasting 30–40 seconds – unless you can't cope with the pain or are concerned about anything, in which case ring the maternity ward or go up sooner. If you've had a baby before, you should contact your midwife when your contractions are seven minutes apart, as second and subsequent babies often arrive more quickly than first.

Who'd have thought?

Only 3 per cent of UK babies are exclusively breastfed at five months of age.

What the netmums say

'Deciding when to go to hospital'

The first time round I stayed at home for as long as I could bear the pain, and when I went in I was 4cm dilated so they admitted me. With Theo, I phoned when my waters broke, and asked if they minded if I went in later in the evening when I had put my son to bed and my husband was home. As I was just short of 37 weeks they practically ordered me to come in straightaway: they actually threatened to send an ambulance if I couldn't arrange a lift in! I managed to phone a friend, and was in half an hour later – I was having contractions, even though I couldn't feel them, and was 3cm dilated already.

Jen from Hertfordshire, mum to Jack, four and Theo, 17 months

I wasn't coping at all well with the pain, so I got my partner to take me in after only a few hours of labour. Luckily they didn't turn me away, and I managed to get an epidural after another couple of hours: then I was in heaven! I still wish I'd managed to cope at home for a bit longer – I felt a bit of a wimp caving in so soon – but once I'd been admitted I stopped worrying about it. After all, if the hospital agreed to take me, I must have gone in at the right time.

Jeanette from Hull, mum to Ellie, two

I've only got the one baby, so I didn't know what to expect when labour started. Consequently I ended up going to the hospital twice and being sent home again both times before getting my partner to ring later in labour and get the go-ahead. By that time I was having contractions almost every seven minutes. It was such a relief that our hospital is only five minutes' drive away as I was almost 8cm dilated by the time we arrived! Another half hour and I could have ended up with my partner delivering the baby in our bathroom! I'm not really confident that I'll know when to go in next time around either as I don't think we or the hospital got it quite right this time…

Anne-Marie from Croydon, mum to Anneliese, 14 months

Sleep in late pregnancy

By now you're probably wondering if you'll ever have a good night's sleep again – and maybe even panicking about sleep because you know what's coming once your baby's born! This, of course, will make matters even worse. Apart from feeling uncomfortable, your mind may begin to race at night towards the end of pregnancy as you mentally check and re-check that everything is as ready as can be, and anticipate the major life changes that are about to happen. As your baby's space becomes more and more restricted he may jab or kick you hard in his attempts to move around and may be more active at night. These movements can give you quite a start and – especially if aimed under your ribs – can be quite painful, too.

There are things you can do to improve your chances of a good night's sleep, though, and if all else fails, just try to rest and relax: practise your breathing exercises, visualisation and meditation, and you might just drop off unexpectedly. Here are some other tried-and-tested ideas:

- take a little exercise between dinner and bedtime: even a short, brisk(ish) walk will release endorphins ('feelgood' hormones) that will help to relax you
- have a warm bath with a few drops of lavender oil added to the water: lavender is supposed to have soporific qualities
- make sure you have a light snack before you get into bed: some mums find a small glass of warm milk soothing, and there's research to suggest that milk contains a chemical that can help induce sleep. (However, as you'd have to drink a vat of the stuff to feel any effect, it's thought that it's the satisfying feeling milk gives you that can help you nod off!)
- use a body pillow or other pillows to support your bump and your back: you might even be better off sleeping alone at this stage of pregnancy as you'll be taking up quite a lot of the bed in any case, and you will be less likely to overheat if you're on your own
- if the weather's warm, have an oscillating fan by the bed to keep you cool: this really can make all the difference
- replace your usual bedcovers with something lighter to prevent night sweats and overheating
- try having a special relaxation or sleep CD playing softly, or choose 'mood music' that is specially selected to soothe and relax you.

Your mission this week: Sort out what to do with your pets

If you have any pets, think about making arrangements for them to be looked after while you're having your baby. You might find it less stressful if they're away from the house altogether in the early days at home with your new baby, too. Although your partner might feel he can manage the pets, you don't know how long you could be away from home if you're having a hospital birth, and it would unfair to miss their feeding times: they're likely to be out of sorts when the baby arrives as it is, so it's important to stick to their normal routine as closely as possible in the run-up. If you can't arrange for them to go elsewhere to be cared for, or if you think this would be too unsettling for them, ask a trusted neighbour or friend to come in to feed them while you're not there.

If your pets will be in the house with your new baby, make sure you find a way of keeping them away from him: with dogs, set up a stairgate to the kitchen so you can shut them in there – you could always give them the run of the garden, too, in good weather. With cats, you'll need to ensure they don't jump into the cot with your baby so buy a protective cat net for the cot and/or pram, or shut the door on your baby when he's in a different room from you, but keep the listening half of your baby monitor with you at all times so you can hear him if he needs you. Never leave your newborn baby alone in a room with one of your pets: even the most rigorously trained pet can act unpredictably.

Look no further

I suddenly need to pee all the time again. Why?
It's quite usual for this to happen – although it is, admittedly, a damned nuisance! It coincides with your baby's head engaging and your uterus dropping and bearing down on your bladder. Don't be tempted to drink less in an attempt to pee less: you need all the fluids you can get throughout your pregnancy as you're vulnerable to becoming dehydrated. Do try to avoid long drinks during the last hour or so before bedtime or a journey where you can't get to a loo, though, or you'll certainly regret it!

I'm really worried my waters will break in public. Is there anything I can do to avoid this?
Unfortunately not: the rupture of the membranes (amniotic sac) occurs completely spontaneously and there are no warning signs that it's about to happen. Whilst you can be reassured that for the majority of mums it happens

as a gradual leakage rather than a tidal wave, it's true that a few do experience a sudden gush that can't be stopped – which could, of course, be hugely embarrassing if you happened to be in the middle of a supermarket, church service or library! The best advice is to wear a heavy-duty sanitary pad or even an incontinence pad whenever you stray away from home so that this will at least help contain the flow; you might even want to keep one on at all times if you're worried about your own carpets or furniture. Apart from that, if the worst does happen, remember you're an obviously pregnant lady and people will understand. Just focus on the fact that you need to call your midwife as soon as possible after your waters break because of the risk to you and your baby of infection. Expect to leak more water whenever your baby moves or you have a contraction: not all the amniotic fluid is lost at once when your waters break.

I'm already panicking about being left on my own with my baby. How will I cope?

This is a very common fear, but hardly a surprising one. Of course it seems like an impossibly responsible task now to manage the single-handed care of a newborn, but you really will be surprised how much you manage to take on once your baby arrives. Even if you feel as if you're all fingers and thumbs at first, you'll find a rhythm and soon get into your stride. Make the most of any paternity leave your partner is planning to take: use the time to find the best ways to manage babycare together so that once he's gone back to work he's equipped and confident enough to take over from you when he comes home. Take up all offers from friends and family to come and help you or just keep you company. Don't forget your midwives are still at the end of the phone and should be making regular visits for between 10 and 28 days after your baby has been born. There will be a regular baby clinic near your home, plus a postnatal class for you to join where you can meet other new mums – some from your antenatal class – and discuss any worries and concerns with the midwives who run it. If you do start to feel very low, alone or unable to cope, do discuss this with a health professional, who will be able to help you.

Who'd have thought?

Jack and Grace were the most popular baby names in England and Wales for 2007.

* Source: National Statistics

Week 38 *21 days to go!*

Don't forget: Pick up your TENS machine

If you're renting a TENS machine or other birthing aid, you'll probably need to arrange to pick it up or take delivery of it this week, as most devices are for hire for two weeks before your due date until two weeks afterwards to allow for early or late babies. Once you've got the machine home, it's a great idea to give it some 'dry runs' so that you and your birth partner know exactly what you're doing when the time comes to use it during labour; you can't do yourself any harm by using TENS early and often as it's a completely drug-free device (see p. 93).

Hey baby!

OK, so your baby may have put on weight – he's now around 3.1kg (almost 7lb), but for once his length won't have changed this week and he's still about 35cm (around 14in) from crown to rump and around 47cm (almost 19in) from top to toe. He's shifting uncomfortably in his confined space and, although he might grow a little longer over the next couple of weeks, the only things that are able to grow significantly are his hair and his finger- and toenails. These nails are hardening as well as growing in length now, too. In fact, some mums have reported being scratched by their babies during delivery! Lanugo (the fine, downy hair covering your baby) usually starts falling out around this time, although some full-term babies still have a little smattering at birth.

All about you

This week your baby is considered to be at full term, and he'll no longer be premature if he arrives any time from now. ('Full term' means any length of pregnancy from 38–42 weeks.) As if you've taken your cue from your baby, you'll have stopped growing around now as well. 'About time!' you might be thinking – and you'd be forgiven for that! It doesn't mean you'll get any more comfortable between now and the birth though. Around this time you might be starting to see labour and the delivery of your baby as a preferable option to staying pregnant for much longer: this resigned feeling of 'Let's just get it over with' does tend to come to lots of mums in the end. The top of your uterus is around 38cm (just over

15in) from your pubic bone and around 18cm (just over 7in) from your belly button.

Electronic Foetal Monitoring

If labour is stressful for a mum-to-be, imagine the impact on her baby! During every contraction your baby's blood supply via the placenta is temporarily cut off as the muscles of the uterus squeeze tight. Most babies cope really well; others less so – and there are some predisposing factors that can mean your medical team might suggest continuous Electronic Foetal Monitoring (EFM). This involves attaching two sensors to your belly with elastic straps: one picks up your baby's heartbeat and the other tracks the pattern of your contractions; the results appear as a continuous printout so that the two results can be compared concurrently. (Imagine a lie detector machine and you'll be able to visualise the printout!)

Your baby might need EFM if:

- he has had growth problems during pregnancy
- you have pre-eclampsia
- you have diabetes
- you have heart problems
- you've got an epidural set up
- you've been induced
- you've experienced vaginal bleeding
- you're having twins
- you've had any infections in pregnancy
- you've previously had a Caesarean
- you're in premature labour
- you've gone very overdue (by more than a fortnight).

If you are offered EFM but the sensor trying to detect your baby's heartbeat can't pick it up well (if, for example, you have a substantial layer of fat over your belly that muffles the sound), your midwife might suggest attaching a scalp monitor, which clips on to your baby's head via your cervix, and which can deliver a more accurate result. If your baby seems distressed, your obstetrician may want to take a sample of blood from your baby's scalp using a needle passed up through your cervix. The procedure is called foetal blood sampling, and although it's thought that it might cause some pain to the baby it should be over with quickly, and the sample can then be analysed to see how much oxygen is getting to your baby. If your baby is found to be very lacking in oxygen, you will probably be advised to have an emergency Caesarean.

If your labour is uncomplicated, normal monitoring will be done using the usual Doppler hand-held listening device, and your midwife will check on your baby every 15 minutes during the first stage and every five minutes in the second stage.

What the netmums say

'Having EFM'

When I was six days late I went in for a routine appointment to check on the baby. Foetal monitoring was a part of this, and during the test, which began at 12 noon, they discovered that my son's heart rate kept dropping. I was moved to the labour ward for more detailed monitoring and I was kept on the monitor until I was taken for a Caesarean at 8 p.m. Fortunately, other than the couple of hours when they started inducing me (before they changed their minds and decided a section was for the best) I wasn't in labour, so I wasn't in discomfort. However, being heavily pregnant I needed the toilet frequently and it wasn't always convenient to come off the monitor. The monitoring really did make a difference to the outcome, as the cord was wrapped around Alex's neck and body. Had I not been in for the appointment, I would have gone into labour like that and not have known anything was wrong, so I'm glad this test was conducted.
Lisa from Glasgow, mum to Alex, 11 months

Who'd have thought?

There's no scientific evidence to support the fact that eating spicy foods can trigger labour, so go ahead and have a curry – but don't expect to follow it with a baby instead of a pud!

Nesting instinct

Lots of mums-to-be experience a primal urge to 'feather the nest' in preparation for their baby's homecoming. For some, this nesting instinct kicks in on and off from around the fifth month of pregnancy, but when it happens this late in pregnancy it's thought to be a sign of imminent labour.

The urge can drive mums to do some quite irrational things, from folding and re-folding baby clothes dozens of times to reorganising the food in kitchen cupboards; flinging out perfectly serviceable towels and bedding in an attempt to have everything 'new' in time for the baby's arrival; staying up into the early hours of the morning scrubbing the insides of drawers and even embarking on last-minute decorating. In most cases there's no use trying to fight it: you'll find yourself incredibly driven! You might want to draw the line at stripping wallpaper, however, or undertaking anything drastic: don't forget you could go into labour at any time – and then you'd have an unfinished job, which would surely be worse! Whilst you're at it, you may as well re-check the contents of your hospital bag (see p. 307)!

What the netmums say

'The irresistible urge to "nest"'

I had been furiously cleaning all day when, for some reason, I decided that I absolutely must clean the outside of my downstairs windows. So off I went, cloth in one hand, squirty stuff in the other, even though it was 10 o'clock at night, in total darkness and freezing cold. Unfortunately, when I woke the next morning and opened the curtains I realised that they would just not do, so I nipped out in my dressing gown and finished them off properly!
Rebecca from Southampton, mum to Evie, two and Louie, eight months

With my second pregnancy, my nesting instinct kicked in quite early at about 26 weeks! I started having these mad cravings to get on my hands and knees and sterilise the floor with anti-bacterial liquid – so I went ahead and indulged! My bathroom got a right seeing-to – and in the hectic early weeks after the birth when I had two little ones under 17 months, it was a godsend to know that I'd got it done and dusted. But I wasn't the only one who got 'nesting': my partner went home and started scrubbing the bathroom wall tiles with a brush to prepare for me and my daughter to arrive home from hospital. He's never done it since and, to be honest, they weren't dirty to start with. It just goes to show that some men feel the pregnancy as much as us ladies!

Alicia from London, mum to Kyrus, two, Demiyah, one, and 14 weeks pregnant

I'm not really into gardening, but when pregnant with Brendan I completely gutted and re-did the whole garden. I was the same with Nicole, and did the whole garden again. This time my husband has recently re-turfed and tidied up the whole garden, so there's nothing left to do out there. Instead I've been re-painting all the walls, doors and skirting boards for that clean-as-new look!

Gillian from Preston, mum to Brendan, four, Nicole, 18 months, and 22 weeks pregnant

As I'm a self-confessed slob, my partner kept asking me when the urge to clean was going to set in. I'm ashamed to say it never did – although I did have a burning desire to get someone else in to do it for me. Does that count? I did, however, have a compulsion to wash all the little baby clothes I'd bought in the gentlest soap flakes and fold them neatly into the nursery drawers. I wish I hadn't: half of them were too small for the baby and I could have taken them back!

Debra, South Yorkshire, mum to Finn, four and Louis, two

Who'd have thought?

Around one in five pregnant women in England is induced. However, the rates vary a lot depending on whereabouts you are in the country, and even within regions, depending on each hospital's policy.

Your mission this week: Play with your baby gadgets

Try out all your babycare gadgets, such as your steriliser; your pram/pushchair combination; the drop-down cot side (try it out one-handed – that's how you'll be operating it once your baby is here); your car seat (try it out with a sizeable doll, teddy or someone else's baby!); your baby-listening device and anything else you've bought but not yet experimented with. Set up your cot mobile (if you've bought one); put the cot in place in your room (as government advice is to share a room with your baby for the first six months); buy in some formula milk and bottles if you're planning on bottle- or mixed feeding; get your basic supplies for at home and in your changing bag, including nappies and wipes (see *Newborn essentials and frivolous luxuries*, p. 193).

What are the signs of foetal distress in labour?
Whilst it can be normal for a baby's heart rate to drop during a contraction as long as it picks up again as the contraction is coming to an end, if the monitoring strip shows that it dips and doesn't come back up to normal this could mean a baby is in distress. Sometimes changing a mum's position and giving her more fluids and oxygen, which in turn are passed to the baby, will help, but if not her baby will have to be delivered quickly, often by Caesarean.

Another sign of distress is when monitoring shows a repeated, gradual deceleration in heart rate after contractions, not returning to normal until well after each contraction ends. If the baby doesn't respond to the treatments outlined above, then quick delivery will become paramount for his or her safety.

Analysing a foetal monitor strip is a complicated business and the results can only be interpreted by a highly trained professional, so you can be assured that the decision to intervene and deliver your baby swiftly won't be taken lightly.

Can I use my TENS to ease my backache before labour?
Yes, TENS isn't just used for pain relief in labour – it's used by patients experiencing all sorts of pain, who don't want to be taking heavy-duty drugs and who want to be in control of their own pain relief. Although it's more effective against some types of pain than others, backache is one of the complaints people often find relief from by using TENS. The system works in two ways:

- by selectively stimulating 'non-pain' nerve fibres which then send signals to the brain blocking other nerve signals carrying pain messages
- by stimulating the production of endorphins, also known as 'feelgood' hormones, which can help combat pain.

TENS is non-addictive, has no side effects, and the pain relief can be rapid and long-lasting, so do go ahead and use it whenever you need it: you'll also be well practised by the time you need it for labour.

Now that my baby's considered full-term, can I start trying to lose some weight?
It's really not advisable to try to lose weight in pregnancy unless you have been advised to do so by your doctors – and this is only likely to happen if you are very obese. Keeping at a steady weight is important in supplying your baby with all the nutrition he needs to stay healthy in your uterus, and he still has some growing to do in terms of weight gain. Having said that, eating a healthy diet of around 2,000–2,300 calories per day, made up from low-fat, low-sugar, high-fibre foods, lean meats or vegetable protein, fresh fruit and veg will stand you in good stead for losing weight after your baby is born: you'll have the basic dietary requirements in place and all you'll need to do is reduce your calorie intake – but even then only after you've finished breastfeeding. During breastfeeding, your calorific intake should be between 2,300–2,500.

Who'd have thought?

Researchers at St George's University, London, have discovered that some men do, indeed, suffer from 'phantom pregnancy'. During a controlled study, expectant dads complained of cramps, back pain, mood swings, food cravings, morning sickness, fatigue, depression, fainting, insomnia and toothache. The condition, labelled Couvade syndrome but not recognised by doctors, is thought to be triggered by anxiety about the pregnancy.

Week 39 14 days to go!

Don't forget: Read up on breastfeeding

Now's a good time to read all you can on breastfeeding techniques so that you are au fait with it, so look for a good book dedicated to the subject, with a troubleshooting section so that if or when things go wrong you'll have a handy source of reference. Yes, your midwife should be at the other end of the phone for you if you need her, but when your baby doesn't seem satisfied and it's 3 a.m., you might want to refer to another source of information. There's no arguing that breastfeeding is best for your baby, and the vast majority of mums are physiologically able to do so – even those with inverted or flat nipples; some mums prefer not to, though, and that's fine too. Don't let anyone make you feel guilty about your decision. For some basic breastfeeding tips see p. 361.

Hey baby!

At around 3.25kg (just over 7lb) your baby is almost at the average birth weight of 3.3kg (7lb 4oz). He may have grown an extra centimetre in length this past week so that he now measures around 36cm (almost 14.5in) from crown to rump, and 48cm (just over 19in) from top to toe. Another surge of hormones will mean that your baby's genitals look disproportionately large at birth, but this will settle down a few days after birth so that they're eventually in the correct proportion to the rest of his – or her – body. If you do have a boy, expect your partner to be most impressed by the size of his crown jewels! (Of course, you don't have to enlighten him to the fact that they're going to shrink back down…) In a baby girl, the labia may seem overly engorged.

All about you

The top of your uterus remains around 38cm (just over 15in) from your pubic bone and around 18cm (just over 7in) above your belly button. Now that you're in your final weeks of pregnancy, you probably won't put on much more, if any, weight. On average a mum gains around 11kg (24.2lb) by the end of pregnancy. You might have a roadmap of stretch marks and veins all over your body, especially over your breasts, thighs, abdomen and buttocks. You may feel as though your baby could drop out any day now. You're probably finding it difficult to get comfy in any position, day or night, for any length of time. You might find that walking feels better than sitting or standing. If you're going to be sitting, standing or lying down for any length of time, make sure your lower back, legs and feet are well supported.

Getting through the last weeks

By now you might be thoroughly bored and disenchanted with being pregnant. What did your feet look like again? What sort of an unruly tangle has your bikini line got into down there? When will you ever be able to aspire to wear your skinny jeans again (maybe never – unless you're one of those back-to-a-size-zero-moments-after-the-birth skinny minnies the rest of us love to hate, to be brutally frank!). It's easy to start focusing on all the negatives around now – like the loss of a spontaneous social (and love) life; a shortage of money; impending sleep deprivation – but there are things you can do to try and make the time pass more pleasurably and more quickly:

- plan your days – and we mean really plan. Obviously it's not worth buying tickets to the Opera when you could go into labour any day (and who wants to squeeze into a scratchy, sweaty, velour theatre seat with little or no leg room at this stage in any case?); but having a focus to each day will mean you get up looking forward to stuff instead of brooding, clock-watching and imagining you will be the first woman to match a blue whale for length of gestation as well as balletic possibility! So invite friends for lunch (strictly cheese and biscuits or something equally easy); plan a picnic in the park with your antenatal chums (ditto); go for a swim and a sauna at your local leisure centre or health club (see if you can get a free day pass from a member friend); go to the cinema (yes, even if you have to go alone); plan a day of watching your favourite movies on DVD; aim to read an entire book in a day. Don't plan anything too taxing, energetic or far from home, but you get the idea
- make another shortlist of baby names, even if they're completely outrageous. It'll make you laugh when you look back on it later, and you just might come up with something that sticks!
- write an account of all your long- and short-term hopes and dreams for your life with your baby so you can refer to it in the years to come. You won't necessarily achieve all your aspirations – and your baby's personality might dictate this to some degree! – but it's a lovely starting point for your relationship. You could put it down on paper in the form of pledges: 'I will

try not to say "Because I said so" every time my child challenges my authority'; 'I will keep a part of every weekend exclusively for family fun'; 'I'm going to try to make myself the most approachable parent ever', and so on
- give yourself a mini project that you can abandon without consequence: catalogue your CDs and DVDs; stick all your old photos into albums at last; start making a cot quilt using old fabric remnants and offcuts from fabric stores; sketch out some ideas for a wall frieze; knit a basic baby blanket, for example. None of these projects is costly or crucial – and you could always take any of them up again later if you felt like it!

What the netmums say

'Helping the time to pass more quickly'

I spent my last weeks attempting to get my baby out by having long walks, spicy foods and so on. Most days were spent shopping for last-minute baby things or cleaning the house (my friends were all working during the week so I couldn't rely on them), but I did something every day to try to keep the time moving.
Kari from Exeter, mum to Jennifer, three months

When I was pregnant with Morgan that last month, I used to take my dog out for walks about three times a day to the local park. When I wasn't walking the dog I was trying to get out and about as much as I could. I'd also take afternoon naps when I was home. With Paige I used to try and keep myself busy with Morgan, taking him out as much as I could, although it did get difficult as the local buses seemed to change from buggy-friendly to not, which was quite a struggle.
Julie from Leeds, mum to Morgan, 17 months and Paige, three months

I worked up to a week before my due date. I had SPD [Symphysis Pubis Dysfunction, see p. 117], but I walked the four-mile round trip to work daily. I spent a lot of my down-time with my pooch, too – he was very loving – and I read books that I knew I wouldn't have a chance to read later on.
Amanda from Barnstaple, mum to Tristan, 23 months

Who'd have thought?

Giving birth to twins doesn't mean you have to go through the whole of labour twice: it's only the pushing phase that you'll have to repeat, and while it means double the effort, it'll also mean double the reward in the long term.

Breastfeeding basics

Here are some of the key points about breastfeeding that you can refer to quickly in the early days (although, as suggested before, it's a great idea to find a good book on the subject for the longer term):

- have a drink, a snack, a muslin cloth and the phone close to hand so you won't have to interrupt the feed
- make yourself as comfortable as possible: sit in a comfy but supportive chair and use a V-shaped pillow or a selection of pillows and cushions to support your whole back and your shoulders. Some mums also like to have their feet up or one foot supported
- have a pillow across your lap to lie your baby on
- lean over your baby and bring him to your breast: he should start rooting (nosing around) for your nipple
- wait until your baby has his jaws wide open before dropping your breast into his mouth (imagine he has a flip-top head and you'll get the idea!)
- make sure your baby gets a good mouthful of breast tissue as well as your nipple: it's only by working the tissue with his jaws that he can 'pump' the milk out of your milk ducts. Latching him on to your nipple alone will only leave you sore and cracked and your baby dissatisfied. You should be able to see the muscles of his jaw and temple working, which indicates that he's feeding effectively
- to unlatch your baby from your breast, slip your little finger between your breast and the side of your baby's mouth to release the suction
- try to feed from each breast at every feed
- if your baby seems uncomfortable or breaks off to cry, it's possible he's got wind (although this is less common in breastfed babies than in bottlefed). Sit him propped on your lap, supporting him under the chin and chest with one hand, and rub or pat his back until he burps

- if you do experience problems with breastfeeding, ask your midwife for assistance or find a local breastfeeding counsellor. (Your local NCT branch should be able to put you in touch with someone in your area.)

What the netmums say

'My best breastfeeding tips'

I got a lovely rocking chair with footstool attached that I put in our bedroom, then into the nursery when we moved our babies in there. It's so important to be comfy, as you could be feeding for hours and it would be so miserable if you were in any discomfort. It's not necessarily the solution for everyone, but it's important to find something that makes you as comfortable as possible.
Carly from Bridgend, mum to Hollie, three and Jake, one

My breasts became engorged for the first few days after my milk came in, and I'd read somewhere that putting Savoy cabbage leaves inside your bra helps to reduce the feelings of swelling and hotness. Poor hubby had to go to three supermarkets before he could find the right thing, and even then he forgot to cut out the central stalks to make it easier to fold the leaves, so I ended up preparing it all myself. It did work for a short while at a time: apparently it's to do with some enzyme in the cabbage. I'd definitely recommend it as it's a fairly cheap and easy remedy.
Lesley from Westerham, mum to Daniel, 18 months

I wanted to express milk as well as breastfeed as I wanted my partner to be able to feed one baby whilst I fed the other, rather than me having a twin at each breast all the time! I tried expressing by hand and by electric pump: one I found too hard and slow; the other was very vigorous and too fast! In the end I found that a hand-operated pump suited me best. In other words, try the cheaper options first: the electric pump was a complete waste of money in my case!
Elaine from Derby, mum to twins Michael and Miranda, seven months

Your mission this week: Organise your visiting list

Everyone is going to be impatient to meet, hold and coo over your new baby as soon as they hear about the birth, and you don't want to find yourself in the position of trying to beat them all back with a huge stick! Because of this it's a good idea to have a discussion now with your partner about who should come and see you when; if you leave it until after the birth you'll probably be in no emotional state to think rationally about other people's feelings. Take into account whether any parents or close friends have to travel from a distance and whether or not they can stay with you or another relative. Keep in mind that both sets of parents – if you both have parents – will probably want to be first to see their new grandchild: can you bear it if they all descend on you at once or will you have to come to a decision as to who to see first? Try to come to a compromise everyone will feel happy with: perhaps if one set of parents is first to see the baby in hospital, the others can be first to visit at home? It can be surprising how snooty people can be about how you draw up your priority list, even when you're talking about close family and friends.

Of course, there's nothing to say that you can't take the first week out to spend almost exclusively with your baby and your partner: this is known in some circles as a 'babymoon'! Take to your bed, gather all your essential provisions around you, dispatch your partner to fetch and carry food and drinks... then relax and really get to know your newborn.

Look no further

How will my baby look at birth?
You might be a bit surprised about your baby's appearance when he's born: it certainly won't be like in one of those saccharine TV dramas where the baby is handed to his mum, all perfectly clean, wrapped and looking about three months old, straight after being delivered! He will probably be covered in blood and some of the creamy-white, waxy vernix that protected his skin inside you. He might have some bruises or 'stork marks' from his descent down the birth canal, a few scratches from his own fingernails and a misshapen head, especially if he's had to be delivered by ventouse or forceps. He might be bluish until he has filled his lungs with oxygen, or bright red from the pressure of delivery. Your midwife might need to clear his airways of mucus by using a gentle suction tube in order to help him breathe. All of these little quirks of appearance will settle and disappear within a few days,

weeks or months of the birth, though, and your newborn will very soon resemble that bouncing TV babe!

Can I condition my nipples for breastfeeding?
There are lots of myths surrounding 'toughening up' your nipples in advance of breastfeeding, with some recommending using lanolin-based creams and others advising massaging colostrum (the creamy substance that leaks from your breasts and forms your baby's first nutrition after birth) into the skin. Actually, your nipples will toughen a little bit once you start feeding, and any discomfort you experience is likely to be due to poor positioning of your baby at the breast. The best preparation is to go over our 10-point *Breastfeeding basics* plan (see p. 360) a few more times in advance of the birth.

I can't get my head around breastfeeding. Is it OK to use bottles?
Whilst it's universally recognised – even by milk manufacturers – that breastfeeding is best for your baby, formula milks have become so sophisticated that they now mimic breastmilk pretty well in terms of nutritional content. What formula milks can't confer is the immunity from infections breastfed babies enjoy or the intellectual head start that's widely purported to be linked to breastfeeding.

One wide-ranging European study, carried out by the Department of Clinical Immunology in Sweden, found that breastfed babies enjoyed greater immunity from acute or prolonged diarrhoea, respiratory tract infections, otitis media (middle ear infection), urinary tract infection, and neonatal septicaemia (blood poisoning). Evidence also points to this extra protection lasting for years after breastfeeding has ended.

Another study, Proceedings of the National Academy of Sciences, found that babies who are breastfed are at an intellectual advantage over their bottlefed peers if they also inherit a version of a gene that is involved in the growth of the brain. Because 90 per cent of people do have this gene, there's also a 90 per cent chance that your baby could benefit.

If you are planning to bottlefeed – and it's important that you do whatever feels right for you – do make sure you've practised with all the equipment you'll need in advance (see p. 194) as it's quite fiddly and involved until you get into a rhythm, and will probably seem like a daunting prospect if you don't have a few dry runs beforehand.

Week 40+ 7 days+ to go! (Can you hear that clock ticking...?)

Don't forget: Write a list of labour day tips for your partner

OK, so you might imagine the more organised birth partner will have drawn up his or her own list of action points for labour day by now, but if yours happens to be your (male) life partner, he is by all accounts a little untypical if he's got himself this sorted. (If, by any chance, your other half prides himself on detail and has a typed-up list with tick boxes to check, our apologies – and hey, how do you feel about getting him cloned?)

Hopefully you'll have got all the obvious essentials sorted, such as organising for someone to look after any older children you may have, and how you're going to organise the switch-over. It's worth having a contingency in place for this, too, just in case your chosen carers are indisposed on the big day. Once this is all sorted, you can get down to the nitty-gritty.

Try to think chronologically about what will happen when, and organise your list accordingly. You don't want to put 'Ring my mother' at the top, for instance! Maybe something like 'Pack drinks and snacks in coolbox' could be a good starting point, as it's something that can't be done until the last minute. Other things on your list could be:

- throw away dead flowers and empty bins
- change the bed (if there's time!)
- set house alarm and leave upstairs light on
- change answerphone message to 'We're at the hospital and we'll call you when we can, so please don't ring our mobiles'
- put baby seat in the car
- ring the hospital to alert them you're on your way
- call anyone else you've asked to attend the birth
- make sure hospital notes are in the bag.

Once you're at the hospital, your birth plan will hopefully be enough guidance for your partner (even if the medical side of things doesn't pan out exactly as you'd hoped!). You'll already have discussed whether or not you'd like him at the head end of the bed for the delivery, what sort of massage might be soothing and other such details.

What the netmums say

'How my birth partner performed on the day'

My husband was my birth partner the first time, although we hadn't actually thought it through and he knew I wouldn't mind if he chickened out at the last minute. In the end, he was so stressed he was making me stressed, too, so I kicked him out when I was about 6cm dilated and did the last five hours on my own while he sat with some other dads and watched telly! Second time round I was more prepared and had my sister, who's a mum, and a good friend, who's a nurse and also has children. It was wonderful: we laughed the whole night through. It was a rare night out for them both away from their children, and we had so much fun.

Jen from Hertfordshire, mum to Jack, four and Theo, 17 months

My husband was my birth partner and he was fantastic, but it does make me giggle when I think back. He became obsessed with making sandwiches – apparently this is something that was suggested in our antenatal classes. Anyway, we had a massive pile, along with currant buns, apples – it was quite a picnic. Unfortunately most of it had disappeared by the time I was able to eat! Otherwise he was amazing: right at the end when I thought I couldn't go on, he whispered in my ear: 'You can do it this time, babe.' It helped me find the remainder of my energy, and out popped Evie.

Rebecca from Southampton, mum to Evie, two and Louie, eight months

My partner was also my birth partner and he was so good, I couldn't have wished for anyone better. I insisted on being discharged from the hospital the same evening I gave birth, so we eventually got home about 11.30 p.m. and he let me sleep all night and looked after our newborn himself.

Fae from Hayes, mum to Ayden, 16 months

> **Who'd have thought?**
> One in eight babies in the UK is born premature or sick – that's 80,000* babies every year.
> *Source: BLISS (www.bliss.org.uk)

Hey baby!

Your baby is now 'cooked' and ready to be born, weighing around 3.4kg (7.5lb). He measures around 37.5cm (15in) from crown to rump. From top to toe his total length is around 50cm (just under 20in). Don't expect to hear the 'ping' any time soon, though, as around two-thirds of babies are overdue – and your baby might get a bit bigger again. With any luck your baby's head is now fully engaged in readiness for the birth. He's likely to be fidgeting slightly but unable to move much within the confines of your uterus. If you're at all concerned that you've not felt him move in a while, then do contact your medical team who should be happy to monitor you to check on your baby's wellbeing.

All about you

You're likely to be sticking out in front in such a way that you're preceded into any room by your bump! The top of your uterus is now around 36–40cm (14.5–16in) from your pubic bone, and around 16.5–20.5cm (6.5–8in) from your belly button. Maybe you don't even care by now: who could blame you! It's hardly going to make much difference to the outcome of your pregnancy at this point, is it? What you might be interested to know, though, is that your cervix might already have started effacing (thinning out) in preparation for dilating. This is exciting news as it means labour could be imminent!

Going overdue

Going beyond Week 40 – as so many first pregnancies do – could mean that your dates were miscalculated from the outset. Don't get too despondent, though: most hospitals won't allow mums to go beyond 42 weeks because staying in the uterus for too long can actually be harmful to an unborn baby. This is because the placenta eventually becomes calcified and stops functioning.

It can be a bit of an anti-climax to get to the 'end' of pregnancy and still have no signs of labour, especially if your antenatal chums are delivering babies left, right and centre – and, of course, there's no way of knowing now whether you'll end up going to 42 weeks and having to be induced, or whether your baby will put in a last-minute appearance spontaneously. You might find that you start to doubt your body's ability to recognise when it's ready for labour, but don't fret: it's coped with the whole of pregnancy to date, and even if you do end up being induced it doesn't cancel out all you've achieved so far. Remember, too, that you'll soon have your baby home, and pregnancy will be a distant memory.

It's important to get as much rest as possible now, preferably with your feet higher than your hips, as you are more likely to get oedema (swelling due to fluid retention) again from now on. You'll have more regular check-ups after your due date so don't worry that you've been forgotten about. Be alert for any vaginal bleeding from now on as this could mean that the placenta has started to detach from the wall of your uterus, and this would mean your baby would need to be delivered fast.

What the netmums say

'Going past my due date'

By Charlotte's due date I was fed up with being pregnant: I just wanted to get it over with and be able to see my feet again! Charlotte was due on 26 February, which came and went without any signs of her arrival. I went to the midwife who booked me in for an induction 10 days later, 7 March. I tried loads of things they say induce labour – raspberry leaf tea, walking, sex – and she finally arrived on 6 March after 27 hours of labour! So the threat of induction did work eventually.
Georgina from Devon, mum to Charlotte, 17 weeks

With my first child I went nine days overdue: he arrived 48 hours after a cervical sweep was done. My second child was 10 days overdue and again I went into labour just 48 hours after having a sweep. I loved everything about being pregnant: I had very easy pregnancies and didn't want them to end. I was uncomfortable, but I was willing to wait as long as possible to deliver as I didn't want to be induced.
Katy from Bracknell, mum to Mikey, four and Jay, three

Being induced

If you don't go into labour this week or by the end of Week 42, there's a very real possibility that you'll be offered an induction. Lots of mums dread this, as it does mean that your contractions will come much thicker and faster, and will probably be much more severe and painful, than in mums who go into spontaneous labour. It's not only going overdue that may mean you are offered an induction, though: your medical team will also be keen to deliver your baby if you have a serious medical condition such as pre-eclampsia; diabetes; high blood pressure or heart disease. Other circumstances when induction might be suggested include when your medical team decides that your placenta is beginning to fail or when your waters have broken but you're not having contractions.

As with all procedures offered in pregnancy, you don't have to accept induction, even if you are more than 42 weeks pregnant. You might have a bit of a fight on your hands if you do decide to refuse – and, as always, you need to weigh up the reasons why it's being suggested and why you're against it before you can decide what you consider is best for your baby – but if you feel very strongly that you don't want to be induced, remember that it's your right to say no.

Having a 'sweep'

The first thing your midwife will usually try is a 'sweep' of your membranes, which literally means sweeping a finger around your cervix to get it to release the hormone oxytocin which is associated with triggering labour. It's uncomfortable for most mums, doesn't work for all and can take up to 48 hours to have an effect – but if it works it's worth it!

Who'd have thought?

We're having more babies than ever: the number of live births in England and Wales increased for the fifth year in succession in 2006. There were 669,601 births in 2006 compared with 645,835 in 2005, which is an increase of 3.7 per cent*.

*Source: National Statistics

Prostaglandin pessary

If a sweep doesn't get things going, you might be offered a pessary of prostaglandin – a hormone that kick-starts contractions. This is a bullet-shaped tablet of gel that's inserted into your vagina. It can take a few hours to be effective, and the procedure might be repeated a couple of times.

Artificial Rupture of Membranes (ARM)

If your waters still haven't broken yet and a sweep and pessaries haven't worked, the next thing your midwife will try is breaking your waters by hand. This is done using an implement shaped a bit like a large crochet hook which is passed up through your cervix to puncture the amniotic sac. This will allow your baby's head to sit against your cervix, encouraging the cervix to efface (thin out) and begin to dilate.

Syntocinon drip

If you still don't find yourself in active labour, you might be offered a Syntocinon drip: Syntocinon is a synthetic form of oxytocin and works quickly because it goes directly into the bloodstream. This form of induction brings labour on big time, so is usually only used if all else has failed.

What the netmums say

'Being induced'

I was induced in Week 42 as they were concerned that Jamie was going to be a big baby and I'm only small. They started me off on the Monday evening with a pessary, which only produced mild contractions. I had another pessary on the Tuesday, but still with only a slight result. I was becoming really tired by now. On the Wednesday, I had my waters broken at around 1 p.m. and as a result my contractions stopped! At 2 p.m., a Syntocinon drip was set up. This really kick-started labour, which for the first couple of hours was manageable on gas & air. However, after cranking the dose up a few times, it was really starting to get painful, so I had an epidural. At around midnight I was able to start pushing. I was exhausted but at least the end was in sight. After over an hour of pushing, Jamie's heart rate started to drop, so a senior midwife performed an episiotomy and ventouse delivery and finally Jamie was born at 1.16a.m. on the Thursday morning, weighing a respectable 8lb 3oz – not the 9lb 5oz they were anticipating! Whilst it was a very long and drawn-out process, I still feel it was a positive experience: I had the most amazing midwife who was so in tune with me and I don't think I could have done it without her! Would I have another induction? Yes, I probably would. At least when they start you off, you know that the end is in sight and you are being closely monitored at all times.

Ruth from Lancaster, mum to Jamie, two

I was due to be induced once I reached 40 weeks + 10 days, so I turned to my friend, who's a reflexologist, to see if she could start me off. She said it worked for some women but not for others, but I was willing to try anything! She came over on a Friday evening and I sat on the sofa watching *Eastenders* with her at my feet. It was so relaxing and the baby was wriggling around like crazy, so I think she enjoyed it too! I did notice the bump drop down and change shape during the treatment, which was a strange feeling. Because I'd been sitting for half an hour I was ready for a trip to the loo: when I got there my waters broke and soon after my contractions started! Seven hours later my beautiful baby girl was born following a perfect labour. I'm not suggesting reflexology will work for everyone, but even if it doesn't it certainly is the perfect way to relax in the run-up to labour!

Jenny from Essex, mum to Elisha, four

Your mission this week: Try to trigger labour

Try out some of the much-talked-about methods of kick-starting labour: some have a degree of foundation in medical truth; others don't, but most of them are great fun, even if they don't work! How about a hot curry, followed by a bit of nipple-tweaking, maybe culminating in penetrative sex? Then you could enjoy a nice cup of raspberry leaf tea before retiring for the night. Bliss!

There aren't any scientific studies that support the 'spicy foods' theory, but there's plenty of anecdotal evidence, so if you enjoy a poky curry, go ahead and have it! As far as sex is concerned, it's thought that the prostaglandins in semen act in the same way as the pessaries used in induction, and that having an orgasm (which is crucial to the success of this, so do insist on it!) triggers the release of oxytocin – the hormone which triggers contractions. Although no one's quite sure why, this only seems to work when your baby is ready to be born, and isn't thought to trigger premature labour. Having said that, some mums who've experienced premature labour before may be advised to abstain from intercourse just in case. Although raspberry leaf tea isn't thought to trigger contractions as such, it seems that it does help to tone and stimulate the uterus, and it's thought that it can make the second stage of labour shorter and easier in some mums, too.

Go ahead and do whatever appeals to you – and if nothing works, well at least you'll have passed a bit more time!

Look no further

I've heard that cuddling a newborn could start off labour. Is this true?
Yes, for some women cuddling a baby can have the same effect as nipple tweaking in that it triggers the release of oxytocin – the same hormone which is not only responsible for kick-starting contractions, but which stimulates your breasts to 'let down' your milk for your baby (so be prepared for the resulting leaks before you take hold!). Some mums only need to hear a baby crying for their breasts to start leaking – so it makes sense that hanging out with newborns could also start your contractions off. But don't expect to be allowed to camp out in the maternity unit, though – you'll have to find your own friends' babies to cuddle!

Who'd have thought?

Cutting a newborn's umbilical cord too soon after birth can be detrimental to his wellbeing, according to Dr Andrew Weeks, a senior lecturer in obstetrics at the University of Liverpool's School of Reproductive and Developmental Medicine. Dr Weeks says that leaving the cord intact for a few minutes can increase the baby's iron levels and reduce the risk of anaemia.

Supposing I forget all my breathing techniques on the day?
Well, your birth partner should be able to coach you – but if, on the day, he or she is overwhelmed with all that's going on in the labour suite (which does happen!), don't panic: your midwife is also an expert in breathing techniques and will be able to coach you through. Resources in many hospitals are limited now, though, so that most mums are unable to have continuous one-to-one midwife care in labour, so although your midwife will help with your breathing as and when she can, unless you're having a home birth you can't rely on her being there throughout and may find yourself alone with your birth partner for some parts of the first stage of labour. For this reason, it's really worthwhile practising the techniques often in the run-up to the birth, so that you're less likely to forget them: the better prepared you are, the less likely you are to panic; and if you can practise the techniques, you'll be less likely to clench all your muscles with each contraction. It's a good idea, too, to type the techniques out in advance so that you have a printed sheet to refresh your memory.

What happens immediately after my baby is born?
If your baby is in good condition and responding well, he can be placed straight on to your tummy after the birth. Whilst you greet him for the first time, lots of things will be going on: he'll be wiped clean, covered with a blanket and the umbilical cord will be clamped and cut. (Your partner should be invited to cut the cord if you've stipulated this on your birth plan.) At one minute after birth, your baby is assessed for heart rate, breathing, muscle tone, reflexes and colour. This is called an Apgar test. He's given a score out of 10, and the test is repeated five minutes after birth. A score of three or less means your baby will need resuscitating and possibly other life-saving measures. A score of four to six means he might need help breathing, either through having some suction to clear his airways or through giving him a little oxygen. A score of seven and upwards after five minutes is considered normal. A lower score at this point means your baby will probably need some extra medical help for any of several reasons, but your doctors will discuss this with you if it happens. Your baby will be weighed and measured between his two Apgar tests. He'll also be given vitamin K for blood clotting unless you've declined it (see p. 295–6).

Who'd have thought?

Your baby's skull is made up from mobile 'plates' of bone, which don't fuse together until after the birth. These plates can slide and move slightly to allow your baby's smooth passage through the birth canal, and account for why his head might appear a bit misshapen straight after delivery.

What the netmums say

'Whether my birth went according to plan'

I'd planned to use hypno-birthing techniques and maybe a little gas & air during labour, and for the most part it went to plan. But then I ended up having a ventouse, then forceps delivery on only gas & air! Believe me, if I'd known I'd have had not one but two epidurals! My midwife was so proud of me: she couldn't believe I'd delivered a 9lb 1oz baby with so little pain relief and all that intervention!
Sarah from Sheffield, mum to Isaac, one

With my eldest I didn't have a plan, which was probably a good thing as it would've gone right out of the window! Second time round, though, I actually wrote out a plan with the help of my midwife, as I was so worried and scared about having another bad experience – and it went like clockwork! My waters broke at 36 weeks and I went into hospital with my birth partners to find that I was 3cm dilated. Then I did lots of walking around and breathing, had an epidural when it got too much, then had a planned episiotomy [cut] and a lovely delivery. I was home by lunchtime the next morning: I think I was extremely lucky!
Jen from Hertfordshire, mum to Jack four and Theo, 17 months

I was unable to get into any antenatal classes but, with the help of my midwife, I decided to try for an active water birth with none of this lying on the bed pushing! I planned to try to get by with gas & air, but I wasn't averse to an epidural. The only thing I was adamant about was that I did not want pethidine! I went into labour naturally on my due date, ended up not even making it to the delivery suite, let alone the pool, as my labour progressed very quickly, and found myself lying on a bed pushing, with pethidine for pain relief. It was the opposite of my plan but it turned out to be perfect! I loved my labour!

Kari from Exeter, mum to Jennifer, three months

I can't say I had a plan at all except to be as calm and relaxed as possible – and it worked brilliantly both times. My first labour lasted less than five hours with only gas & air and pethidine. I had no cut or stitches and was up and about almost straightaway. My second labour was even better: I went into hospital with quite strong contractions at 2.30 a.m. and my second daughter was born at 4.48 a.m. I was home by 8.30 a.m., and my first daughter was still in bed: it was great to go and wake her up to meet her new baby sister. I've been very lucky!

Aimee from Northamptonshire, mum to Morgan Olivia, nearly three and Bethany Ann, nearly one

Who'd have thought?

According to a recent series of Canadian studies, a skin-to-skin cuddle with your newborn can not only help regulate his heart rate and body temperature, it can also act as a natural painkiller! The practice is known as 'kangaroo cuddling'.

How are you feeling?

Tick the box that most closely represents how you feel about the given statements, then look back to the charts in previous chapters to see how you've changed over the months.

Physically	Emotionally
One more day of being pregnant and I will EXPLODE! Strongly agree ☐ Agree ☐ Neither agree nor disagree ☐ Disagree ☐ Strongly disagree ☐	OK, I'm getting really scared now! Strongly agree ☐ Agree ☐ Neither agree nor disagree ☐ Disagree ☐ Strongly disagree ☐
My contractions keep starting and then stopping again Strongly agree ☐ Agree ☐ Neither agree nor disagree ☐ Disagree ☐ Strongly disagree ☐	I'm sort of looking forward to what labour will be like Strongly agree ☐ Agree ☐ Neither agree nor disagree ☐ Disagree ☐ Strongly disagree ☐
I'm all swollen up again Strongly agree ☐ Agree ☐ Neither agree nor disagree ☐ Disagree ☐ Strongly disagree ☐	I don't want to lose touch with my friends Strongly agree ☐ Agree ☐ Neither agree nor disagree ☐ Disagree ☐ Strongly disagree ☐
My breasts are so heavy I feel I need someone to hold them up for me Strongly agree ☐ Agree ☐ Neither agree nor disagree ☐ Disagree ☐ Strongly disagree ☐	I suddenly feel like a child again Strongly agree ☐ Agree ☐ Neither agree nor disagree ☐ Disagree ☐ Strongly disagree ☐
My pelvis is aching with the pressure of my baby Strongly agree ☐ Agree ☐ Neither agree nor disagree ☐ Disagree ☐ Strongly disagree ☐	I'm just bursting with anticipation about meeting my baby Strongly agree ☐ Agree ☐ Neither agree nor disagree ☐ Disagree ☐ Strongly disagree ☐
I'm not sure if I'd recognise a 'show' if I saw it Strongly agree ☐ Agree ☐ Neither agree nor disagree ☐ Disagree ☐ Strongly disagree ☐	The end of pregnancy will be such a relief Strongly agree ☐ Agree ☐ Neither agree nor disagree ☐ Disagree ☐ Strongly disagree ☐

Quick quiz

What have you learned about pregnancy?

1 How much nausea is normal in pregnancy?

a. A little

b. A lot at the start, but tailing off

c. None

2 Which of the following are common complaints amongst mums-to-be?

a. Stretch marks

b. Constipation

c. Oedema (swelling due to fluid retention)

3 Which of the following are methods of pain relief you might be offered in hospital?

a. Gas & air

b. Pethidine

c. Epidural

4 Which of the following is an indication that labour's underway?

a. Having a 'show'

b. Your waters breaking

c. Regular contractions, increasing in intensity and frequency

5 Which of the following interventions can you refuse in labour?

a. Pain relief

b. Induction

c. Episiotomy

Answers: a, b and c are all correct!

Mostly a, b, or c: You can't have failed to get a perfect score this time as all the above answers are right!

Now that you've met your baby...

Well, we're guessing that you've got your hands full at last (of the most gorgeous little bundle) and are somewhat preoccupied with having finally become a mum. Congratulations to you all! The rest of your journey into parenthood will unfold bit by bit and you'll find your way, even if you encounter a few bumpy bits along the road.

Pregnancy is never entirely straightforward, but it's fair to say that it's only now that the real work begins.

Here are a few things for you to remember, especially when the going gets tough:

- newborns don't come with manuals and there's no such thing as a 'perfect' or 'natural' parent. Everybody around you might suddenly claim to be an 'expert', but you just follow your own instincts and you won't go far wrong
- yes, breast is best – but if you can't get on with breastfeeding despite your best efforts (or if you just really don't want to), then there's no need to feel at all guilty about bottlefeeding
- being a parent is the single most important job you'll ever undertake – but it can also be the most rewarding
- when you're awake in the wee small hours feeding your baby and feeling like you're the only person in the world who's awake – remember you're soooo not alone! And if you don't believe us, log on to www.netmums.co.uk and you'll find plenty of Netmums who are up, about and ready to chat to you!
- the Netmums will be your companions throughout parenthood and beyond. For more practical help, advice and real mums' experiences to see you through the first 12 months, read *Baby's First Year: The Netmums Guide to Being a New Mum*.

What the Netmums say

'That first moment of meeting'

With my eldest, I was in so much shock after a traumatic and painful delivery that I just didn't focus on him to start with. I just remember arms and legs and dark eyes. I had to go to theatre afterwards, and when I came out a couple of hours later, the midwife handed him back to me. My first thought was, 'Are you sure he's mine?' as he was nothing like I'd expected: he looked just like my father-in-law. Then I had an overwhelming sense of love, and burst into tears. I remember the midwife smiling and leaving the room, shutting the door really gently. Second time around, it was instant. The midwife passed him to me before they even cut the cord. He wasn't crying but his bottom lip was wobbling – he was so perfect, I just loved him straightaway.

Jen from Hertfordshire, mum to Jack, four and Theo, 17 months

When I had Lily-Mae the midwife put her straight on my chest while my partner cut the cord. I'd never felt so scared in all my life, but a few minutes later I had this huge, overwhelming wave of love and joy, and I didn't stop crying for about an hour.

Sarah from Derby, mum to Lily-Mae, eight-and-a-half months

Connor was put straight on to my chest while my hubby cut the cord, and I was in shock and disbelief, but also elation: I was so dumbfounded, I couldn't believe I'd done that. I remember my first thought being, 'Oh, my God, he's perfect', and I just kept saying it over and over in my head. I was so shocked that he was a real little person, and that I had given birth to him. Actually, I still can't believe I did that!

Erin from Leeds, mum to Connor, 11 months

I didn't get to see my son straightaway as he was rushed to Special Care. It took me ages to bond with him, although I don't know whether it was through the shock of labour or the fact that he was blue and not breathing when he was delivered: I think I was frightened to bond with him in case anything bad happened. With my daughter, I had her placed on my chest and it was instant love. My husband hadn't been keen on having a second baby, so I gave her to him to hold and he looked so scared! However, now he just loves her so much. I think he was panicking in case he couldn't love another baby like he loved our son.

Gail from Glasgow, mum to Brodie, six and Zoe, four

When Aleisha first came out I got that instant rush of love, but it quickly turned to horror as she went purple and got rushed off for a few minutes. But then it was back to excitement as I put her straight to my breast for a feed. I couldn't get over how beautiful she was and I couldn't believe she was mine.

Louise from Barnsley, mum to Aleisha, six

Glossary of Medical Terms

Italics denote other Glossary entries.

A

AFP (alpha-fetoprotein) A protein normally produced by the liver and yolk sac of a *foetus*

Afterbirth Another term for the *placenta*

Albumin A protein which is sometimes found in urine as an indicator of a urine infection or, if accompanied by other symptoms, *pre-eclampsia*

Amniocentesis An invasive diagnostic test for chromosomal and genetic abnormalities which involves passing a needle through the abdomen and into the *amniotic sac* in order to extract *amniotic fluid* for analysis

Amnion The innermost of two membranes that make up the *amniotic sac*

Amniotic fluid The fluid within the *amniotic sac*, which surrounds a *foetus* in the *uterus*. Also known as *waters*

Amniotic sac Thin membrane sac enclosing the developing *foetus*

Anaemia A medical condition caused by not having enough red cells in the blood

Anaesthesia A drug that induces partial or total loss of sensation

Analgesic A drug to relieve pain

Anomaly scan An *ultrasound scan* to check for major developmental defects in a *foetus*

Anterior lie When a *foetus* is lying with his/her spine to the front of the *uterus*

Anti-D immunoglobulin A drug given by injection to pregnant mums who have a blood type known as *rhesus negative*

Apgar score An assessment score of a newborn for skin colour, breathing, muscle tone, reflex responses and heart rate

Aquanatal classes Classes which offer light aerobic exercise performed in water and led by a qualified instructor with a special interest in pregnancy

Areola The darker area of skin surrounding the nipple

Artificial Rupture of Membranes (ARM) When a midwife breaks your waters by puncturing the amniotic sac with a special implement, which she passes up through your cervix

Assisted delivery The delivery of a baby using artificial means such as *forceps* or *ventouse*

B

Bilirubin A reddish-yellow pigment present in human bile that is a by-product of red blood cells

Birth plan A written projection of a pregnant mum's ideal birth, including choices for pain relief, *induction*, *episiotomy*, delivery and more

Blastocyst The name for the mass of subdividing cells that emerges after fertilisation but before implantation

Blood pressure The measurement of the force with which blood leaves and re-enters the heart's chambers

Blood sugar Glucose in the blood

Blood test A screening test during which blood is extracted for analysis via a needle

Braxton Hicks contractions Involuntary tightenings of the *uterus*, felt by some mums from early to mid-pregnancy onwards, which differ from true labour *contractions* in intensity and regularity

Breakthrough bleeding Any unexpected vaginal bleeding

Breech baby Term for a baby presenting in one of several head-up positions

Butterfly mask A characteristically butterfly-shaped stain (also known as *chloasma*), which can appear across the face in pregnancy, caused by an over-production of the pigment melanin

C

Caesarean section Major abdominal surgery whereby a baby is extracted from the mum's *uterus* via a surgical incision

Candida albicans See *thrush*

Cannula A fine plastic tube inserted into a vein for the purpose of administering drugs

Carpal tunnel syndrome A condition where pressure on a nerve in the wrist causes pain, pins and needles, weakness and numbness in the hand

Catheter A length of plastic tubing inserted into the bladder through the urethra for the draining of urine

Cephalo-pelvic disproportion (CPD) Where a baby's head is too large to pass through the mum's pelvis

Cervical incompetence Anatomical weakness of the *cervix*, causing the *uterus* to lose its contents, typically around mid-pregnancy

Cervical stitch A non-absorbable stitch put in around an *incompetent cervix* to hold it closed throughout pregnancy and removed for delivery

Cervical sweep Procedure whereby a midwife runs a finger around the *cervix* in an attempt to release the hormone *oxytocin*, which can trigger labour Also known as a *sweep of the membranes*

Cervix The neck-like opening of the *uterus*

Chloasma See *Butterfly mask*

Chorion The outermost of two membranes, the chorion will surround the *amnion* and become the *placenta*

Chorionic villus sampling (CVS) A procedure whereby a needle is passed through the abdomen in order to take a sample of the chorionic villi – tiny hair-like projections on the *placenta*

Chromosome A structure in all living cells consisting of a single molecule of DNA bonded to various proteins. Chromosomes carry the genes determining heredity

Colostrum The creamy substance rich in antibodies and minerals produced by the breasts to nourish a newborn as a forerunner to true breastmilk

Contractions The regular shortening and thickening of the uterus for the purpose of expelling the *foetus*

Cordocentesis A procedure whereby a needle is passed through the abdomen into the *uterus* where the umbilical cord meets the *placenta*, in order to extract a sample of blood for analysis

Cravings See *pica*

Crowning The stage of labour when a large part of the foetal scalp is visible at the opening of the vagina

Cystitis Inflammation of the bladder

D

Deep Vein Thrombosis See *DVT*

Diabetes, gestational See *gestational diabetes*

Diamorphine A pain-relieving opiate drug usually given by injection

Diastasis Symphysis Pubis (also known as *Symphysis Pubis Dysfunction*) The separation of normally joined pubic bones, caused by the hormone *relaxin* combined with the weight of the *uterus*

Dilatation and curettage (D&C) A medical procedure performed under general anaesthetic after around 10 per cent of miscarriages, to remove any retained particles of pregnancy

Doppler An electronic hand-held device often used to listen to the foetal heartbeat, and which works by sending out low-frequency ultrasound waves which 'bounce' back to translate into sound

Doula A paid birth assistant – usually a mother herself – who supports a pregnant mum through labour and birth and then helps out at home for a specified period

DVT (*Deep Vein Thrombosis*) A condition where a blood clot forms in a deep vein, usually in the leg, sometimes leading to complications such as pulmonary embolism

E

Early Pregnancy Assessment Unit (*EPAU*) A specialist unit managing early pregnancy problems such as vaginal bleeding and abdominal pain

Eclampsia A serious condition of pregnancy which can occur during or just after labour and is characterised by convulsions induced by high blood pressure. Left untreated, eclampsia can lead to maternal and foetal death

Ectopic pregnancy An unsustainable pregnancy in which an *embryo* implants somewhere in the abdominal cavity other than the *uterus*

ECV (*External Cephalic Version*) A technique whereby an experienced obstetrician tries to turn a baby into a head-down position by external manipulation of the mum's bump

EDD (*Estimated Due Date*) The date on which a baby is calculated to be due, based on the date of the first day of the mum's last menstrual period (*LMP*)

EEG See *Electroencephalography*

EFM Electronic Foetal Monitoring, where the foetal heart rate is monitored either via an electronic monitor strapped to the mum's belly or via an electrode passed up through the cervix and clipped to the foetal scalp

Elderly primigravida A first-time pregnant woman who is 35 years old or over

Electroencephalography (EEG) A test that measures brain activity

Electronic Foetal Monitoring See *EFM*

Embryo The term given to a fertilised egg until Week 10 of pregnancy, from which point it is referred to as a *foetus*

Endometrium The thick, blood vessel-rich tissue which lines the *uterus*

Endorphins *Hormones* released from the pituitary gland in response to certain triggers, which can act as natural painkillers and mood enhancers

Engagement When the foetal head drops into the pelvis in readiness for birth. Also known as *lightening*

Entonox (also known as '*gas & air*') A 50/50 mix of oxygen and nitrous oxide administered via a breathing pipe as analgesic pain relief in labour

EPAU See *Early Pregnancy Assessment Unit*

Epidural Anaesthetic pain relief administered into the epidural space between the vertebrae, providing a partial or total block of sensation in the abdomen and lower limbs

Episiotomy An incision made to the *perineum* in order to facilitate vaginal delivery

ERPC Evacuation of Retained Products of Pregnancy, or the removal of any remainder of pregnancy after miscarriage

Estimated Due Date See *EDD*

External Cephalic Version See *ECV*

F

Fallopian tubes The two very fine tubes leading from the *ovaries* to the *uterus*

Foetus The name given to a developing baby from Week 10 of pregnancy until delivery

Folate Naturally occurring form of the water-soluble vitamin B9. Folates occur naturally in certain foods or can be taken as *folic acid* supplements

Folic acid See *Folate*

Fontanelles The *soft spots* on a foetus's scalp which allow the bony plates of the skull to flex during birth, allowing the baby's head to pass through the birth canal. These don't close completely until around the second birthday

Forceps Instruments used to cradle a foetus's head to rotate the baby and facilitate delivery, usually in conjunction with an *episiotomy*

Fundus The top portion of the *uterus*, at the opposite end from the *cervix*

G

Gas and air See *Entonox*

Genetic disorder A condition caused by abnormalities, usually present from conception, in genes or *chromosomes*

Gestational diabetes A form of (Type II) diabetes mellitus which affects some pregnant mums, but which usually disappears within six weeks of birth. Women who develop gestational diabetes are more likely to develop diabetes mellitus permanently later in life

Glucose A simple sugar

Glucose Tolerance Test (*GTT*) A test given to pregnant mums showing signs of *gestational diabetes*, which involves testing blood-sugar levels before and after ingesting a *glucose*-loaded solution

Gravida Pregnant woman

GTT See *Glucose Tolerance Test*

H

Haemoglobin A special protein inside red blood cells enabling them to carry oxygen to the organs

Haemorrhoids Also known as *piles*, these are varicose veins in the anus and rectum

Heartburn A burning sensation in the gullet, just below the breastbone, usually caused by the regurgitation of stomach acid

Heparin An anti-coagulant drug given by injection to prevent or help disperse blood clots

Hepatitis B An inflammatory disease of the liver

Hormones Chemicals released by cells that affect cells in other parts of the body

Human chorionic gonadotrophin (hCG) The *hormone* produced in pregnancy by the *embryo*, indicating the presence of human life

Hyperemesis Gravidarum (HG) Excessive, sometimes debilitating, vomiting in pregnant mums

Hypertension Medical term for raised blood pressure

Hypoglycaemia Low blood-sugar levels

I

Incompetent cervix Anatomically lax *cervix* which tends to open during pregnancy, causing *miscarriage*

Incontinence The inability to control the flow of urine or the expulsion of faeces

Indigestion Pain in the upper abdomen or a feeling of over-fullness after eating relatively little. May be accompanied by wind or *heartburn*

Induction The artificial stimulation of *labour* by manual and/or chemical means

Insulin A *hormone* synthesised in the pancreas for controlling levels of glucose in the blood

L

Labia The lips of the vagina

Labour The period of time from the onset of *contractions* to the delivery of a baby

Lanugo The fine down covering a *foetus* from the second *trimester* of pregnancy to regulate body temperature

Lightening See *engagement*

Linea negra/nigra A dark vertical line caused by the pigment melanin that appears on the abdomen during pregnancy

LMP Last menstrual period

Lochia Discharge that follows childbith

M

Meconium First stool of a *foetus* or newborn, composed of matter ingested in the *uterus*

Morning sickness The term used to refer to vomiting and nausea in pregnancy. In practice it can occur at any time

Multigravida Term referring to a woman who is in her second or subsequent pregnancy

N

Neural tube Precursor to the central nervous system in a *foetus*

O

Obstetric cholestasis A potentially serious liver condition of pregnancy affecting around 2 per cent of expectant mums

Obstetrician Doctor specialising in all aspects of pregnancy and maternity care

Oedema Swelling of bodily tissues caused by fluid retention

Oestrogen The primary female sex *hormone*

Oligohydramnios Too little *amniotic fluid*

Ovaries Female reproductive organs producing eggs

Ovulation The release of an egg from one or other *ovary* during the menstrual cycle

Oxytocin A *hormone*, produced by the pituitary gland, which stimulates the *uterus* to contract

P

Paediatrician A doctor specialising in care of newborns and infants

Palpation The term given to the examination of the pregnant abdomen by a midwife

Pelvic disproportion See *Cephalo-pelvic disproportion (CPD)*

Pelvic floor The girdle of muscles supporting the pelvic organs, including the bladder, *uterus* and intestines

Perineum The area of tissue that lies between the vagina and anus

Pethidine Injectable opioid pain relief for labour

Pica The medical term given to *cravings* for non-edible substances in pregnancy

Piles See *haemorrhoids*

Placenta An organ grown specifically during pregnancy to support the life of the *foetus* until birth

Placenta praevia Where the placenta lies low down, obstructing the cervix

Polyhydramnios An excess of amniotic fluid

Posterior lie When a *foetus* is lying with the back of its head facing the mum's spine

Pre-eclampsia A potentially dangerous condition of pregnancy characterised by high blood pressure, *oedema* and protein in the urine. Left untreated it can develop into *eclampsia*

Presentation The part of your baby which is facing downwards in the *uterus* in readiness for birth

Primigravida A first-time pregnant mum

Progesterone One of the female *hormones* associated with conception and the continuation of pregnancy

Prostaglandin A substance that acts like a *hormone* and is found in many bodily tissues and especially in semen

Prurigo A benign itchy rash of pregnancy

Psoriasis Inflammatory skin disease

R

Relaxin A *hormone* produced in pregnancy to relax ligaments and joints in preparation for childbirth

Restless Legs Syndrome (RLS) A sporadic condition, often made worse in pregnancy, which results in an uncomfortable or unpleasant urge to move the legs

Rhesus negative The description of blood which lacks a substance known as D antigen on the surface of its red cells. This can have implications for an unborn baby, although usually only in second and subsequent pregnancies if left untreated

RLS See *Restless Legs Syndrome*

Round ligament pain Pulling pains in the abdomen as the ligaments of the *uterus* stretch during pregnancy

Rubella The medical term for German measles

S

Scans See *ultrasound scan*

SCBU See *Special Care Baby Unit*

Show The term used for when the mucus plug covering the opening of the *cervix* comes away as a prelude to *labour*

Soft spots See *fontanelles*

Special Care Baby Unit (SCBU) A dedicated neonatal hospital unit offering intensive care to vulnerable or sick newborns

Spinal A one-off dose of spinal anaesthesia which numbs the lower body in the same way as an *epidural*, but is quicker to set up, lasts for less time and cannot be topped up

Stillbirth The delivery of a baby who has died in the *uterus* or during labour and birth

Stretch marks Red, sometimes angry-looking lines which can appear down and across certain areas of the body of pregnant mums where the skin has stretched most. These do eventually fade after birth to less obtrusive, silvery marks, although they don't disappear

Surfactant A substance produced in a baby's lungs that helps to keep them open during breathing

Sweep of the membranes See *cervical sweep*

Symphysis Pubis Dysfunction See *Diastasis Symphysis Pubis*

T

TENS (Transcutaneous Electrical Nerve Stimulation) A portable machine that transmits electrical impulses via electrodes to offer distraction from the pain of *labour*

Thrush An overgrowth of yeast that leads to discharge, itching and soreness around the vagina. Also known as *Candida albicans*

Toxoplasmosis Parasitic infection that can affect foetal brain and eye development

Transvaginal scan A detailed scan of the *uterus* and *placenta* using a microscopic camera mounted on a slim probe which is inserted into the vagina. Often used in early pregnancy where an external *ultrasound scan* would be ineffective

Transverse lie Where a *foetus* is lying head to feet across the *uterus*

Trimester The term given for each of the three sections of pregnancy

U

Ultrasound scan Scan performed externally by passing a hand-held monitor across the abdomen of a pregnant mum. Soundwaves bounce through the *uterus* and back to the scanner, producing on-screen images of the *foetus* and *placenta*

Umbilical cord The collection of blood vessels that connects a *foetus* to the *placenta* and allows nutrients and waste products to filter to and from the *foetus* via the *placenta*

Urethra Anatomical tube through which urine passes out of the body from the bladder

Uterus The large, muscular organ which is home to a growing *foetus*

V

Vena cava Either of two large veins that return oxygen-depleted blood to the right atrium of the heart

Ventouse An electronic suction cup device used to facilitate a baby's passage down the birth canal

Vernix A creamy, sticky substance that covers a *foetus* in the *uterus*, protecting the skin

Vitamin K An anti-haemorrhaging vitamin administered to most newborns at birth to prevent a serious bleeding condition

W

Water birth A choice for *labour* and delivery where the labouring mum spends all or part of the time in a birthing pool

Waters Another term for *amniotic fluid*

Wharton's jelly A thick, mucous tissue which protects and insulates the blood vessels of the *umbilical cord*

Appendix: Useful Sources of Information

Medical information

Active Birth Centre
tel: 020 7281 6760
web: www.activebirthcentre.com

Amnio-PCR
Can give you results in 48 hours, although you usually have to pay for this test
web: www.amniopcr.com/patients/summary

Antenatal Results and Choices (ARC)
Offers counselling to help you come to a decision before, during and after the antenatal testing process
tel: 020 7631 0285
web: www.arc-uk.org

APEC (Action on Pre-Eclampsia)
tel: 020 8863 3271
web: www.apec.org.uk

Association for Improvements in the Maternity Services (AIMS)
tel: 0870 765 1433
web: www.aims.org.uk

Association of Breastfeeding Mothers
Offers guidelines on expressing and storing breastmilk
web: www.abm.me.uk

Birth Trauma Association
Offers a free service run by volunteer mums
web: www.birthtraumaassociation.org.uk

Bliss
This special care baby charity provides support and care to premature and
sick babies across the UK
web: www.bliss.org.uk

Boots maternity rental products
For maternity TENS machine rental
web: www.bootsmaternityrentalproducts.co.uk

Car seats
RoSPA's dedicated website has advice and information
web: www.childcarseats.org.uk/choosing

Daycare Trust
web: www.daycaretrust.org.uk

Diabetes UK
tel: 0845 120 2960
web: www.diabetes.org.uk

Doulas
web: www.doula.org.uk
          www.britishdoulas.co.uk

Down's Syndrome Association
tel: 0845 230 0372
web: www.downs-syndrome.org.uk

Home birth reference site
web: www.homebirth.org.uk

Independent Midwives Association
web: www.independentmidwives.org.uk

The Miscarriage Association
tel: 01924 200 799
web: www.miscarriageassociation.org.uk
email: info@miscarriageassociation.org.uk

The Multiple Births Foundation
tel: 020 8383 3519
web: www.multiplebirths.org.uk

National and local child care information
web: www.childcarelink.gov.uk

National Association of Family Information Services (NAFIS)
web: www.familyinformationservices.org.uk

National Childbirth Trust
web: www.nct.org.uk

National Childminding Association
web: www.ncma.org.uk

Netmums
web: www.netmums.com

Newlife Foundation for Disabled Children
tel: 01543 462 777
web: www.newlifecharity.co.uk

NHS Direct
tel: 0845 46 47
web: www.nhsdirect.nhs.uk

Obstetric Cholestasis Support
web: www.ocsupport.org.uk

Royal College of Midwives' Campaign for Normal Birth
web: www.rcmnormalbirth.org.uk

SANDS (Stillbirths and Neonatal Death Society)
tel: 020 7436 5881
web: www.uk-sands.org

The Twins and Multiple Births Association (TAMBA)
tel: 0800 138 0509
web: www.tamba.org.uk

Vaginal Birth After Caesarean (VBAC)
Provides information for women who have previously had a caesarean section but who are considering vaginal birth
web: www.vbac.org.uk

Government information

Child benefits
All parents are entitled to child benefit, regardless of their income. If you had a hospital birth and received a Bounty pack, you will find an application form inside it. Otherwise, you can apply online at the HM Revenue & Customs site
web: www.hmrc.gov.uk/childbenefit/online.htm

General Register Office
For information about registering your baby's birth
web: www.gro.gov.uk

Healthy Start scheme
You may be able to receive free formula milk and vitamin supplements if you
qualify for certain benefits
web: www.healthystart.nhs.uk

Maternity entitlements
For information on maternity pay and benefits
web: www.direct.gov.uk

Sure Start
Government programme to deliver the best start in life for every child,
bringing together early education, childcare, health and family support
web: www.surestart.gov.uk

Birthing techniques

Mongan method
web: www.hypnobirthing.co.uk

Natal hypnotherapy
web: www.natalhypnotherapy.co.uk

Self-hypnosis
web: www.birthwithoutfear.co.uk

Comfort items and maternity body jewellery

Comfort items

Bump to 3
Has devices that allow you to expand your maternity clothes, as well as lots of other baby and mum items
web: www.bumpto3.com

Bumpband
Elasticated fabric bands that act like a sling under your belly
web: www.bumpband.co.uk

Chillow Pillow
Chilled pillows, no refrigeration or power required
web: www.chillowpillow.co.uk

Maternity Pillow
Full-length body pillows to support your back and bump
tel: 01633 430 467
web: www.maternitypillow.co.uk

Sleep bras
web: www.mothernaturebras.co.uk
        www.babiesrus.co.uk

Maternity body jewellery

You can buy extra long bars, made from flexible plastic, as well as plastic 'retainers' suitable for pregnancy wear
web: www.bellybar.co.uk
        www.bodyjewlleryshop.com
        www.ouchbodyjewellery.co.uk

Baby's First Year: Chapter 1

Baby's First Year is the next book in the Netmums parenting series. It's the definitive guide to helping you through the first 12 months of your baby's life, which is an exciting and happy time, but a testing one too. The adventure – and all its challenges – is only just beginning. Children aren't born with instruction manuals. New parents need all the help they can get.

Chances are that when your baby's born there's a lot you're scratching your head about. And while there may not always be a perfect answer to your questions, good advice is crucial. Taking you through baby's first year month-by-month, this book tells you what you can expect at every stage of your child's development and gives advice on every aspect of caring for your new baby, from feeding and sleeping patterns, to teething and baby-proofing your home. Plus there's advice on how you can look after yourself, so you can be sure you're emotionally and physically fit for every milestone of your baby's first year.

Helping you make the most of a challenging and wonderful time, *Baby's First Year* is an indispensable bible for the first year of your baby's life. Chapter 1 is given here so that you can get a sense of what life with your baby is going to be like and a sense of how helpful it's going to be to have the latest expert thinking and peer advice to hand.

The First Month

Welcome to your first month of motherhood

Congratulations – you're a mum! The long, difficult haul of pregnancy and birth is over and your reward for sticking it out is a wonderful new baby, and the precious gift of motherhood. To say it takes time adapting to such a challenging new role is an understatement. For many new parents, this early period can be as bewildering, scary and exhausting as it is joyous. The first six to eight weeks of your baby's life is a learning period – you don't have to worry about anything else but getting through it as best you can. Take things super-slow, accept whatever help is offered and concentrate on getting your strength back, and on getting to know your baby. This is, after all, your 'babymoon'...

Health, Growth and Development

Baby milestones

At birth, your baby will typically:

- show a 'Moro response' (or reflex) by throwing out his arms and arching his back when startled by a sudden movement or noise
- display a 'rooting' reflex, turning towards a touch on the cheek, or the side of the mouth, and suck instinctively when offered a nipple or teat
- demonstrate a number of newborn reflex behaviours – he will take steps if held upright with his feet on a firm surface, bend his legs under his body when placed on his tummy, as if trying to crawl, or grasp hard on something placed close to his palm. (He won't be able to do these things after a few days, and will need to re-learn them later on in his development)
- be sensitive to light and sound, turning towards a major source of light and appearing startled by a sudden loud sound
- be able to focus on and see things within 20–25cm, showing particular interest in your face, or anything with a sharp outline or a bright, bold colour
- move his arms and legs
- gaze up at the adult holding him
- vocalise his feelings and needs by crying in a number of different ways
- have a sense of smell and taste.

Your health visitor

At some point after ten days, your midwife will sign off responsibility and your health visitor will introduce themselves. They will make one or more home visits, and provide you with a personal child health record (often known as the 'red book'), in which healthcare professionals, and you, can make a note of all significant health and development information in your child's early years. They will weigh your baby at home at least once before they are five days old and will also let you know where and when to find your nearest baby clinic – these run regularly in health centres and GP surgeries and will usually be the place to go for routine tests and immunisations, and for weighing and measuring sessions (they're also a good place to meet other parents).

Although in the past parents have been encouraged to have their babies measured weekly, it's now considered pointless to go so frequently (it may even cause unnecessary anxiety), so it's recommended that full-term babies are measured no more than six times in their first year.

When help isn't immediately at hand

If you are in doubt about any aspect of your baby's health (or about your own) and you are unable to see or talk to your midwife, health visitor or GP, you may be able to get the help you need by calling NHS Direct, which offers 24-hour advice. We've included this number in the Useful Addresses appendix at the back of the book.

It's official: Registering your baby's birth

Don't forget that, by law, you must register your baby's birth within 42 days (or 21 days, if you live in Scotland). You may be able to do this at the hospital before going home, or you may have to visit a register office to do so. There's more information about registering your baby's birth on the website of the General Register Office (www.gro.gov.uk).

When you register your baby's birth, you'll be given a birth certificate and a pink registration card which you'll need to fill in and sign before taking it to your doctor's surgery, so that your baby can officially become a patient there. It's a good idea to get this done as soon as possible, just in case your baby needs to see a GP before his first routine check at around six weeks.

Weird and wonderful: what your newborn baby may look like

Let's face it, newborn babies can be weird-looking little things! There'll probably be an explanation for any physical oddity you may notice: the main ones are listed below, and there's further detail in the Medical A–Z appendix at the back of the book. (If in any doubt about a feature of your baby which seems unusual, you should check with your midwife, health visitor or GP.)

The cord stump The remains of the umbilical cord (the link between the baby and the placenta during pregnancy) will be attached to your baby's tummy for a little while after the birth but shrivels up and drops off within a fortnight or so. In the meantime it needs to be kept clean and dry as they're prone to infection – when you wash or bathe them, always make sure the area is carefully dried afterwards by gently dabbing it with tissue or a soft, clean towel. Once they drop off, it can take another week or so until the area is healed. It's normal for them to appear a little weepy during this time, but if you're worried, ask a health professional to check it.

The head Babies' heads are often a bit misshapen, or 'moulded' at first. They may be slightly pointed, flattened or swollen as a result of birth, particularly if forceps or a ventouse were involved (these can also leave marks that will fade after a few days) but this will usually be temporary. The bones in a new baby's head are not yet joined together and a careful feel will reveal the fontanelles – two soft spots. The smaller of these closes by about six weeks, the larger closes by about 18 months.

Eyes These commonly look 'squinty' early on as babies haven't yet learned to control the muscles round the eyes. If they are yellowish it may indicate jaundice (see *Skin*, below). Sometimes they may have a crusty discharge which suggests a mild infection known as sticky eye (NB this is not the same as conjunctivitis) which can be treated with drops.

Skin This may well be blotchy, spotty, patchy, dry, or uneven in colour. Because it's so sensitive, it's prone to all sorts of rashes and spots, including milia (milk spots) which are harmless tiny white spots on the nose or cheeks and are extremely common. It's also common for babies to be slightly jaundiced in the early days because of the immaturity of their livers – this is shown with a yellowish tinge. In most cases it's harmless, but your midwife will be keeping a close eye on it. You may also notice traces of vernix (particularly in premature babies), which is the greasy white substance that protects a baby's skin from amniotic fluid in the womb. Don't be tempted to wash it off – any left on the skin after birth will absorb naturally, and until then it can help keep the skin moisturised.

Birthmarks These are also common and they come in many different forms. Sometimes a red mark will be a simple result of pressure on the skin during the birth and these will quickly fade.

Hair They may have lots or very little at birth, and in any case, it is very likely to fall out over the coming months (and what grows back may be an entirely different colour or texture). It's not unusual for babies to have a fine covering of body hair, which is the same soft fuzz – called lanugo – which they were protected by in the womb, particularly if they were born pre-term. It drops out over time.

Nipples and genitals These may be swollen due to an overflow of mum's hormones finding its way into the baby. It's just a temporary thing. (You may also notice a little blood in a baby girl's nappy for the same reason.) Boys' testicles come down into the scrotum just before birth but occasionally, one may remain undescended. This is usually temporary, but may sometimes need a small operation to correct. Your doctor, midwife or health visitor will be alert to the possibility during your baby's routine examinations.

Feeding
Breast, the best
You'll most likely have made a decision on how you hope to feed your baby before he was born. The majority of new mums breastfeed initially, and there's no doubt that it offers the best possible start for a baby. Almost all women have the physiological wherewithal to make a success of breastfeeding – although a minority may not be able to breastfeed for specific medical reasons – and those who encounter difficulties have a very good chance of getting through them if they persevere, and with the right help.

At the outset, breastfeeding can be really hard work, it's true: your nipples can get extremely sore until they toughen up, and whilst you work out how to get the positioning right and, in the early weeks, the sheer amount of time that babies want to suckle can be draining. On top of that are the emotional factors: the worry that they're getting enough milk, and the guilt if you don't think they are. Feeding your baby in the best way you can is the top priority for any new mum, so if for one reason or another you're struggling to, it can lead to misery.

Once you're over the early hurdles, though, breastfeeding invariably becomes easy and even, for many mums, a great pleasure. You should get all the advice and support you need to get started from your midwife or health visitor. You'll also need moral support and plenty of practical help from your partner, and from other close relatives and friends, too – for example, you'll need someone who's prepared to bring you sustenance while you're pinned to the sofa for long stretches of time (or by keeping the fridge well stocked with snacks and drinks for when you need them). So make sure everyone around knows about your decision to breastfeed, and that you've got their backing.

The benefits of breastfeeding

- Breast milk is 100 per cent natural and contains all the nutrients your baby needs. It provides the perfect food and drink for him. It's also free.
- It's easily absorbed and digested so he is less likely to have colic or constipation.
- It's rich in antibodies which help protect against infection – research shows that breastfed babies are less likely to develop gastrointestinal and respiratory illnesses and ear infections.
- Certain allergic conditions, such as eczema, may not be as severe.
- Children and adults who were breastfed are less likely to be obese.
- Some research suggests that breastfeeding may lower the risk of cot death.
- Mums who breastfeed lower their chances of developing breast cancer and some ovarian cancer, and have less chance of developing osteoporosis (weakening of the bones).

- Breastfeeding helps the uterus contract back to normal in the days after birth, and helps you lose your baby-weight because it uses up calories.
- It's ultra-convenient. The milk is 'on tap', and there's no bottle-washing, sterilising and preparation to worry about, or equipment to lug around when you're out and about. You don't need to venture into a cold kitchen for night feeds, either.
- You get lots of cuddly, skin-to-skin contact with your baby while feeding them.
- Once established and comfortable, breastfeeding gives you the perfect excuse for sitting down and relaxing with your baby for long stretches of time. (And you should make the most of this time with your first baby – you may not be able to give subsequent babies the luxury of devoting so much time to them when you have older children to tend to!)

Get ready

Be prepared for breastfeeding in good time for the birth by reading up on it, and make sure you have what you'll need in advance: several well-fitting nursing bras, a good supply of breast pads, and plenty of loose, comfortable tops which either lift up easily or open at the front. Don't forget to have a good stock of bibs to hand, or better still, a multi-pack of muslins.

Give them the gold top

For the first few days after birth, the breasts provide a special sort of milk called colostrum, a rich, creamy and yellowish substance which is particularly nutritious as it's thick with antibodies and nutrients that help provide resistance to infection.

On the third or fourth day after birth, a new mum's breasts fill up with regular breast milk – be prepared, as it can come as rather a surprise to wake up with very tender boobs that are close to bursting. Most (but not all) women find there's a certain amount of leakage to cope with, especially at first. You may need a sense of humour and a good supply of breast pads for a while. It can also be an extremely uncomfortable period. Make sure you have a bra that's well-fitting and supportive and try a cold or hot pack, available from chemists, to relieve pain. Putting Savoy cabbage leaves in your bra is an old-fashioned remedy which can actually help (although there's no medical evidence to explain why!).

Are you sitting comfortably?

Before you begin breastfeeding, make sure you're comfortable and relaxed (not easy at first, admittedly, but you'll get there). You may prefer to hold your baby across your lap – if so, pillows to support your back and arm and a footstool or pillow to elevate the baby so he's level with your breasts can be a great help. (You can buy a special, boomerang-shaped breastfeeding pillow, but the ordinary sort piled up will do fine). Some mums find the 'rugby ball' position works well – holding the baby under your arm with their legs tucked round your body. Others like to breastfeed lying down, especially those with very large breasts, or if they are very sore after birth (particularly after a Caesarean, which can make breastfeeding challenging at first).

Getting the 'latch on' right

Finding the right positioning and getting your baby to 'latch on' properly is key to getting the baby to feed well, and avoiding the agony of cracked and sore nipples. It may not come naturally at first – for either baby or mum – but can be mastered with practice and perseverance. Much like having new shoes, you need to accept that your nipples will hurt for a short time while they get 'worn in'. However, extremely sore, cracked or bleeding nipples almost certainly mean you've yet to get the positioning right.

Start with the baby's nose opposite the nipple and allow his head to tilt back. Move his mouth gently across the nipple until he opens his mouth wide, which is known as the 'rooting reflex'. Bring your baby towards the breast quickly, making sure his whole body is closely tucked in, in a straight line, facing yours. Aim the nipple towards the roof of his mouth and allow him to get a big mouthful of breast – you may need to support your boob underneath with your hand to guide it in. He is on correctly if his chin is resting firmly against the breast and his lower lip is rolled outwards. You'll know when the milk is on its way because you'll feel a tingling 'let down' reflex as it gathers behind the nipple and areola, and you'll know when he is feeding because he'll be taking big, rhythmic gulps and his ears will be wiggling slightly!

If they aren't latched on properly and they obviously don't have enough nipple in their mouths, start again – don't tug the nipple out as if it was a cork from a bottle though, or it will hurt like hell. Break the suction cleanly by inserting a finger into the corner of their mouth.

A two-course meal

Let your baby feed for as long as he wants. Milk comes out of the breast in two stages – first the thirst-quenching foremilk, and secondly the fat-rich hindmilk. So always let him empty the first breast you offer (you can tell when the breast is empty simply by the look and feel of it, or by squeezing it slightly to see what's left) before moving him on to the second. He may not empty that one as well, so be sure to offer that one first at the next feed. Some mums find it helpful to put a safety pin into the bra strap on the side of the breast they need to start with to help them remember.

Supply and demand

These days, it's recommended that babies are allowed to 'demand feed', which means offering them the breast whenever and for however long they want. It's the best system for feeding because breastmilk is made on a supply and demand basis, so the more you feed them, the more milk you'll make. (Which is why if you stop breastfeeding for any length of time it can be hard to start again.)

Don't be surprised, in the early days, by just how much 'demanding' your baby may do. A lot of new mums are rather overwhelmed by how often they find themselves whipping their boobs out and how long they must sit there feeding. (Sometimes your baby may not even be that hungry, just hankering for the comfort of a suck.) This is just a temporary phase, though – after six to eight weeks they will generally settle down into a more widely spaced and regular feeding pattern, as they become adept at suckling so can take what they need in a shorter time, and as their stomach capacity grows.

Feeding yourself

You don't need to eat especially well to ensure the production of your milk, but it's advisable to eat a balanced diet, at regular intervals throughout the day, and it's recommended that breastfeeding mums consume an extra 400 or so calories a day than they would normally. The Food Standards Agency now recommends that all women take 10mg a day of a vitamin D supplement while breastfeeding.

You'll need (and will probably want to) drink lots of fluid, preferably water, as breastfeeding can be dehydrating. But it's wise to keep an eye on your intake of caffeine and alcohol, because small quantities of these things can filter through to the milk and may affect your baby. That doesn't mean you need to be a saint – a glass of wine or two, a couple of times a week, or three to four cups of coffee each day are fine, particularly if they're going to relax you and improve your state of mind.

Foods that may be a problem

Some babies seem to be affected by the food their mums eat whilst breast-feeding: likely culprits include spicy dishes, vegetables such as cabbage, broccoli, onions and sprouts, and acidic citrus fruits or juice – if they seem windy, uncomfortable, or colicky, it may be eased by a little attention to your diet.

Occasionally a baby may have an allergic reaction to something his mum has eaten, resulting in a rash, diarrhoea, or flu-like symptoms. Common allergens include cow's milk protein, wheat, eggs, nuts and soy. You'll need to take advice from your GP if you suspect your baby is affected in this way.

Burping the baby

After a feed you can help to bring up any excess air your baby may have swallowed, which could otherwise cause him discomfort, by 'burping' him. Place him over your shoulder, face down on your lap, or in a well-supported sitting position, and gently pat or rub his back. You may or may not get an audible reward for your efforts!

Give up smoking, if you can

It's not a good idea to smoke if you're breastfeeding, as traces of chemicals including nicotine can pass through to your baby – and heavy smoking is believed to affect milk production. However, you shouldn't be put off breastfeeding just because you're a smoker, as it still represents a healthier way to feed your baby.

Smoking in the house is a bad idea all round with a new baby, because it increases the risk of cot death and makes them more prone to colic and illness. If you're a smoker and you weren't able to give up during pregnancy, perhaps you could now? At the very least, be sure to always smoke outside the house, away from your baby.

Are they getting enough milk?

Many mums worry that their baby isn't getting enough breastmilk because they can't see what's going in. If a child is feeding regularly and producing plenty of wet nappies, he will be doing OK and, if not, you should seek the advice of your health visitor or GP. But don't be tempted to stop trying – health professionals will rarely advise a mum to ditch breastfeeding in favour of formula, although if there's a genuine problem they might recommend it as a supplement.

In the longer term you'll be able to see if your baby is thriving by his progress on height and weight charts. (Bear in mind that all babies, however they are fed, are expected to lose between 5 and 10 per cent of their birth weight over the course of the first week or so, before beginning a gradual gain after that.) Be guided and advised by the health professionals looking out for you. However, a mum's own intuition is the best gauge of her baby's health and progress: you will need to have faith in your own feelings!

What to do when it's not working

If you encounter problems with breastfeeding, try not to panic. Keep on trying as best as you can and get advice as soon as possible from your midwife, health visitor or GP, from a local breastfeeding counsellor, or by calling a breastfeeding helpline (there are several, and we've included their numbers in the Useful Addresses appendix at the back of the book).

Common breastfeeding problems

Blocked Duct This occurs when milk builds up in a duct causing a hard, painful lump in the breast. Again, a good feed can help relieve it, or you can try and massage the lump. If left, blocked ducts can lead to mastitis (see below), so are best tackled.

Engorgement This happens when the breasts become painfully full of milk, usually because of a delay in emptying them. The best way to resolve the problem is to feed your baby, but if they're too full for him to get a hold of, you may need to massage your boobs and express a little milk to relieve the fullness first. Like a blocked duct, engorgement can lead to mastitis.

Mastitis. A painful inflammation of the breast, which may be caused by an infection, usually the result of a cracked nipple, or because of engorgement or a blocked duct. You can help prevent it by feeding your baby whenever he wants, so the breast is being regularly emptied, and by making sure your positioning is right to avoid cracked nipples. You may notice a patch of the breast which is red, hot, sore or swollen, or flu-like symptoms. If you suspect mastitis, you should seek treatment from your GP, as severe cases will require antibiotics. It's perfectly safe – in fact, it's advisable – to carry on breastfeeding during a bout.

Sore or cracked nipples If you get these, you need help from a health professional or breastfeeding counsellor, to check that you're correctly positioned and that the baby's latching on properly. Inevitably, once nipples get sore, it's painful to keep on feeding. So get all the help you can in getting the position right – and meanwhile, you could try holding him in the rugby-ball style, or lying down (or however you haven't been doing it up until then). Expressing may be the only way to keep the milk coming if your nipples are really sore.

A traditional 'cure' for sore nipples is to wipe a little breastmilk on them after each feed and this is no old wives' tale, as breastmilk contains healing antibodies. You can also buy creams, although you can only put these on when you're sure you're going to get a break from feeding for a while, to allow them to absorb. Nipple shields may help, but they make it harder for the baby to suck – and there's also the worry that your baby will come to prefer the shield's teat to the real deal. Keep your nipples clean and dry and try getting fresh air to your breasts whenever possible, and keep breast pads changed regularly. Very sore nipples may occasionally be a sign of thrush. See the Medical A–Z for more information.

What the netmums say

'Breastfeeding'

One thing I did in the very early days was to keep a breastfeeding journal. I'd note down the time, how long she fed for and on what side. It really helped me keep on top of the feeds and helped make sure I fed her enough and evenly on both sides. The funniest thing for me was leaky boobs. Who knew a woman could produce that much milk?
Sophie from Glasgow, mum to Ava Charlotte, 18 months

I was determined to breastfeed, however I found it incredibly difficult and painful, and then developed mastitis in both sides. At that point I decided to give both me and my son a break and move to formula. The failure to breastfeed properly was devastating and I felt tremendous guilt for a long time (still do, if I'm honest).
Sharon from Rotherham, mum to Edward, two

I was determined to breastfeed, and had I not been so stubborn about it I might have given up many a time. How much has she had? Is she still hungry? She's only feeding ten minutes from each side, is she getting enough hindmilk? Is she latching on properly? These were the thoughts that occupied me constantly. I could cope with the pain, which only lasted a couple of weeks and was greatly helped by the cabbage leaves I kept in the fridge, but it was whether she was feeding enough that bothered me. If I'd taken a step back I would have realised that week after week she was putting on weight and thriving, so my breastmilk must have been giving her enough!
Alex, from Kings Langley, mum to Niamh, seven months

I don't think midwives are entirely honest in telling you just how frequently a newborn baby will feed! I felt like all I did all day was feed him, change his nappy, and feed again.
Debra from Rotherham, mum to Finn, four, and Louis, two

Choosing not to breastfeed

A minority of mums choose not to breastfeed (or may be unable to for a specific reason) from the off. And statistics show that, of those mums who start, a high proportion give up well before the six months that's recommended by the Department of Health.

Although bottlefeeding with infant formula milk can never be as beneficial as breastfeeding, it's a very good alternative as long as scrupulous attention is paid to hygiene and the making-up instructions. If you decide it's the right option for you, don't waste a moment feeling guilty about it.

The benefits of bottlefeeding

- It's not difficult to master and there's no pain involved.
- It's not such a tie – other willing adults can do it, taking the pressure off Mum and allowing them to enjoy the closeness of feeding, too.
- You know exactly how much milk they're getting.
- Formula milk is more filling and feeds tend to be quicker (once they've finished, they're finished – breastfed babies like to linger a while), so there'll be longer spaces between feeds.
- They will probably wake less frequently at night and are more likely – a couple of months down the line – to sleep through the night.
- You don't have to keep tabs on what you eat or drink.
- You never have to bare your boobs in public.
- It will be easier to go back to work if and when you want to.

What you'll need to bottlefeed

If you plan to, or if you switch to bottlefeeding, you'll need to have a constant supply of infant formula milk, at least six bottles with teats and lids, and the appropriate equipment for cleaning and sterilising them.

Sterilising everything properly is absolutely vital during the first year, when a baby's immune system is still weak, to keep bacteria at bay and prevent him from becoming ill. You can use a steam steriliser (some of which are designed to work in the microwave), a container of cold water with a sterilising solution, or put the bottles, teats and lids through a very hot cycle

(80 degrees) in a dishwasher. (You can sterilise effectively by simply boiling what you need in a pan of water for 10 minutes.)

Before sterilising you need to clean bottles and teats very thoroughly with hot soapy water and a bottle brush, making sure all traces of formula are gone, as these can harbour bacteria. You should always make sure that the surface you make up formula feeds on is clean, and wash your hands thoroughly beforehand.

Problems with formula feeding

Constipation is sometimes a problem with formula-fed babies. Make sure you are giving them the right formula type for their age. Most brands come in a 'hungry baby' version, for instance, which is not suitable for newborns and may well cause them to become bunged up. It's now recommended that formula-fed babies are given supplements of vitamins A, C and D if they are drinking less than 500mls of formula a day.

Occasionally, a baby may show an intolerance or allergy to normal formula milk. If you suspect this is a problem, you'll need to get advice from your GP about possible alternatives – don't attempt to experiment on your own.

If you qualify for certain benefits, you may be able to get free formula milk and vitamin supplements under the government's Healthy Start scheme. Ask your health visitor, or look online at www.healthystart.nhs.uk. Don't forget that all parents are entitled to child benefit, regardless of their income. If you had a hospital birth and received a Bounty pack of information, you will find an application form inside it. Otherwise, you can apply online at the HM Revenue & Customs site. www.hmrc.gov.uk/childbenefit/claiming.

Bringing it up again

Babies fed on either sort of milk may bring up a surprising amount of vomit after a feed. This is known as 'possetting' and is perfectly normal. You can help avoid it by keeping him still and upright for a while after a feed. If the amount he brings up is excessive, if he is doing it very frequently, or if the vomit is projectile, you should ask your health visitor or a doctor for advice.

Mixed feeding

Many mums successfully combine breast and bottle feeding, but if you want to do both you should put off introducing a bottle until your baby is six weeks old, to give breastfeeding a good chance to get established and to avoid him becoming confused between nipple and teat.

Sleeping

Sleeping like a baby?

New babies' sleep patterns vary enormously, but on average they will spend 16–18 hours out of 24 asleep during their first month and will typically spend large chunks of the day napping (this can be a good time for you to catch up on a bit of sleep, too). One thing is certain: you are highly unlikely to get an uninterrupted night's sleep in the early weeks and, in most cases, for quite a long time after that! It's just one of the parts of parenthood you have to come to terms with.

Very young babies wake up at night because they're hungry: they have tiny tummies and they need regular top-ups. A breastfed baby may wake up to four or five times a night in need of a feed at this stage (a bottlefed baby probably less so), and they will only stop crying if you give it to them. The upside is that they also sleep a lot during the day, in theory allowing you to catch up on a bit of the rest you've missed the night before.

Early days (and nights)

In the first month, there probably won't be any semblance of a routine to your baby's sleep and there's little point in rigorously trying to introduce one. Newborns don't understand the difference between day and night and, besides, most parents like to keep them permanently close by at this stage, which is why a portable Moses basket or carrycot is useful. So go with the flow – let him nap whenever and for however long he wants to, and simply accept it when he is awake. You may find your baby is more content and comfortable at this stage being 'swaddled' – wrapped firmly in a blanket, to emulate the snug environment of the womb.

However, even at this early stage, it's worth getting him used to the idea of being put down for sleep while still awake. That's because later on, when you're aiming to get him sleeping through the night, you'll need him to be able to drop off independently. It's never too early to start practising this!

(Babies have six states of alertness: deeply asleep, light sleep, drowsy, quiet alert, busy alert and crying. As you get to know your baby you'll be able to recognise when he is getting drowsy as he'll be yawning and stretching, and his eyes will be gradually taking longer to open and shut. This is the best time to place him in his cot to sleep.)

It's also a good idea to get him used to a sleeping against a certain amount of background noise, too, so don't tiptoe round your baby when he's asleep, or talk in whispers – it's just not realistic to aim for total quiet every time you put him down.

Safest in their own bed

It's also important to encourage them to sleep in their own cot, crib, or basket right from the start, so they learn it's a happy and comfortable place to be. (Lovely as it is to have them curled up against you when they're little it's a precedent you might want to think twice about setting.) Another thing you can do now is to teach him that night-times are for sleeping, and not for partying – keep night-feeds brief and to the point (if possible!), your voice low, and the lights dim.

Some people choose to have their baby in bed with them because they feel it's convenient and pleasurable. Many more find their babies end up in with them anyway, because it's the easy option when you're tired. It can certainly make night feeds easier if you're breastfeeding. But most health professionals, as well as experts from the Foundation for the Study of Infant Deaths (FSID), believe it's safer for a baby to sleep in his own cot for the first six months, because co-sleeping is linked to a greater risk of cot death.

Goodnight, sweetheart: All you need to know about safe sleeping

Since a major awareness campaign was launched in 1991, the number of cot deaths in the UK has fallen by 75 per cent. But 300 babies a year still die suddenly and unexpectedly in their sleep, for no obvious reason.

According to the Foundation for the Study of Infant Deaths, there are a number of things you can do to reduce the risk:

- Always place your baby on his back when you put him to sleep. You will need to give him lots of opportunities whilst he's awake to spend time in other positions, to avoid a misshapen head (there's more about this condition, plagiocephaly, in the Medical A–Z at the back of the book) but whilst he's asleep, he should always be put down on his back.

- Put him with his feet at the foot of the cot, and with his covers firmly tucked in, to prevent him from wriggling down under the covers.

- Never give your baby a pillow.

- Don't let him get too hot. Babies' rooms should be 16–20°C, which isn't especially warm. In most weathers, you won't need to keep the heating on overnight and you should never put him close to a radiator or other source of heat. Always keep his head uncovered when he is asleep. Check body heat by touching him to see he is not too hot, or sweaty – if necessary, remove a layer of bedclothing. Use lightweight layers of blankets, not a duvet or quilt. Baby sleeping bags are a safe option, as long as they are the right size, lightweight and hoodless.

- Make sure your baby's mattress is kept clean and dry. It's best to buy one new when you're preparing for a new baby. This is because there is evidence to show that babies are at risk from bacteria that can proliferate in an old mattress.

- Don't smoke anywhere near your baby, or allow anyone else to.

- Never fall asleep with your baby on a sofa or armchair.

- Put your baby to sleep, at night and for naps, in their own crib or cot.

- Keep his crib or cot in your room for the first six months.

- Never bedshare with your baby if you or your partner is a smoker, if you have been drinking alcohol, if you have taken medication or drugs that make you drowsy, or if you are very tired, or obese. Don't bedshare with a baby who was born before 37 weeks, or weighed less than 5.5lbs at birth, or is less than three months old.

- Consider giving your baby a dummy for night-time sleeps and daytime naps, too, for at least the first six months (but only once breastfeeding has been well established). Recent research has found this may help lower the risk of cot death, although it is unclear why.

- Seek immediate advice if your baby seems unwell.

General Care

Handle with care

Picking up, holding and carrying, and dressing a baby all sound like simple enough things, but unless you've cared for one before, it's by no means obvious how you do them and, since newborns seem so small and fragile, it's nervewracking trying to get it right.

Babies like to be held firmly and securely, so it's important that you feel confident in doing so – and besides, it's the only way you're ever going to get a really good cuddle with him. As with so many other aspects of babycare, practice makes perfect.

Lifting and holding

When lifting and holding the key thing is to keep your movements slow and gentle, and be sure to keep your baby's head and neck supported, as he is not strong enough to do this for himself in the first month or so. You can hold a new baby in the traditional way, with their whole body resting on an arm, or you can let them lie against your chest with their head nestling into your neck, supporting their bottom or back with your other hand. In time, as their neck muscles strengthen, they'll enjoy looking over your shoulder while in this position.

Putting your baby's clothes on (and taking them off)

Babies often dislike being dressed and undressed. If so, it's important to be able to do it quickly and gently – and why those simple sleepsuits make the best choice of clothing when they're tiny. Make sure they're as warm as possible when dressing or undressing, putting them on a warm surface and if they are unsettled, covering them with a towel or muslin. Most babies dislike having things pulled over their heads as it covers up their eyes, noses and mouths, so aim to do this with speed – scoop your thumbs into the neck of the garment and stretch it before pulling it on or off. With sleeves, be sure to pull the garment rather than your baby's arms in order to get them in. And where poppers are concerned: you'll get there in the end!

Nappy talk

Poo-filled nappies are one of the less pleasant aspects of babycare. Think of them as reassurance, though: if they're producing regular poos (or stools to give them their correct medical name), and the colour and consistency comes within the normal range, it's a good sign that feeding's going OK.

During his first few days, your baby's poo will consist of meconium, a dark, sticky substance that's built up in his intestines during pregnancy. It looks disgusting and can be hard to clean off, but it means his bowels are working correctly. It soon changes, becoming yellow or greenish, rather runny, and often seedy in breastfed babies, but firmer and less brightly coloured in bottlefed babies. Poo tends to be less smelly (and less frequent) in breastfed babies, too. Don't be surprised or concerned by very runny or 'explosive' poos, as these are quite normal.

Keeping regular

How often they poo varies. Breastfed babies may go several times a day or they may go for several days without one – this is nothing to be concerned about, as they are very unlikely to suffer constipation. Bottlefed babies are more prone to constipation and really need to go at least once a day to avoid a build-up. They can be given a little cool, boiled water to soften their stools up, if necessary. There's more on constipation in the Medical A–Z at the back of the book.

Wet nappies are an important sign that your baby's feeding well, so keep an eye on them – as a general rule they should be producing five to six wet nappies a day (it can be hard to gauge when a disposable nappy is wet as they're so absorbent – they'll feel heavier, though). Always let a health professional know if they don't seem to have had a wee for more than a couple of hours, or if you are concerned that they may be constipated, have diarrhoea, or that their stools do not look normal. Any health visitor or GP will be very happy to check for you.

Disposable versus reusable nappies

Reusable nappies are:

- generally reckoned to be better for the environment – even if you consider the energy and detergents required to wash and dry them
- cheaper in the long run – it's estimated they could save around £500 over the course of several years' nappy use
- well designed these days, so they are easily put on, stay in place and don't leak
- natural – they don't contain chemicals, as disposables do

Disposable nappies are:

- much more convenient – especially when out and about as they are readily available in all supermarkets and chemists
- highly absorbent, so can take lots of wee before causing discomfort
- more affordable in that there's no large initial outlay

Time for a change

Change your baby as soon as possible after they've done a poo or when they've become wet, to help avoid nappy rash. A good tip is to make sure you have everything you need to hand before you start – mat, wipes, clean nappy and change of clothes if necessary. Be sure to clean the whole bottom area thoroughly using plain, warm water and cotton wool, or wipes. (These are undoubtedly convenient, but rather cold! Some also contain ingredients which may exacerbate nappy rash, so always stick with the alcohol and fragrance-free varieties.) Always wipe girls from front to back to avoid the spread of germs, and gently clean around the penis and balls – but avoid pulling back the foreskin – when changing boys. Gently pat dry afterwards with tissue or a soft towel. A barrier cream like Vaseline can help prevent against nappy rash but shouldn't be necessary if you've cleaned and dried properly.

Finally, don't forget to wash your hands before and after every nappy change.

What the netmums say

'... about nappies'

I'd been so saturated with information about pregnancy and then when they put Sam in my arms I thought, 'Damn, nobody has told me anything about the baby'. I didn't have a clue. Luckily the midwives were really good and showed me how to change a nappy, dress, feed and bathe him. However, we did have problems. When he was a few days old I noticed that every nappy I put on him leaked. I was changing his clothes about eight times a day and was totally baffled! Eventually I realised this was because I was fastening his nappies with his willy pointing up!

Elaine from Lincoln, mum to Samuel, four months

We wanted to use real nappies but I totally regretted going down that route with a demanding baby. I could never put him down and washing nappies was an added stress. It got easier as he grew older but I wished I hadn't bothered using them in the first couple of weeks, and just enjoyed my new baby.

Claire from Letchworth, mum to Oliver, four and Daisy, two

Topping and tailing

Whilst it's OK to put them in a bath right from the start, even whilst they've still got their umbilical stump, many babies dislike being submerged at first – you may find it easier just to avoid it in the first few months and simply 'top and tail' them once a day. (Most babies come round to the idea of a bath eventually.) To do this, undress them in a warm room, wrap them in a towel and put them securely on a changing mat or on your lap. Gently wipe their face with dampened cotton wool or a soft sponge, and (in the early weeks, at least) use cooled boiled water to clean their eyes (wipe inside to outside to avoid infection, using a new piece of cotton wool each time). Clean gently around the ears with a bit of cotton wool or a sponge, but not inside them – *never* be tempted to push a cotton wool bud into the ear canal; there's no need, anyway, as the insides of babies' ears are self-cleaning. The same goes for noses. Give their neck and hands a wipe, keeping them as warm as possible with bits of the towel in the meantime. Don't forget to pay attention to the folds of skin under their chin and their armpits, because old milk can gather here, go nasty, become very smelly, and cause soreness.

Bathing your baby

After a few weeks you'll probably feel more confident about bathing – and although most babies are wary of the bath at first, many come to adore a splash around in some warm water. They don't need a bath every day, but it can become a useful stage in a bedtime routine, so if they're willing, make it a regular thing.

Begin by half-filling the bath with warm water – be sure to put the cold in first then add hot, and test the temperature before you put the baby in. It should be mildly warm. Undress and wrap him in a towel, then wash his face as with topping-and-tailing method. If you want to wash his hair (and it's not particularly necessary at this stage), do so while he is still wrapped up in a towel by holding him over the bath by pouring a little water carefully over his head. Then lower him into the bath, carefully supporting his head and shoulders with one arm, keeping the other free to wash, rinse, tickle and splash him. Try to keep the distance between the undressed baby and the bath as short as possible, so he's not dangling in cold air longer than necessary.

Once they're out, pat them completely dry, especially in all their creases. Finish off with a nice clean nappy, and a fresh sleepsuit – then cuddle him thoroughly, to make the most of that lovely, clean-baby smell. It won't last long!

All about you

Although experiences vary greatly, giving birth takes a major physical toll on the vast majority of women and, during the first month, your other focus will be on getting your own strength back. Your midwife will make a number of visits (and should also be available over the telephone) to help with this process, and to keep an eye on any possible complications.

In the immediate weeks after birth, your body will probably be feeling the consequences of birth in many different parts.

Your body after birth

- **Lochia, or postnatal bleeding** A discharge of leftover blood, mucus and tissue from the uterus (womb), this is like a heavy period which will continue for up to ten days, after which the flow should lessen, although it may still carry on for several weeks more. It usually starts off bright red (and will often have clots in it), changing to pink or brown and then a yellowish white. You'll need some heavy-duty maternity pads, which are longer and softer than ordinary pads. (Tampons aren't recommended because of the risk of infection).

- **Afterpains** Similar to labour or bad period pains, these are caused by contractions of the uterus as it shrinks back to normal size after the birth. They're often particularly noticeable whilst breastfeeding (and if you breastfeed it can help to speed the shrinkage process up) but should only occur for up to seven days after the birth. If necessary you can take a painkiller such as codeine or paracetamol – but double check with your midwife, first.

- **Soreness, scars and stitches** Some level of pain and discomfort down below is inevitable after a vaginal birth (or after a C-section if you experience normal labour beforehand). The perineum (the bit between the vagina and the anus) will commonly be bruised and sore (even if it didn't tear during birth, it's still had a battering) so sitting down can hurt for a while. To avoid infection, keep it clean and change your maternity pad regularly, being sure to wash your hands before and afterwards. It may hurt to wee for a while, too – try waiting until you're in the bath, or pouring a jug of warm water over your bits when you're on the loo. Pain and discomfort is likely to be even worse if you had stitches after the birth because of a tear or episiotomy and these can take up to four weeks to heal. You may find some relief from a warm bath or shower, a chilled gel-filled pad, a local anaesthetic spray or cream, an over-the-counter painkiller such as ibuprofen or a homeopathic remedy such as arnica (check with your midwife before taking anything). Lie down as much as possible and use a soft pillow to sit on (you can hire the specially designed 'Valley Cushion' from the NCT). If you've had a very serious tear, you may be referred to an obstetric physiotherapist for extra help. Stitches will usually dissolve within a fortnight. If you've had a C-section, recovery times vary. The pain tends to be acute for a few days afterwards but will then subside. You may be very immobile for a while and need lots of help – it is major surgery, after all. You'll also need painkillers to get you through the first week or so – and loads of practical help when back home, especially if you're breastfeeding and are struggling to even pick up your baby.

- **Painful boobs** Your breasts can expand to bursting point when your milk comes in and if you delay a breastfeed when it's due. (If you've decided not to breastfeed, there will be an uncomfortable or painful period while the milk dries up naturally over the course of a day or two. Painkillers and a supportive bra can help.) Nipples may be extremely sore while breastfeeding and an effective 'latch on' is established.

- **Aches, pains and exhaustion** It's not unusual to feel as though you've emerged from a big fight after birth. General pain and achiness in the pelvis, chest, tailbone, back and legs are all normal.

- **Saggy tums and stretched skin** Immediately after birth you'll lose up to a stone in weight, and inevitably you'll have a very saggy stomach as a result. Postnatal stretch marks which can occur on the tummy, breast and thighs affect some women, but not others (the cause is thought to be a simple matter of genetics). They fade over time and become silvery but will never disappear completely, so if you have them, you may just have to embrace them as a proud mark of motherhood. Meanwhile, a good moisturiser will ease any itchiness.

- **Poo, wind and piles** Bowels can be sluggish after a delivery, and this physiological problem can be worsened by psychological ones. You may feel as though your stitches are going to burst open (they won't!) and it may help to hold a pad or wad of tissue over your wound to protect your stitches, for psychological reassurance as much as anything. If you're badly constipated, your doctor or midwife may advise you to take a stool softener such as lactulose solution – this is available over the counter, but check with your doctor or midwife first. Eating a balanced diet with lots of fruit and veg and drinking lots of liquid will help keep your movements soft and less likely to cause a problem. Excessive wind is common, because the muscles and nerves around the bowels can be stretched and even damaged by childbirth. Occasionally, postpartum faecal incontinence (leaking poo) may occur for the same reason. Haemorrhoids (piles) are varicose veins just inside the anus and are extremely common after birth, caused by the pressure of pushing during delivery. Over-the-counter or prescription creams and plenty of fibre and fluids can help.

- **Sweating and weeing.** You may notice you're doing a lot more of both these things, as the body releases all the extra fluid that's stored up in pregnancy. (The good news about this is that if you suffered from puffy ankles, face and hands in the build-up to birth, they will soon begin to go down.) It's essential that you have a wee within eight hours of birth to avoid urinary tract infection, which is why your midwife will always check to make sure you've emptied your bladder.

- **Weakened pelvic floors and leaky bladders (stress or urinary incontinence)** Loss of muscle tone in the perineal area can affect the bladder and cause leakage – doing your pelvic floor exercises will help if this is a problem. These exercises also improve the flow of blood to the vaginal area which speeds up the healing process.

- **Sheer exhaustion** You've given birth, you're emotionally overwhelmed, and you're caring for a new human being 24/7. You're going to be very, very tired for a while!

When complications become serious

Post-pregnancy complications may occasionally lead to a serious medical condition. Your midwife will be alert to possible symptoms, but you should seek immediate treatment if you develop any of the following:

- sudden or extremely heavy and bright-red blood loss or very large blood clots, particularly if accompanied by racing heartbeat, faintness or dizziness; feverishness or shivering; or bleeding that smells unpleasant

- swelling, tenderness or pain in the legs
- sharp chest pain or shortness of breath
- severe or persistent headache, dizziness, vomiting, or blurred vision
- swelling, redness or oozing at the site of a Caesarean incision
- difficulty or pain in urinating
- persistent pain in the abdomen or perineal area.

Ups and downs

It's not just the way you feel on the outside that can take a battering after birth – your state of mind will also need some TLC. Whilst you may well feel intermittently high, there may also be times when you feel very low. These postnatal mood swings – probably caused by a combination of hormonal changes, anxiety, and exhaustion – are experienced, to one extent or another, by just about all new mums. They can be heightened if you've been through a particularly difficult delivery, if you're finding breastfeeding hard going, or if you're really struggling with one or more of the physical consequences of birth, or if you are isolated from friends and family, or your partner is not around much, perhaps because he has had to return to working long hours.

Often called 'the baby blues', this period of changeable emotions won't last long and is best tackled by getting as much rest, sympathy, and practical help as you possibly can. The development of full-on Postnatal Depression (PND), on the other hand, is something to watch for as you may need some professional help to get through it.

You will probably feel a very strong rush of love for your baby very soon after birth – but you may not. For some mums (and dads), the bonding process can take a while and those deep feelings of love may take several weeks or more to kick in.

What the netmums say

'Baby blues and bonding'

I'd been constantly told that as soon as I saw my baby I would feel an overwhelming sense of love, so I felt awful when this didn't happen. I didn't feel that bond – I just felt numb. It wasn't until about Week 4 that all of a sudden I just couldn't bear to be apart from him. Now I'm absolutely loving it, although I still feel like I've got a constant hangover from the lack of sleep! But none of that matters when he looks at me and smiles.

Carly from Norwich mum, to Finley, four months

I think I had the baby blues, to be honest. I felt totally overwhelmed with the responsibility of a new baby and wondered what on earth I'd let myself in for! I honestly couldn't imagine how I was going to get my life back again. I felt really unwell with mastitis when Rebecca was two weeks old and rang my health visitor a couple of times in tears because of the pain. It's scary trying to care for a baby 24/7 when you're unwell. The breastfeeding didn't come as naturally as I'd expected and I felt like a leaky cow a lot of the time but when it went well, I felt great. I found it easier as each month passed and by the time she was four months, thought it was a doddle!

Linda from Bristol, mum to Rebecca, 12 and Sam, 11

Bless her, I did NOT enjoy my baby for the first month, and it took me a while to bond. I felt terribly guilty, and used to pretend that I loved her. I was all blown up with water retention, leaky breasts and painful episiotomy scars. And I didn't think I was ever going to get a good night's sleep again. But now, she is the light in my life, my gorgeous baby girl. With my next baby I'm going to relax, and enjoy the first few weeks if I can.

Sally from Matfen, mum to Lily, 17 months

The first few weeks for me were so amazing. I hadn't bonded with my bump at all and didn't really feel like I was going to have a baby, so when my son was born and put on my chest I felt such a rush of love for him (and amazement that I had a baby). I know it will be a feeling that I will never forget or ever be able to describe how amazing it was. The first few days I just watched him sleep but felt a bit afraid of holding him in case I dropped him, then three days later I couldn't stop crying as every horrible thing that might happen to my baby went through my mind. By the time he was two weeks old I'd got over that and felt like a pro. I was so

confident that I was the best mum for my baby and I felt on top of the world.
Jenna from Wolverhampton, mum to Jude, 15 months

A helping hand

If there's one piece of advice you need to follow in the first month, it's to take it easy. Do the bare minimum of housework (aim to keep food preparation areas and toilets reasonably clean and the floor clear enough that you don't trip over things), and live on ready meals and speedy snacks, and delegate anything that doesn't involve looking after yourself or your baby to someone else.

Most new parents will have at least a couple of good friends or relatives who are willing to help in some way – exploit them, and let them know how much you appreciate their help. (And don't forget to ask for it – people may not realise you're in need, or they may not want to offend you by offering.) At the same time, you may need some peace and privacy in this period, so if your mother-in-law's bustling is causing you stress, or the constant flow of visitors getting you down, you'll just have to politely say so. A 'do not disturb' note on the front door should do the trick. But whatever you do, don't try and go it alone in this month – if you're a lone parent or if your partner has a demanding job and isn't able to take time off, take help wherever else you can find it.

Grab a kip, when you can

Sleep deprivation is unavoidable, but any amount of rest and relaxation that you can come by is worthwhile – if your baby is asleep, ignore the fact that there's ironing to do (who needs neat-looking clothing, anyway?) and grab a 'power nap' while you can. Eating well is also important now – home cooking might be a tall order, but simple nutritious snacks such as a wholemeal sandwiches, jacket potatoes, beans or egg on toast, fresh cartons of soup, oatcakes and cheese, yoghurts, salad and fruit should see you through.

Don't forget to get out in the fresh air whenever possible, as it can be a real tonic for your physical and mental health – being stuck permanently inside can send anyone a little stir crazy. Just don't try and go too far, or do too much.

What the netmums say

'Sleep deprivation'

I do remember the sleep deprivation making me feel a bit mad and down. I don't think I had 'baby blues' – it was just tiredness making mountains out of molehills. I never felt anything but overwhelming love for the baby but my husband got the rough end of my tongue several times in those first weeks. I remember finding it hard to achieve anything other than feeding and sleeping and even going to the loo or having a shower was hard to fit in.

Amanda from Otley, mum to Dylan, six, Fraser, four and Bethany, two

I was surprised how much my newborns slept! When people spoke about being sleep deprived, I assumed they meant they were up all the time, day and night. I found that napping in the day when my son slept meant I didn't feel so out of it.

Jenna from Wolverhampton, mum to Jude, 15 months

Index

breathlessness 168, 246
breech babies 87, 285, 286, 289, 300–3, 327
  assisted delivery 302–3
  'complete' breech 300
  elective Caesarians 301–2
  'footling' or 'incomplete' breech 300, 301–2
  'frank' breech 300
  Netmums' experiences 301
  turning the baby 300, 301, 308–9
  vaginal delivery 302
buggies 191, 194, 252
'bump'
  belly massage 77, 100, 120
  bump size 77, 79, 206
  bump supports 310, 392
  itchy 239–40
  strangers touching 169–70
  unwelcome remarks about 77, 198–9

C-section *see* Caesarean deliveries
Caesarean deliveries 96, 285–90, 334
  anaesthetic 285, 286–7, 293
  elective 12, 286–7, 288, 290
    advantages 286
    for breech babies 301–2
    situations 286
  emergency 98, 251, 278, 285–6, 289, 292, 301, 348
    situations 285
  emotional recovery 288, 289–90
  epidurals 97, 98, 286, 287
  gestational diabetes and 209
  Netmums' experiences 289–90
  percentage of births 285
  physical recovery 287, 289, 417
  soreness, scars and stitches 416–17
  twin and multiple births 12, 286, 293
  vaginal birth after 293, 390
caffeine 26, 175, 402
calamine lotion 229, 240
calcium 178, 230, 231
Candida albicans 151
car seat 190, 308, 351, 388
carpal tunnel syndrome 203–5, 217
  Netmums' experiences 204–5
carrycots 190, 408
catheterisation 97, 98, 303
cephalo-pelvic disproportion (CPD) 293

cervical sweep 363, 364
cervix 247
  cervical incompetence 57, 311
  cervical mucus 4
  dilation 248, 249, 253, 263, 312, 362
  mucus plug 125–6, 247–8, 341
chamomile 144
changing bag and mat 192
cheese 26
chewing gum 35
chickenpox 142–3
chickenpox syndrome 142
child benefits 390, 407
childcare 267, 389
  arranging 20, 141, 142
  contingency arrangements 267
  nurseries 20
childminders 20, 141, 267, 389
  parents or in-laws as 143
chloasma 121
chlorine 229
chorion 4, 215
chorionic villus sampling (CVS) 60, 70
  Netmums' experiences 61
cleft lip/palate 173
Clomid 59
clothes
  baby 189, 191
  see also maternity clothes
cod liver oil supplements 25
codeine 416
colic 398, 402
collagen 91
colostrum 97, 157, 207, 359, 399
complementary therapy 233
compulsive behaviour 72
concentration difficulties 72, 82
conception 3–4
  success rate 20
constipation 45, 234, 417–18
  baby 398, 407, 412
  iron supplements and 247
contact lenses 162
contractions
  Braxton Hicks contractions 181, 202, 203, 253, 268, 340
  see also labour, contractions
cool-water spray 188, 240, 267, 305
cord blood sampling *see* cordocentesis